Subjective Well-Being and Security

Social Indicators Research Series

Volume 46

This new series aims to provide a public forum for single treatises and collections of papers on social indicators research that are too long to be published in our journal *Social Indicators Research*. Like the journal, the book series deals with statistical assessments of the quality of life from a broad perspective, It welcomes the research on a wide variety of substantive areas, including health, crime, housing, education, family life, leisure activities, transportation, mobility, economics, work, religion and environmental issues. These areas of research will focus on the impact of key issues such as health on the overall quality of life and vice versa. An international review board, consisting of Ruut Veenhoven, Joachim Vogel, Ed Diener, Torbjorn Moum, Mirjam A.G. Sprangers and Wolfgang Glatzer, will ensure the high quality of the series as a whole.

For futher volumes:
http://www.springer.com/series/6548

Dave Webb • Eduardo Wills-Herrera

Editors

Subjective Well-Being and Security

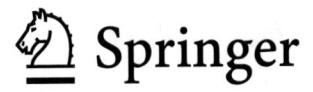 Springer

Editors
Dave Webb
35 Stirling Highway
6009 Crawley
Western Australia
Australia
dave.webb@uwa.edu.au

Eduardo Wills-Herrera
Calle 21, No. 1-20
Room SD 945 Bogotá
Colombia
ewills@uniandes.edu.co

ISSN 1387-6570
ISBN 978-94-007-2277-4   e-ISBN 978-94-007-2278-1
DOI 10.1007/978-94-007-2278-1
Springer Dordrecht Heidelberg London New York

Library of Congress Control Number: 2011942516

Printed on acid-free paper

Springer is part of Springer Science+Business Media (www.springer.com)

I dedicate this book to my parents, Cliffe and Beryl Webb, who by example and with love taught me the importance of security and well-being. Thank you for always being there.

Dave Webb

I dedicate this book to my lovely wife Ana Maria and my lovely sons Santiago and Antonio whose support and patience during this time have been very precious for me and have added to my personal well-being.

Eduardo Wills-Herrera

We also dedicate this book to all the people around the world who are experiencing reduced well-being for whatever reason. We hope in some way that this volume leads to positive change in their lives.

Contents

Chapter 1
Introduction

Dave Webb and Eduardo Wills-Herrera

Humankind today is facing challenges that question traditional thinking and research concerning the development of nations, communities, and individuals. For instance, fear of crime constitutes one of the main worries for individuals in cities, regions, and nations. Similarly, global threats such as climate change, the depletion of natural resources, recurrent economic and financial crises, increased inequality, and societal insecurity, all point to the heightened importance of finding new ways of understanding and acting to reduce the insecurity and non-sustainability of existing models and processes of development. Many challenges lie ahead: climate change, increasing terrorism, and violence against individuals, minorities, and nations, recurrent financial crisis in the business world, civil conflict, natural environmental disasters, catastrophies, interconnected corruption and narco-trafficking, human trafficking, and so on. These globalized phenomena highlight the interconnectedness of threats, risks, and dangers which in turn create many challenges for security, human development, and well-being. The aforementioned are global and independent of the place where people live.

Increasing feelings of insecurity and non-sustainability of development processes are related to how development has historically been understood as economic growth and globalization. In this special issue, we recognize that human beings need much more than economic satisfaction in order to flourish. In contrast to seeing development as economic growth only, we propose in this special volume to understand development as a guided process of change by which each individual and social group advances autonomously in what they understand as their promotion of human and social well-being (Wills-Herrera et al. 2011). Under

D. Webb (✉)
University of Western Australia, 35 Stirling Highway, Crawley, WA 6009, Australia
e-mail: dave.webb@uwa.edu.au

E. Wills-Herrera
School of Management, Universidad de los Andes, Bogotá, Columbia
e-mail: ewills@uniandes.edu.co

D. Webb and E. Wills-Herrera (eds.), *Subjective Well-Being and Security*,
Social Indicators Research Series 46, DOI 10.1007/978-94-007-2278-1_1,
© Springer Science+Business Media B.V. 2012

this vision, economics is seen and understood as a life dimension, not as exclusive or as the most important. Consequently, security becomes one of the main life domains that has to be considered, understood, and researched in this new perspective of development.

Security and development were, until recently, treated by traditional objective approaches of economic growth and nation-state defense of sovereignty (Haq 1999). Today we propose multidimensional approaches for understanding the development of individuals and communities stressing the contribution of other nonmaterial and noneconomic values to the well-being of individuals, such as feelings of security, family ties, social interconnectedness and social capital, perceived health, aspirations, spirituality, and engagement, among others. Satisfaction with these life domains is encompassed under the umbrella term of well-being. The progress of societies should be seen as a guided process of social change by which each individual in her/his freedom and autonomy can meet the conditions of the life she/he wants to live well.

Well-being then, is one such concept that introduces new ways of thinking about the development and progress of societies. It calls for an understanding of both objective conditions and subjective appraisals of individuals and communities concerning their well-being. Objective conditions and indicators for development have dominated the literature for several decades (Gasper 2010). However, in recent years, the importance of subjective indicators is also evidenced by the success of the leading journal in the area, "Social Indicators Research," as well as a significant number of edited books focussing on many areas of social indicators research. The social indicators movement began some years ago (Noll 2002) as a systematic search for alternative measures for understanding the development and progress of societies.

Subjective well-being (SWB) is associated with the idea of human development. In the literature, it is recognized that human development needs to be considered from a more subjective point of view, (Veenhoven 2000) challenging the notion that economic growth will automatically promote the well-being of all individuals concerned. The increasing importance of this movement can be tracked in the efforts that multilateral agencies such as OECD (*see* the recent OECD Better Life initiative http://www.oecdbetterlifeindex.org/topics/life-satisfaction/ as well as the UNDP Human development Index) are making to redefine the concept of the progress of societies (Rojas (ed) 2011) as well as the increased concerns of governments of individual countries, such as France and Bhutan, which are calling for increased efforts in scientific missions that can redefine what development means (see for instance Stiglitz et al. 2009; McDonald 2010).

SWB has been proposed as the construct and measurement of well-being indicating a type of development "of, by and for the people" (Sen 1999). It is a bottom-up measure directly assessed by the people in contrast to other definitions of development and well-being that have been developed in a top–down approach by academic, elite, and political groups. It encompasses a subjective appraisal, including cognitive and affective dimensions. It is important to note that we speak of SWB because it is appraised as perceived and felt by an individual. But we also think that the individual transcends his/her own subjectivity in accordance to his relations with others in community or society.

SWB is directly evaluated by the concerned citizen in a process in which each individual considers those aspects of life that each one has reason to value. It has become one of the most popular measures of quality of life (e.g., Diener and Seligman 2004). It implies an evaluation of how people evaluate their lives both positively and negatively (Kim-Prieto et al. 2005). It enquires how people subjectively perceive their well-being in different contexts such as cities, cultures, and regions. This subjective appraisal includes both cognitive and affective dimensions. SWB has more specifically been measured in a number of ways. Diener and colleagues (1985) approached SWB with a single global question included in the "Satisfaction with life as a whole" scale (SWLS). Other authors (Brief et al. 1993) have approached it in a bottom–up way, rating satisfaction with life across different life domains (*see also* Cummins et al. 2003). Cummins and colleagues consider life satisfaction across initially seven life domains and more recently eight life domains with the addition of spirituality and religion. The collective assessment of life satisfaction is aggregated to form the personal well-being index (PWI), which has now successfully been implemented in 23 consecutive survey waves in every State of Australia. The PWI measure has also validly been applied in many other countries. The idea of PWI is to approach parsimoniously the minimal sets of domains of the construct. Consequent studies have shown seven domains and an additional domain (satisfaction with spirituality) has been proposed, adding significantly to explained variance e.g., (Wills 2009). With these new "subjective" scales it is possible to understand how different dimensions such as personal security, safety, community, health, standard of living, etc. all add to a person's sense of well-being from the standpoint of his/her personal feelings and evaluations.

In that way, development is not evaluated by objective external experts or members of dominant groups within each country but by each individual. The evaluation of a well-lived life and its corresponding domains is done with universal measures such as SWB, which have shown their reliability and validity in scientific research and which allows comparisons at the interpersonal and intercultural levels as well as comparisons between nations and cities.

Individuals and communities evaluate their SWB in different contexts and settings such as cities, rural areas, regions, and nations, and in this appraisal they evaluate their subjective feeling of security or insecurity. Satisfaction with security becomes one of the crucial dimensions that influence development and well-being. As such, new understandings of the concept of security should be proposed.

At this stage it is worth highlighting that while thus far we have been talking about well-being, essentially, this concept is often discussed under a broader quality of life label and discussed synonymously with life satisfaction and happiness, though many authors highlight the subtle differences that exist between each. That said, this is not the place to dwell further on this topic since many excellent sources exist to which the interested reader can go. Indeed, *Social Indicators Research, Applied Research in Quality of Life* and *The Journal of Happiness Studies* represent three such leading journal resources. A significant body of literature exploring many facets of quality of life (QOL) research exists. Examples include the following: research on well-being (e.g., Cummins et al. 2003; Diener et al. 2010), life satisfaction (e.g., Cummins 1996), and happiness (e.g., Veenhoven 2000).

In brief, security/insecurity and well-being are then closely related. Research has established that among the domains that contribute significantly to the well-being of individuals are satisfaction with security (Cummins et al. 2003) and future security. Considering security from a subjective perspective introduces a new way of thinking about the concept as differentiated from traditional thinking which has tended to focus on militarism and sovereignty (Haq 1999).

In this order of ideas, a discussion remains about how to conceptualize and measure both concepts and to understand how they are related in different contexts. Consequently, exploring new ways of conceiving, defining, and studying development, well-being, and their relationship to security/insecurity at the individual, group, organizational, and national levels becomes an urgent agenda item for the academic community. In regard to measurement, discussion about their subjective or objective nature constitutes an interesting avenue for empirical research. The reader should note that in discussing security, by implication we include consideration of insecurity too. We also make no assertion here in this introduction regarding the uni or bivariate nature and structure of these concepts.

But how should we understand security and safety? Human security is a new concept that has emerged in this respect. It is closely related to the human development approach that follows the insights of several authors, for example, Sen (1999, 2006), Haq (1999), and Jolly and Ray (2007). With the eruption of different global crises a limited definition has been challenged by scholars from the human development stream (Gasper et al. 2008) because a narrow military conception of security excludes considerations of other types of threats and fears coming from other areas such as food security, health security, political security, environmental security, and so on. Human security is not limited to the negative dimension of the absence of violent conflict in social organizations, but it includes the construction of safeguards and opportunities for people's strengths and aspirations. The human development movement including the idea of human security highlighted the importance of relating issues of security with the lives of people and their corresponding well-being

Earlier concepts of security (Haq 1999), which focus predominantly on militaristic security, seem highly inappropriate since they emerged in the context of the cold war and were mainly used in relation to Nation–State security. These definitions were closely tied to a State defense of sovereign interests. It usually portrayed activities to protect a given country, a location, a building, or a person by the military forces. These insecurities in turn are felt by individuals and groups in different contexts and situations such as rural area, cities, villages, communities, and so on. Interdependent potential threats can be felt by actor's today at all different levels and units of analysis, and, not necessarily alone within national borders. The human security literature highlights the important point that perceptions of insecurity, fear of crime, and concern about personal safety may have a greater negative influence on life satisfaction than actual objective victimization.

This wider consideration includes not just protection from harm and injury (see for example the Introduction to the Human Security Issue (Anand and Gasper 2007) in the *International Journal of Development*, March, 2007) which connected the themes of human security, development, and well-being based on the previous human development reports made by the United Nations Development Program (UNDP). Potential access to water, food, shelter, health, employment, and other requisites that are associated with citizen quality of life independent of where citizens are located is recognized as being among the many crucial security concerns. In this sense, a broadened consideration of security brings together the following concepts: development, human development, quality of life, and well-being. As noted by Myers (1993: 31): it is the collectivity of citizens' needs, overall safety and quality of life that should figure prominently in the nation's view of security.

Both safety and security, together with how they relate to other concepts such as well-being, are currently studied across multiple disciplines, using multiple methodological approaches and at multiple levels of analysis. Additionally, SWB and security are employed to guide public policy as well as other actions, the goal being to increase the well-being of global individuals and societies.

Contemporary thinking about security should include the many interactions between the social, political, cultural, epidemiological, and economical systems, which are often studied and treated separately in past research. The concepts safety and security are often considered interrelated and sometimes treated as synonymous. For example, while in the English language it is possible to differentiate between them, in others it is not. In Spanish and Catalan for instance, only one word *seguridad* representing the two exists. This may imply certain cross-cultural differences which deserve exploring and indeed this volume explores this question too in its content.

This volume of the SIR Community Indicators Series considers how security and well-being are defined, operationalized, measured, and related to other important concepts. This is achieved using multiple lenses, methodologies, and levels of analysis in the different chapters of this book. Similarly, in the context of security, multiple areas of major crime and their impact on well-being as well as security receive attention. Both concepts are analyzed and understood in new and creative ways that challenge traditional definitions of security and development.

Some years ago, we could not have imagined preparing a separate volume on security and well-being. However, in recent years the interconnectedness of these two concepts has been brought to the forefront of attention by different streams of research, particularly those emerging from the SWB domain. According to Roberts (in this issue) a review of more than 6,000 publication abstracts conducted a decade ago by Michalos and Zumbo (2000: 246) revealed that scant attention had been devoted to studying the interconnections between measures of individual criminal victimization, insecurity, and quality of life. Five years later, Møller (2005) supplemented this search by examining approximately 600 journals published by Kluwer between 1997 and 2004, and identified that only three articles (in addition to the Michalos and Zumbo (2000) paper) had probed the insecurity and crime-quality of life relationship.

In this issue, we are interested in exploring new meanings and approaches to security and well-being, and particularly in relation to both objective and subjective measures associated with individual citizens, groups, and communities in different contexts.

1 Papers in This Issue

This volume of the SIR series explores many important questions in its diverse content. For example: Are objective indicators of security the same as perception-based assessments? How are these constructs correlated and why? Also, how are safety and security related? At the same time, how do the different levels of analysis aggregate for a more comprehensive explanation of these concepts not only in English-speaking contexts but also non-English speaking?

To address these and other important questions, we (the editors of this volume) invited a number of noted international scholars from diverse fields of enquiry and representing different countries, to submit a chapter addressing key issues relevant to SWB and security from different disciplinary and interdisciplinary approaches.

Considered together, the contents of this volume represent a timely and significant contribution to knowledge in the area. By way of example, within this volume the reader will find SWB discussed in the context of many major crime-types including: terrorism, human trafficking, the drugs trade, murder, rape, robbery, and so on to name a few. These are considered broadly in Australia, Latin America, Europe, and South Africa, again to name a few.

As crime, fear of crime, and terrorism have become major pathologies connected to living in both cities and rural regions (e.g., Di Tella et al. 2008), it is important that they be considered not only in respect to their psychological consequences but also in terms of associated economic and political ramifications. In this volume, interesting comparative results are presented in separate studies for cities and regions in Portugal (Chap. 5, this volume), Croatia (Chap. 4, this volume), and Colombia (Chap. 8, this volume). We now introduce a brief overview of what the reader will find in this volume.

In Chap. 2, Cummins explores whether satisfaction with safety adds significantly to the comprehensiveness of a measure of SWB. In his discussion, he highlights the importance of considering how homeostatic forces at the individual level come into play for preserving equilibrium levels of SWB such that the fears of individuals are reduced. Similarly, using the personal well-being index (PWI) which advances the development of a barometer to measure satisfaction with life among Australians (Cummins et al. 1994), Cummins highlights the importance of the need to consider the perceived likelihood of a terrorist attack. This observation reaffirms the importance of taking into consideration globalization variables since Australia, where the author resides, has not suffered any direct major terrorist attack in recent years. This is not the case in other nearby locations that are frequently visited by Australian holiday-makers. Drawing on panel data results obtained across 23 surveys implemented between 2001 and 2010, the author reveals that satisfaction with safety seems to have little relevance to SWB, certainly within Australia. Cummins offers three reasons for this finding: (1) a strong link evidenced between safety satisfaction and homeostatically protected mood (HPMood) implies that safety satisfaction is driven by levels of HPMood, (2) the paucity of variance contributed by the measure, and (3) people's strong adaptation to situations where their sense of security is threatened. Nevertheless, the author proposes that this conclusion does not necessarily apply to specific threatened groups within nations, nor for that matter to constituent nations, and for this reason recommends it be retained as a domain of consideration. This conclusion adds to the previous articles in the sense that for cities in countries that have high security concerns, such as Portugal, Colombia, and Croatia, satisfaction with safety constitutes an important contributor to SWB.

In Chap. 3, and also in Australia, Aly explores the fear of terrorism and its impact on community and individual wellbeing. Incorporating Australia's first Metric of Fear, her chapter uses responses to media discourses to explore fear among Australian–Muslim communities and the broader Australian community. She reports that the fear of terrorism extends beyond an individual fear, vis a vis being physically harmed in a terrorist attack, to include community fear associated with perceived threat to civil liberties and democratic freedom. For Australian–Muslim communities, the fear of terrorism is very much associated with community identity and their status as a community to be feared.

In relation to the practical application and formulation of public policy, it is important to highlight the disconnection revealed in various papers of this issue between perceptions of insecurity at different levels such as the individual and community level on the one hand, and public opinion and the leaders perception on the other (Chap. 9, this volume). It is possible to call for the development of more convincing indicators of feelings of insecurity at different levels, which in turn can be communicated clearly to the general public. Clear results and information to the public will exert pressure to public actions that are missing in this sensitive field.

People seek security of various types, including bodily or health (Graham 2008), material, psychological, social, and existential and in that process they include their families, friends, co-workers, systems of meanings and esteem and so on. Solving safety needs by individuals was highlighted by the pioneering work of Maslow (1943) as one of the basic human needs to be solved in order to aspire to other high-order needs such as self-actualization and personal growth. In this context, safety at the neighborhood, village and city levels becomes essential. Safety needs reflect order and predictability in the environment and the human desire for security and protection (Maslow 1943). The concept of security that is considered in the content of this issue is citizen-centric with an emphasis on its subjective components. Furthermore, it is multidimensional, interconnected, and articulated at the local, regional, national, and global levels.

Fear of crime and terror is the predominant independent (predictor) variable in this research stream. This variable is measured from a subjective and objective point of view, reaffirming the known result that both variables correlate between themselves but are discriminatory.

In Chap. 4, fear of crime is assessed as feelings of safety under different circumstances and contexts by Franc et al. in Croatia. Examining a large sample of 4000 Croatian citizens in different cities, the authors measure perceptions of safety at night under three different situations: traveling in public transport, being at home and, being on the streets in the neighborhood. The prevalence of different types of crime (delinquency, minor crime, corruption, etc.) and illegal substance abuse (drugs and alcohol) are also taken into account.

In Chap. 5, similarly reinforcing the need for a multi-level perspective, Palma et al. highlight the need for studies at the local, municipal, and regional levels to achieve a more comprehensive assessment of security. Their study contributes to the growing human security literature by measuring both objective (crime against the person, property and the social context) and subjective variables related to personal safety in order to assess the life satisfaction of citizens. Presenting results for a sample of 3,757 citizens across 20 urban communities in Portugal, their results reveal an important effect of fear of crime against property vis a vis individual well-being. A possible explanation offered by the authors is that because crime against property is committed at home as compared to other types of crime, it is more proximal to the victim and hence, has a higher effect than other more distant types of crimes. In addition, Palma et al.'s results reveal that subjective security does not correlate highly with objective indicators such as physical crime against the person, a finding that is corroborated by other studies presented in this volume (e.g., Chaps. 8 and 9, this volume) that were carried out in a Latin American context. These findings pose important and intriguing questions for new research about why objective and subjective measures of insecurity are not highly correlated. Indeed, Cummins's discussion of adaptation processes (in this issue) may go some way to explaining this. Thus, an important conclusion which Palma et al. highlight and which offers support to other authors in this issue (e.g., Chap. 8, this volume) is that the consideration of objective indicators alone is inadequate for explaining levels of well-being both at the urban as well as rural levels.

Another important contribution to the discussion of crime in communities is made in Chap. 6 by Medina and Tamayo. They assess the effect that crime, perceptions of security, and victimization rates have on satisfaction with life in different neighborhoods in Medellin, a city that for decades has been recognized as one of the most dangerous cities in the world due to the heavy influence of cartels. It is important to note that in recent years the crime rate has dropped dramatically due to a shift in public security policy.

In Chap. 7, Roberts presents an exploratory study to investigate the extent and nature of fear of crime in South Africa after nearly two decades of democracy. In addition, he builds on recent empirical studies by exploring the impact of crime-related issues on quality of life in a developing country context. The results pose critical challenges to some of the prevailing stereotypes in respect to those who are most fearful, and provide further support for other national and sub-national surveys that have arrived at similar conclusions. A very important conclusion of this study is that in many instances, there is no significant difference in fear of crime between black and white respondents, with Indian respondents constantly displaying the highest levels of fear. Given this finding, the popular reference to fear of crime in the country as predominantly "white fear" is lamentable (see also Møller 2005) in that it is misleading and neglects the needs of a majority who are less able to adequately voice their concerns. Another important conclusion is that people residing in rural areas tend to experience less fear of victimization than their urban counterparts. In this respect, a significant finding is that it is in the country's informal settlements that fear seems most pervasive. South Africans have shown resilience by not allowing insecurities and experiences of crime to impact to any significant degree on their life satisfaction. However, from the results presented in the chapter, it is readily apparent that the fear equation remains of considerable importance for policy discussion.

In Chap. 8, adopting a multidisciplinary (sociology, economics and social psychology) approach, Wills-Herrera and colleagues study how social capital can moderate the relationships between the perceptions of insecurity of rural producers in Colombia and their level of SWB. With a methodology that uses a multi-level model, the authors show how objective indicators of insecurity in rural areas of a conflict-ridden country such as Colombia are distinct from perceptions of insecurity and how these perceptions can be divided into four sub-categories of insecurity: personal, communitarian, political, and economic. The study shows empirically how to associate in networks and organizations, seen as social capital, and it highlights how the development of associations becomes one of the mains strategies that rural producers can follow in order to attenuate insecurities. It further reveals how perceptions of insecurity are related with adaptation processes such as the strengthening of organizations and belonging to social networks.

Next in Chap. 9, Graham and Chaparro offer an interesting paper considering how insecurity affects well-being (considered as happiness and health), and how the effects can be mitigated by adaptive mechanisms. This represents an important avenue for public policy in the future. The authors also show how victimization has a negative effect on friendships as well as a deteriorating effect on confidence in public institutions. This highlights the important question of how to handle reductions in the well-being of individuals at the same time that society-wide costs are created by way of insecurities?

In Chap. 10, adopting the earlier-mentioned PWI (Cummins et al. 2003), Gonzalez et al. explore perceptions of future security among a sample of young post-compulsory secondary education students in Spain. The results obtained offer a further contribution to our understanding of security, not only in general, but specifically for young persons aged between 15 and 24 years old, via an exploration of its relationship with psychosocial factors such as self-concept, overall sense of meaning in own life, freedom of choice and control over own life and, values aspired to in the future.

Finally, in Chap. 11 we conclude this volume with an exploratory study by Webb and Rodriguez de la Vega. The authors open new and important avenues for SWB research with their consideration of the effects of the growing global crime of human trafficking for the specific purpose of sexual exploitation on the well-being of victims as well as communities in the crime-ridden Triple Frontier region of South

America (Argentina, Paraguay, and Brazil). This important study proposes how local communities can organize themselves to acquire more power and voice to combat these illegal practices, and to make the region more secure for its inhabitants so that their well-being and quality of life can be enhanced.

We are excited to be able to bring together in one volume this collection of research from a group of renowned international authors, whose chapters extend our knowledge about a fundamental dimension of human well-being, namely, security. We hope that these studies inspire others to explore the rich research avenues suggested by the authors in their respective chapters.

References

Anand, P., & Gasper, D. (2007). Special issue on human security, well-being and sustainability: Rights, responsibilities and priorities. *Journal of International Development, 4*, 449–456.

Brief, A. P., Butcher, A. H., George, J. M., & Link, K. E. (1993). Integrating bottom-up and top- down theories of SWB: The case of health. *Journal of Personality and Social Psychology, 64*, 646.

Cummins, R. A. (1996). The domains of life satisfaction: An attempt to order chaos. *Social Indicators Research, 38*(3), 303.

Cummins, R. A., McCabe, M. P., Romeo, Y., & Gullone, E. (1994). The comprehensive quality of life scale (ComQol): Instrument development and psychometric evaluation on college staff and students. *Educational and Psychological Measurement, 54*, 372–382.

Cummins, R. A., Eckersley, R., Pallant, J., Van Vugt, J., & Misajon, R. (2003). Developing a national index of subjective wellbeing: The Australian unity wellbeing index. *Social Indicators Research, 64*(2), 159.

Di Tella, R., Ñopo, H., & MacCulloch, R. (2008). *Happiness and beliefs in criminal environments* (Inter-American Development Bank, Research Department Working Papers WP-662).

Diener, E., & Seligman, M. E. P. (2004). Beyond money: Toward an economy of well-being. *Psychological Science in the Public Interest, 5*(1), 1–31.

Diener, E. D., Emmons, R. A., Larsen, R. J., & Griffin, S. (1985). The satisfaction with life scale. *Journal of Personality Assessment, 49*, 71–75.

Diener, E., Ng, W., Harter, J., & Arora, R. (2010). Wealth and happiness across the world: Material prosperity predicts life evaluation, whereas psychosocial prosperity predicts positive feeling. *Journal of Personality and Social Psychology, 99*, 52–61.

Gasper, D. R. (2010). Understanding the diversity of conceptions of well-being and quality of life. *Journal of Socioeconomics, 39*(3), 351–360.

Gasper, D. R., Van der Maesen, L., Truong, T. D., & Walker, A. (2008). *Human security and social quality: Contrasts and complementarities* (Institute of Social Studies, Working Papers 462, The Hague).

Graham, C. (2008). Happiness and health: Lessons – and questions – for public policy. *Health Affairs, 27*(1), 72–87.

Haq, M. ul. (1999). *Reflections on human development* (2nd ed.). New York/New Delhi: Oxford University Press.

Jolly, R., & Ray, D. B. (2007). Human security – national perspectives and global agendas: Insights from national human development reports [dagger]. *Journal of International Development, 19*(4), 457.

Kim-Prieto, C., Diener, E., Tamir, M., Scollon, C. H., & Diener, M. (2005). Integrating the diverse definitions of happiness: A time-sequential framework of subjective wellbeing. *Journal of Happiness Studies, 6*(3), 261–300.

Maslow, A. H. (1943). A theory of human motivation. *Psychological Review, 50*(4), 370–396.

McDonald, R. (2010). *Taking happiness seriously: Eleven dialogues on gross national happiness.* Bhutan: Center for Bhutan Studies.

Michalos, A. C., & Zumbo, B. D. (2000). Criminal victimization and the quality of life. *Social Indicators Research, 50,* 245–295.

Møller, V. (2005). Resilient or resigned? Criminal victimization and quality of life in South Africa. *Social Indicators Research, 72,* 263–317.

Myers, N. (1993). *Ultimate security: The environmental basis of political stability.* New York: W.W. Norton & Co.

Noll, H. (2002). Towards a European system of social indicators: Theoretical framework and system architecture. *Social Indicators Research, 58,* 47–87.

Rojas, M. (Ed.). (2011). *La Medición del progreso y Del Bienestar: Propuestas desde América latina.* México: Foro Consultivo Científico y Tecnológico.

Sen, A. (1999). *Development as freedom.* New York: Oxford University Press.

Sen, A. (2006). *Identity and violence: The illusion of destiny.* New York: W. W. Norton.

Stiglitz, J. E., Sen, A., & Fitoussi, J. (2009). *Report by the commission on the measurement of economic performance and social progress.* Retrieved March 2011, from http://www.stiglitz-sen-fitoussi.fr/documents/rapport_anglais.pdf

Veenhoven, R. (2000). The four qualities of life: Ordering concepts and measures of the good life. *Journal of Happiness Studies, 1*(1), 1–39.

Wills, E. (2009). Spirituality and SWB: Evidences for a new domain in the personal well-being index. *Journal of Happiness Studies, 10*(1), 49.

Wills-Herrera, E., Orozco, L. E., Forero, C., Pardo, O., & Andonova, V. (2011). The relationship between perceptions of insecurity, social capital and SWB: Empirical evidences from areas of rural conflict in Colombia. *Journal of Socioeconomics, 40*(1), 88–96.

Chapter 2
Safety and Subjective Well-Being: A Perspective from the Australian Unity Wellbeing Index

Robert A. Cummins

Satisfaction with personal safety forms a part of many scales measuring subjective well-being (SWB). Yet it seems intuitive that this item will have a different association with well-being from other commonly included life areas, such as relationship. While high satisfaction with relationships is a positive, constantly reinforcing experience, high satisfaction with safety is neutral. Rather like pain, in its absence, the construct is likely to be ignored. However, if people feel unsafe, then this life area could easily overwhelm their world view and lead to a drastic reduction in well-being. This chapter explores these associations, particularly focusing on data from Australia.

The level of safety in Australia is comparable to that within similar nations. For example, the level of crime is similar to that of Canada and the United Kingdom (NationMaster 2011), and has not changed systematically over the past decade (Australian Institute of Criminology 2009). However, understanding the connection between the sense of personal safety and well-being has become more complex since the terrorist attacks of September 2001. This outrage gave people a new source of fear.

Prior to that date, such acts of destruction were unthinkable in Australia. Now, however, severe acts of terrorism gain worldwide publicity, thereby creating the opportunity for people to feel fearful of terrorist attacks even though no such acts have been perpetrated in their own land. Indeed, this is the terrorists' intention. Acts of terrorism are designed to have far-reaching psychological repercussions beyond the immediate act itself (Hoffman 1998; Wilkinson 2000). So any contemporary analysis of the link between safety and SWB must now include the perceived danger from terrorism.

R.A. Cummins (✉)
School of Psychology, Deakin University, 221 Burwood Hwy, Melbourne,
Victoria 3125, Australia
e-mail: robert.cummins@deakin.edu.au

D. Webb and E. Wills-Herrera (eds.), *Subjective Well-Being and Security*,
Social Indicators Research Series 46, DOI 10.1007/978-94-007-2278-1_2,
© Springer Science+Business Media B.V. 2012

1 Terrorism and Australia

The closest that Australia has come to with respect to deadly terrorist attacks has been in a neighboring country. Bali, in Indonesia, is a favorite Australian tourist destination, and on the 12th of October 2002, bombs detonated in the tourist district of Kuta killed 202 people, 88 of whom were Australians. This was followed some 3 years later by a similar attack. In response to this, since 2003, we have asked people two questions. First, whether they expect a terrorist attack in Australia to happen in the near future and, second, if they do, the strength of their conviction.

The results from these two items and safety satisfaction are interpreted in terms of three constructs. The first is the Homeostatic Theory of Subjective Wellbeing, which proposes that SWB is actively managed by each person to remain positive and stable. The second is the normative range for SWB, established through the combination of data across surveys. The third is the idea of causal and indicator variables. Causal variables, like the fear of an attack, are the symptoms of pathology that may cause an end-state to change. Indicator variables, such as SWB, constitute a measured end-state. It will be demonstrated that the relationship between the perceived probability of an attack and SWB is predicted by each of the above-mentioned constructs.

2 Subjective Wellbeing Homeostasis

The theory of Subjective Wellbeing Homeostasis proposes that for each person, in a manner analogous to the homeostatic maintenance of body temperature, SWB is actively controlled and maintained (see Cummins 2010; Cummins and Nistico 2002, for an extended description). This homeostatic system attempts to maintain a normal positive sense of well-being as a generalized and rather abstract view of the self. This view can be most easily measured by a response to the classic question "How satisfied are you with your life as a whole?," which has been asked in population surveys for over 35 years (e.g., Andrews and Withey 1976). Given the extraordinary generality of this question, the response that people give does not represent a cognitive evaluation of their life. Rather, it reflects a deep and stable positive mood-state that we initially called Core Affect (Davern et al. 2007), but which we now refer to as Homeostatically Protected Mood (HPMood: Cummins 2010). This is a mood-state dominated by a sense of contentment flavored with a touch of happiness and arousal. We propose that it is this general and abstract state of subjective well-being which the homeostatic system seeks to defend. As one consequence, the level of satisfaction people record to this question has the following characteristics:

1. It is normally very stable. Certainly unusually good or bad events may cause measured SWB to change. Such events generate affect as emotion, which can dominate HPMood and give the person a level of affect that lies outside their range of HPMood. However, over a period of time, homeostasis will normally

return SWB to its previous level (Hanestad and Albrektsen 1992; Headey and Wearing 1989).

2. Each person has a level of HPMood that is set genetically. This results in a "set-point" for SWB which lies in the "satisfied" sector of the dissatisfied–satisfied continuum. That is, on a scale where zero represents complete dissatisfaction with life and 100 represents complete satisfaction, people's set-point lies within the range of about 60–90 points and constitutes an individual difference (Cummins et al. 2002).

3. At a population level within Western nations, the average set-point is 75. In other words, on average, people feel that their general satisfaction with life is about three quarters of its maximum extent (Cummins 1995, 1998).

While this generalized sense of well-being is held positive with remarkable tenacity, it is not immutable. A sufficiently adverse environment can defeat homeostasis and, when this occurs, the level of subjective well-being falls below its homeostatic range. For example, people who experience strong, chronic pain from arthritis or from the stress of caring for a severely disabled family member at home, have low levels of SWB (Cummins 2001; Cummins et al. 2007a, Report 17.1). However, for people who are maintaining a normally functioning homeostatic system, their levels of SWB will show little relationship to normal variations in their chronic circumstances of living.

So, how does homeostasis manage to defend SWB against the unusually good and the unusually bad experiences of life? The answer we propose is that there are two levels of defense, and we call these defensive systems "buffers." One set of buffers is external to the person and the other internal.

2.1   Homeostatic Buffers

Interaction with the environment constantly threatens to move well-being up or down in sympathy with momentary positive and negative experience. While such movement does occur, most people are adept at avoiding large fluctuations. They avoid strong challenges to homeostasis through the maintenance of established life routines that make their daily experiences predictable and manageable. Under such ordinary life conditions, their level of mood-state varies by perhaps 10% points or so from one moment to the next: this is the set-point range. Homeostasis works hardest at the edges of this range to prevent more drastic mood changes which, of course, also occur from time to time. Strong and unexpected positive or negative experience will shift the sense of personal well-being to abnormally higher or lower values, usually for a brief period, until adaptation occurs. However, if the negative experience is sufficiently strong and sustained, homeostasis will lack the power to restore equilibrium, and SWB will remain below its set-point range. Such homeostatic defeat is marked by a sustained loss of positive mood and a high risk of depression (Cummins 2010).

So, the first line of defense for homeostasis is to avoid, or at least rapidly attenuate, negative environmental interactions. This is the role of the external buffers.

2.2   External Buffers

The two most important external resources for the defense of our SWB are close relationships and money. Of these two, the most powerful buffer is a relationship with another human being that involves mutual sharing of intimacies and support (Cummins et al. 2007b, Report 16.1). Almost universally, the research literature attests to the power of such relationships to moderate the influence of potential stressors on SWB (Henderson 1977; Sarason et al. 1990).

Money is also a very important external buffer, but there are misconceptions as to what money can and cannot do in relation to personal well-being. For example, it cannot shift the set-point to create a perpetually happier person. Set-points for SWB are proposed to be under genetic control (Braungart et al. 1992; Lykken and Tellegen 1996), so in this sense, money cannot buy happiness. No matter how rich someone is, their average level of SWB cannot be sustained higher than one that approximates the top of their set-point range. People adapt readily to luxurious living standards, so genetics trumps wealth after a certain level of income has been achieved. This limitation is supported by the findings of a recent report (Cummins et al. 2007b) using cumulative data from the Australian Unity Wellbeing Index. The purpose of the analysis was to locate demographic groups with the highest levels of well-being. The highest, reliable, group mean score is 81.0 points. Thus, this seems to be the maximum SWB that can be maintained as a group average even for people who have close relationships and plenty of money.

The true power of wealth is to protect SWB through its capacity to be used as a highly flexible resource (Cummins 2000) that allows people to defend themselves against the negative potential inherent within their environment. Wealthy people can employ their monetary resources to introduce target hardening measures (e.g., intrusion alarms) to protect themselves and their property. Poor people who lack such resources have a level of SWB that is far more at the mercy of their environment.

2.3   Internal Buffers

When people fail to control their external environment and their SWB is threatened, their internal buffers come into play. These comprise protective cognitive devices that are designed to minimize the damaging impact of personal failure on positive feelings about themselves. There are many such devices, collectively called Secondary Control (Rothbaum et al. 1982), and a detailed discussion of these systems in relation to SWB is provided in Cummins and Nistico (2002) and Cummins et al. (2002). They have the role of protecting SWB against the conscious realities of life. They do this by altering the way we see ourselves in relation to some challenging agent, such that the negative potential in the challenge is deflected away from the core view of self. Thus, the role of these buffers is to minimize the impact of personal failure. The ways of thinking that can achieve this are highly varied. For example, one can find meaning in the event ("God is testing me"), fail to take responsibility for the failure ("it was not my fault") or regard the failure [breaking a glass] as unimportant ("I did not need that old glass anyway").

In summary, the combined external and internal buffers ensure that our well-being is robustly defended. There is, therefore, considerable stability in the SWB of populations. As has been stated, the mean for Australia is consistently at about 75 points on a 0–100 scale. The theory of SWB Homeostasis also makes some quite specific predictions concerning the nature of the interaction of SWB with other variables. The first prediction is a generally weak negative correlation between the strength of challenging agents and the level of SWB. The primary purpose of homeostasis is to prevent any such relationship. The second prediction is a nonlinear relationship between SWB and the strength of challenging agents. This is because homeostasis can only maintain a steady level of SWB up to a threshold level of challenge, strong enough to defeat homeostatic control. At this threshold, homeostasis relinquishes control of SWB to the challenging agent, and SWB rapidly decreases (Cummins 2010).

3 Method

The results to be presented throughout this Chapter are available from Cummins et al. (2010). They are based on cumulative data from 23 surveys of the Australian Unity Wellbeing Index conducted between 2001 and 2010. Data are collected by telephone, and each survey involves a new sample of 2,000 people, geographically representative of the adult population based on population density. Each survey contains the Personal Wellbeing Index (International Wellbeing Group 2006), a seven-domain measure of subjective well-being (SWB). Each domain is assessed through a question of "satisfaction" directed to standard of living, health, relationships, currently achieving in life, future security, community connection, and safety.

Thus, "satisfaction with safety" is one of the seven domains of the Personal Wellbeing Index, and these domains, in combination, are designed to represent the first-level deconstruction of "satisfaction with life as a whole" (International Wellbeing Group 2006). In order to create such representation, the wording of all domain items is semiabstract. That is, they are determinedly nonspecific. Because of this nonspecificity, respondents predominantly use mood affect as information when answering the question (for "affect as information" see Schwarz and Strack 1991, 1999). If items were to be made more specific (e.g., How satisfied are you with your safety at work?), then their satisfaction response would reflect a more cognitively driven evaluation.

4 Safety Meaning and Measurement

The term "safety" does not have exactly the same meaning as "security" in English (Merriam-Webster Online 2011); however, the differences are subtle and would almost certainly be lost when translated into many other languages. The term itself is a complex amalgam of affect and cognition (see Liska et al. 1988). Thus, "safety" is not one of the primary emotions represented on the circumplex (Huelsman et al. 1998; Russell 2003; Yik et al. 1999), but it fulfills the criteria of a domain in the Personal Wellbeing Index (International Wellbeing Group 2006) as follows:

(a) Safety describes a broad aspect of life which is amenable to both objective and subjective measurement. This requirement is based on the fundamental principle that quality of life exists as separate objective and subjective dimensions. While the PWI is concerned only with the subjective dimension, this criterion allows the possibility that a parallel objective scale could be constructed.

(b) Safety also fulfills the criterion for a PWI domain in being an unequivocal indicator variable, as opposed to a causal variable, of life quality (Fayers et al. 1997). An indicator variable may be defined as one that can never act alone as a mediator (for a description of the mediator–moderator distinction, see Baron and Kenny 1986). A causal variable, on the other hand, is normally a mediator for an Indicator variable. An example of a causal variable is "satisfaction with your control over your life." Because, the perception of control can mediate the influence of, for example, physical disability on safety, control is not an unequivocal indicator variable.

(c) The final criterion is that, in the presence of the other domains, "satisfaction with safety" makes a significant contribution of unique variance to "satisfaction with life as a whole." It is notable that, in the context of general Australian surveys, safety consistently fails to meet this criterion. It has also been reported to make no contribution in China (Smyth et al. 2010). However, it does so in other countries (International Wellbeing Group 2006) and in some Australian population subgroups (Cummins et al. 2009).

Apart from its use in the PWI, authors have quite commonly considered that "safety" should be considered part of life quality. A search for this term within the Instruments section of the Australian Centre on Quality of Life (2010) identifies ten scales that include such an item. Safety is also widely incorporated in the measurement of other diverse constructs. The majority of such scales are measures of negative experience such as a Deprivation Index (Klasen 2000), Lived Poverty Index (Mattes et al. 2003), school victimization (Benbenishty and Astor 2005), and Job Dissatisfaction (Patmore 2010). Other authors, however, have used safety in the context of positive experience, such as school attachment (Wei and Chen 2010), positive youth development (Shek 2010), and family solidarity (defined objectively: Chua et al. 2010). Despite this wide usage, a critical consideration for the inclusion of this item in any scale is whether "safety" contributes unique information to such scales, or it just shares its variance with other scale items, making no independent contribution to understanding.

5   The Contribution of Shared and Unique Variance

Because safety is one of the seven PWI domains it has a direct relationship with SWB. Moreover, within the context of the PWI, the contribution of safety satisfaction to the PWI can be characterized as comprising two sources of variance.

The dominant source is variance shared with the other domains, and the minor source is variance unique to safety satisfaction.

The shared variance with the other domains means they all tend to rise and fall together. There are two sources of this shared variance. The first is HPMood, which represents the genetically determined, individual difference set-point. The level of affect corresponding to each set-point permeates all domains. Thus, people with high set-points tend to rate all domains as relatively high, and people with low set-points tend to rate all domains as relatively low. This is the dominant source of variance for all domains when the person is operating normally within their set-point range. However, another source of shared variance operates when the person is reporting a level of SWB outside their set-point range.

When SWB is abnormally high or low, normal contact with HPMood is lost. Then, instead of the person experiencing their normal set-point level of positivity, they will feel a level of affect as emotion, either positive or negative, that is being generated by the challenging agent. This will influence the felt level of satisfaction with all domains. For example, sadness due to the death of a close friend is caused by the negative affect associated with this event. If this affect is strong enough to dominate homeostatic control, it will cause a universal reduction in the reported satisfaction of all domains.

When under the control of either HPMood or a challenging agent, each individual domain contributes little unique information. Variation from one time to the next is mainly predicted by the satisfaction level of the other domains. However, even under these conditions, there is another source of information, much weaker than shared variance but unique to each domain. This comes about because the power of shared variance is not uniformly influential across all domains. The reasons for this are:

(a) The domains differ in their level of abstraction. Thus, "future security" is more abstract than "health." The more abstract the item, the more likely it is that people will use their level of HPMood as information (for "affect as information" see Schwarz and Strack 1991, 1999).

(b) The domains will differ in the extent to which they are being influenced by circumstances at the time of measurement. Of course, the emotions attached to acute circumstances just comprise measurement noise. But the chronic circumstances that the respondent is experiencing can exert a systematic and differential influence on domain satisfaction. For example, if the respondent is chronically experiencing the fear of partner violence, then their satisfaction response to "safety" is more likely to contain unique variance related to this issue. Thus, their response will be less likely to simply reflect HPMood.

(c) The domains may compensate for one another, as described by Best et al. (2000). Domain compensation is hypothesized as a homeostatic device that facilitates satisfaction in some domains to compensate for low satisfaction in others. For example, if satisfaction with safety goes down, satisfaction with relationships may go up to help maintain a steady level of SWB.

In summary, any assessment of SWB has a variable contribution from HPMood that is influenced by three sources of variance. The first and second are the shared variance caused by set-points and challenging agents. The variance caused by set-points is the pure reflection of HPMood, is proposed to be under genetic control, and cannot be modified. The shared variance caused by challenging agents diminishes the measured contribution of HPMood, most especially if these agents cause homeostatic failure. The third contribution is unique variance caused by low levels of domain abstraction, domain-specific influences, and domain compensation. Unique variance diminishes the measured contribution of HPMood due to its differential influence on specific domains.

5.1 Theoretical Implications for the Interpretation of Results

There are various predictions that emerge from this flow of reasoning. The first is that the measurement of HPMood can be most accurately assessed in the absence of both challenging agents and unique variance. The absence of challenging agents could be approximated by selecting samples where all PWI values lie within the hypothesized set-point range of 60–90 points (Cummins et al. 2002). The absence of unique variance may, in fact, be approximated by safety since, at least in Australia, it is the domain with the least unique variance. Safety consistently fails to make an independent contribution in general population samples (Cummins et al. 2009, Report 22.0; Lau et al. 2005), and also fails to do so in Algeria (Tiliouine et al. 2006), Hong Kong (Lau et al. 2008, 2005), and other Chinese cities (Smyth et al. 2010). However, it does contribute unique variance in Slovakia (International Wellbeing Group 2006) and other subpopulation groups, such as the elderly people in Hong Kong at the time of the Severe Acute Respiratory Syndrome epidemic (Lau et al. 2008). Because of these positive results it is retained as a domain in the PWI.

The second prediction concerns interpreting changed levels of satisfaction. That is, if some systematic and significant influence on SWB is applied at different levels of intensity, then the above analysis predicts that each level of intensity will exert a systematic and different influence on shared and unique variance. Consider, for example, different levels of income. The strongest level of shared variance should occur at the lowest levels of income. The logic is as follows:

1. Shared variance can be caused by either HPMood or homeostatic failure. The latter is the most powerful potential source since it has the potential to cause the greatest mass movement of domain satisfactions.
2. Because income is a protective buffer through its use as a flexible resource, as income rises, the probability of homeostatic failure decreases.
3. As the probability of homeostatic failure decreases, the proportion of shared variance caused by challenging agents decreases, up to the point that the shared variance is created by HPMood alone.

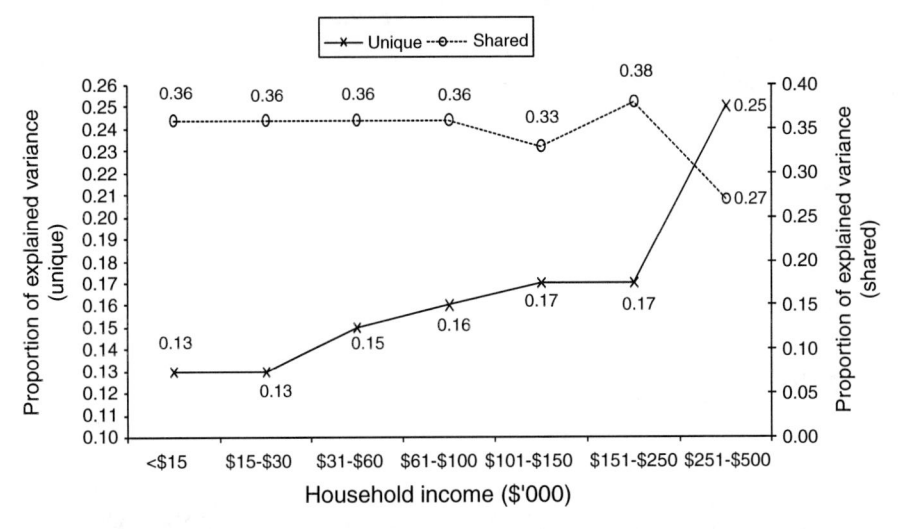

Fig. 2.1 The proportion of unique and shared variance by income

Following a different line of logic, the weakest levels of unique variance should occur at low incomes. The logic is as follows:

1. The unique variance will tend to be negated by the presence of homeostatic failure. Any powerful force moving domains down or up will dominate the individual domain contributions to explained variance.
2. As income rises, and the presence of homeostatic failure is diminished, the domains are more able to exert their own contribution.
3. As income rises, the unique variance of domains most relevant to income will rise faster than others.

5.2   An Empirical Test of the Theoretical Predictions

An empirical test of the above-mentioned predictions is shown in Fig. 2.1. This shows the average level of shared and unique variance at each income level as the seven domains are regressed against "satisfaction with life as a whole." The data are cumulative over nine surveys using the Australian Unity Wellbeing Index.

As can be seen, both trend lines show the predicted changes. Shared variance does not reliably decrease until the highest income is reached. However, the domains progressively capture more unique than shared variance as household income rises above $30,000. This is consistent with the progressive release of domains from the influence of homeostatic failure due to inadequate income.

In order to investigate changes in the individual domain contributions (β), Fig. 2.2 has been produced using the same cumulative data set.

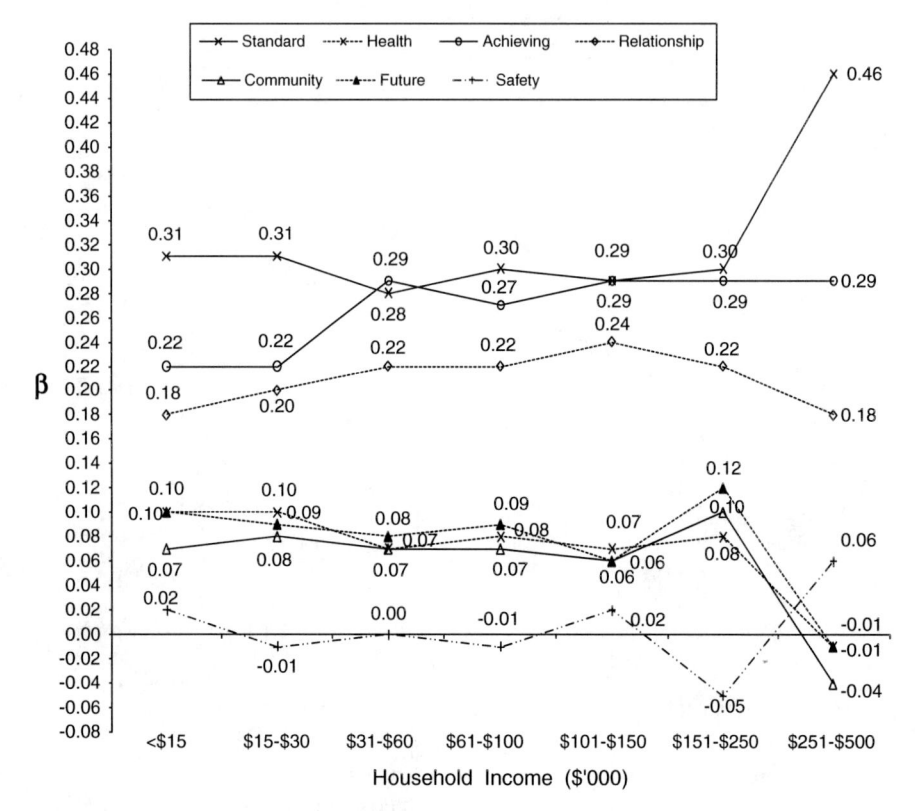

Fig. 2.2 Domain unique variance × income (combined data)

The most dramatic result is provided by the highest income group ($251–500K). Up to this level of income, all of the domains except safety contribute significant unique variance. Then, at this highest level of income, the unique contribution from health, community, and future security all become non-significant, leaving only three domains to make a significant unique contribution (standard, achieving, and relationships).

Three other features of these results in Fig. 2.2 are notable and can be explained in conjunction with Fig. 2.1 as:

1. At the highest level of income, the combined unique variance supplied by these three remaining domains is the highest of all the regressions (see Fig. 2.1).
2. Coincident with this sharp rise in amount of unique variance, the shared variance decreases to its lowest level. However, the overall variance accounted for remains stable at about 50%. In other words, it appears that some shared variance has become unique variance within standard, achieving and relationships. Perhaps these are the only domains required when life is easy?
3. The peak unique variance is achieved at different income levels for each domain. Relationships peaks at $101–150K, achieving peaks first at $31–60K, while standard peaks at $251–500K. This may reflect their different sensitivity to income.

In summary, from the above-mentioned analyses, the results are generally consistent with theory. Perhaps most important, it is evident that the interpretation of changed levels in domain satisfaction will differ depending on what is causing the change. In the case of safety, the very small contribution of unique variance indicates that safety satisfaction is driven by shared variance emanating from either HPMood or failed homeostasis. Thus, changes in safety satisfaction are not part of the driving force behind the differences in the PWI. On the contrary, the level of the PWI, as driven by other factors, accounts for the differing levels of satisfaction with safety. Thus, within this context, safety satisfaction carries very little additional information to that available from the average of the other domains.

6 Linear Statistics Obscure Important Information

From what has been discussed above, it seems that safety satisfaction may not be a useful measurement to make. Not only will it resist change due to its strong bond with HPMood but, when it does change, will also provide no unique information. However, such findings must be reconciled with a large literature showing an otherwise inverse relationship between positive psychological states, such as SWB, and negative psychological states, such as fear.

This reconciliation may be achieved through the application of two related ideas. The first kind involves an assumption that the actual level of fear or anxiety in general population samples in Australia is generally quite low. This implies that homeostasis is effective for most of the samples, resulting in a nonsignificant relationship between the strength of negative affect and SWB. However, this will not apply to all members of the sample. At the extremes, there will almost always be those who say they are 10/10 worried, stressed, or anxious about whatever the question concerned. Their evaluation may have very little to do with the topic under discussion. Instead, their extreme evaluation may be driven by high levels of general anxiety, depression, or extreme personality characteristics.

As a result of these extreme respondents, data from general population samples will be predicted to have the following characteristics. Over most levels of challenge strength, there will be no significant relationship between challenge strength and SWB. However, at very high levels of challenge strength, SWB will evidence an association with the challenging agent as homeostasis fails. As a consequence, when linear statistics are applied to the sample as a whole, these extreme values will cause the appearance of a significant correlation.

As an extension of this logic, if general population samples are subdivided into those with homeostatic defeat (very low SWB) and those with normal SWB, only the former group will show a strong relationship between the strength of the challenging agent and SWB. This has been demonstrated by Kitchen and Williams (2010) using life satisfaction and fear of crime. It is also demonstrated by our Australian Unity data on people's fear of a terrorist attack.

Australia has experienced no major acts of terrorism on home soil. However, this pestilence has afflicted nearby countries. As mentioned in the introduction, bombs

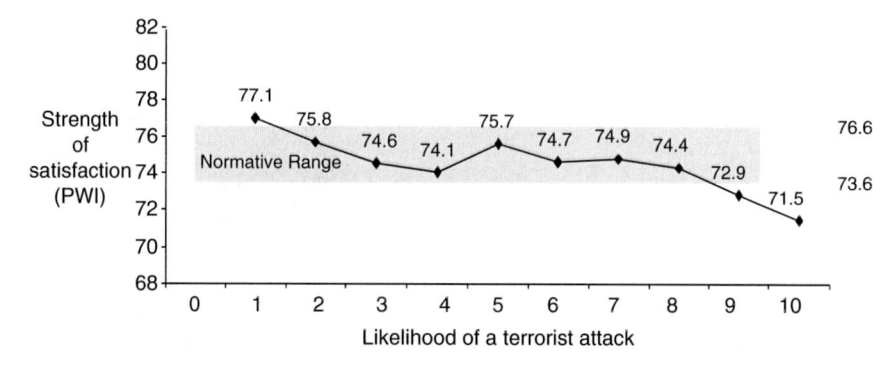

Fig. 2.3 The relationship between SWB and the considered likelihood of an attack

detonated in Bali, Indonesia, in 2002 killed 88 Australians, and this was followed in 2005 by a similar attack. Since 2003, we have been asking people two questions. First, whether they expect a terrorist attack in Australia to happen in the near future and, second, if they do, the strength of their conviction.

Figure 2.3 shows cumulative data, from Surveys 9–21, on the strength of belief that an attack is likely in the near future. The horizontal bar represents the generic normal range of SWB for group mean scores, and the 0.3% of the sample who rate the probability as 1/10 lie above this range.

From a probability of 2/10 to 8/10, SWB does not reliably change and remains in the normal range. Thus, as predicted by homeostasis, most levels of belief, that a terrorist attack is likely in the near future, have no systematic effect on well-being. However, at a probability estimate of 9 or 10/10, SWB goes down.

These results are interesting from two perspectives. First is that using the full set of results, the correlation between the perceived likelihood of a terrorist attack and personal well-being is −.82 ($p < .01$). This is the statistic that would normally be reported, but it is quite misleading. It implies that there is a simple progressive decrease in SWB as the perceived likelihood of an attack increases. However, this estimate is exquisitely sensitive to the extreme values.

The inclusion of data from the people who rate the probability as 1/10 is problematic. These people comprise 0.5% of the sample and so, clearly, most people require a higher level of probability before answering "yes" to the initial question. Moreover, their PWI of 77.1 points is 0.6 points above the normative range. The reason for this high PWI is probably not related to the issue of a terrorist attack. More likely, these people have a personality which is associated with a high set-point. At the other end of the distribution, the two response groups 9 and 10/10 (5.9% and 9.3% of the sample) are also different from the other groups in lying below the normal range. These response groups may contain a higher-than-normal proportion of people with depression, and it may be that this depression is driving their pessimistic view of attack probability.

Whatever the reason for the extreme PWI scores, the inclusion of these response groups profoundly affects the correlation between the probability of attack and SWB. If the correlation calculation includes values from 2 to 10, on the 0-to-10-response scale, then $r = .74$, which accounts for 55.1% of the variance. If the calculation omits the two extreme values and includes the probabilities from 2 to 8, then $r = .34$, which accounts for only 11.9% of the variance. Thus, these results are consistent with the homeostasis theory. They show that, up to an estimated perceived attack probability of 8/10, personal well-being is being actively managed, and the rated probability of an attack has no systematic influence to reduce SWB.

7 Other Reasons Safety Satisfaction Is Resistant to Change

The fear of a terrorist attack in Australia is the fear of a distal threat. Very few people with this fear have had personal experience of such an attack, so it is an imagined fear based on hearsay and media reports. However, even when the threat of attack is more likely than it is in Australia, the effects on SWB are small. For example, Frey et al. (2009) use life satisfaction data from three countries (Great Britain, Northern Ireland, and France) which had experienced terrorism over the period of 1970–2002. They found that an increase of one standard deviation in the number of recorded incidents in Britain and France lowered life satisfaction by 0.40 points and 0.43 points, respectively, on the 0–100 scale. Recorded fatalities similarly decreased life satisfaction by 0.3 points in both countries. These very small effects were significant due largely to the large number of observations (>30,000) in each country.

More proximal to the individual is the living-environment defined by family and neighborhood. People who do not feel integrated into their neighborhood may be especially prone to feeling a reduced sense of safety, so it is not surprising to find that fear is higher among people who are female, elderly, nonwhites (in the USA), poor, lonely, dissatisfied, or alienated (Liska and Baccaglini 1990; Liska et al. 1988). However, despite such findings, one of the predictions from homeostasis is that, generally, safety referenced to neighborhoods will have little impact on SWB. The main reason is that people adapt to their circumstances of living by adapting their behavior to suit their environment (Bannister and Fyfe 2001).

As an example of such adaptation, it is known that parent's perceptions of neighborhood safety in physically rundown neighborhoods (McDonell 2007, urban/rural setting in the USA) exert strong influences on their behavior toward their children. Most obviously, these involve closer monitoring and restricting of their children's behavior outside the home (e.g., Kling et al. 2001), and these tendencies may be enhanced if the parents feel socially isolated (Hill and Herman-Stahl 2002). Constrained social behavior within the neighborhood may also act as a negative feedback loop for the parents, resulting in them avoiding social interaction, which, in turn, accentuates their fear (Liska et al. 1988).

Nevertheless, these are all forms of adaptive behavior in the face of perceived threat, and as long as their behavior engenders a sense of control, safety as such will impact minimally on SWB. This has been confirmed by Michalos and Zumbo (2000) within Prince George, British Columbia. This city is ranked by Macleans (2008) as the fourth most dangerous city in Canada, based on aggregated crime statistics. Nevertheless, these authors found only a weak association between life satisfaction and crime issues, which disappeared with the inclusion of other variables in a multiple regression.

Moving up the danger list, Macleans (2008) ranks Saskatoon as the most dangerous Canadian city. So it makes sense that in samples from Saskatoon selected for low levels of life satisfaction, Kitchen and Williams (2010) found a strong relationship between life satisfaction and high fear of crime. Notably, however, and consistent with the homeostasis theory, the great majority of the population did not show this relationship, showing the effectiveness of their adaptation, as has been discussed.

Progressing still further up the danger list, Moller (2005) examined criminal victimization in one of the most dangerous countries of the world. Within South Africa's Nelson Mandela Metropolitan Municipality, in the Eastern Cape Province, Moller found that fear of crime and concern about personal safety had greater negative influence on life satisfaction than actual victimization. This confirms a wider literature showing that crimes against the person have greater negative influence on subjective well-being and feelings of personal safety than on property and other household crimes (Liska and Baccaglini 1990). However, even in very unsafe areas, poverty and unemployment were found to be greater threats to SWB than crime and safety (Moller 2005).

8 Conclusion

This aim of this chapter has been to examine the connection between safety satisfaction and subjective well-being (SWB). It is concluded that, despite the wide employment of the safety domain within measures of life quality and other constructs, feelings about safety seem to have little relevance to SWB, certainly within Australia. The reasons for this appear to be threefold as: (a) the strong link that such satisfaction has to HPMood, implying that levels of safety satisfaction are strongly driven by levels of HPMood; (b) the paucity of unique variance contributed by the measure, which probably reflects a generally low level of homeostatic threat from this domain; and (c) people's strong adaptation to situations where their sense of safety is threatened. Whether this conclusion applies to general population samples from other countries, especially those with more evident safety threats, requires more research. Notably, however, these general conclusions do not apply to threatened population subgroups in Australia, where safety satisfaction does contribute unique variance. For this reason, it is retained as a domain within the Personal Wellbeing Index.

Acknowledgement I thank Ann-Marie James for her assistance in preparing this manuscript. I also thank Wendy Kennedy and Rubecca Servinis for their comments on an earlier draft.

References

Andrews, F. M., & Withey, S. B. (1976). *Social indicators of well-being: American's perceptions of life quality*. New York: Plenum Press.
Australian Centre on Quality of Life. (2010). *Instruments*. Retrieved January 19, 2011, from http://www.deakin.edu.au/research/acqol/instruments/instrument.php
Australian Institute of Criminology. (2009). *Australian crime: Facts and*. Retrieved January 19, 2011, from http://www.aic.gov.au/en/publications/current%20series/facts/1–20/2009.aspx
Bannister, J., & Fyfe, N. (2001). Introduction: Fear and the city. *Urban Studies, 38*, 807–813.
Baron, R. M., & Kenny, D. A. (1986). The moderator-mediator variable distinction in social psychological research: Conceptual, strategic, and statistical considerations. *Journal of Personality and Social Psychology, 51*, 1173–1182.
Benbenishty, R., & Astor, R. A. (2005). *School violence in context: Culture, neighborhood, family, school, and gender*. New York: Oxford University Press.
Best, C. J., Cummins, R. A., & Lo, S. K. (2000). The quality of rural and metropolitan life. *Australian Journal of Psychology, 52*, 69–74.
Braungart, J. M., Plomin, R., DeFries, J. C., & Fulker, D. W. (1992). Genetic influence on tester-rated infant temperament as assessed by Bayley's infant behavior record: Nonadoptive and adoptive siblings and twins. *Developmental Psychology, 28*, 40–47.
Chua, H., Wong, A. K. W., & Shek, D. T. L. (2010). Social development in Hong Kong: Development issues identified by Social Development Index (SDI). *Social Indicators Research, 95*, 535–551.
Cummins, R. A. (1995). On the trail of the gold standard for life satisfaction. *Social Indicators Research, 35*, 179–200.
Cummins, R. A. (1998). The second approximation to an international standard of life satisfaction. *Social Indicators Research, 43*, 307–334.
Cummins, R. A. (2000). Personal income and subjective well-being: A review. *Journal of Happiness Studies, 1*, 133–158.
Cummins, R. A. (2001). The subjective well-being of people caring for a severely disabled family member at home: A review. *Journal of Intellectual and Developmental Disability, 26*, 83–100.
Cummins, R. A. (2010). Subjective wellbeing, homeostatically protected mood and depression: A synthesis. *Journal of Happiness Studies, 11*, 1–17. doi:10.1007/s10902-009-9167-0.
Cummins, R. A., & Nistico, H. (2002). Maintaining life satisfaction: The role of positive cognitive bias. *Journal of Happiness Studies, 3*, 37–69.
Cummins, R. A., Gullone, E., & Lau, A. L. D. (2002). A model of subjective well-being homeostasis: The role of personality. In E. Gullone & R. A. Cummins (Eds.), *The universality of subjective well-being indicators: Social indicators research series* (pp. 7–46). Dordrecht: Kluwer.
Cummins, R. A., Hughes, J., Tomyn, A., Gibson, A., Woerner, J., & Lai, L. (2007a). *Australian Unity wellbeing index: Report 17.1 the wellbeing of Australians – Carer health and wellbeing*. Melbourne: Australian Centre on Quality of Life, School of Psychology, Deakin University. ISBN 978 1 74156 092 3. Retrieved July 9, 2010, from http://www.deakin.edu.au/research/acqol/index_wellbeing/index.htm
Cummins, R. A., Walter, J., & Woerner, J. (2007b). *Australian Unity wellbeing index: Report 16.1 – "The wellbeing of Australians – Groups with the highest and lowest wellbeing in Australia"*. Melbourne: Australian Centre on Quality of Life, School of Psychology, Deakin University. ISBN 978 1 74156 079 4. Retrieved July 9, 2010, from http://www.deakin.edu.au/research/acqol/index_wellbeing/index.htm
Cummins, R. A., Collard, J., Woerner, J., Weinberg, M., Lorbergs, M., & Perera, C. (2009). *Australian Unity wellbeing index: – Report 22.0. The wellbeing of Australians – Who makes the decisions, health/wealth control, Financial Advice, and Handedness*. Melbourne: Australian Centre on Quality of Life, School of Psychology, Deakin University. ISBN 978 1 74156 133 3. http://www.deakin.edu.au/research/acqol/index_wellbeing/index.htm. Retrieved July 9, 2010.
Cummins, R. A., Woerner, J., M., W., Perera, C., Gibson, A., Collard, J., et al. (2010). *Australian Unity wellbeing index: – Report 23.0 "The wellbeing of Australians - life better/worse, children*

and neighbourhood". Melbourne: Australian Centre on Quality of Life, School of Psychology, Deakin University. ISBN 978 1 74156 141 8. Retrieved January 19, 2011, from http://www.deakin.edu.au/research/acqol/index_wellbeing/index.htm

Davern, M., Cummins, R. A., & Stokes, M. (2007). Subjective wellbeing as an affective/cognitive construct. *Journal of Happiness Studies, 8*, 429–449.

Fayers, P. M., Hand, D. J., Bjordal, K., & Groenvold, M. (1997). Causal indicators in quality of life research. *Quality of Life Research, 6*, 393–406.

Frey, B. S., Luechinger, S., & Stutzer, A. (2009). The life satisfaction approach to valuing public goods: The case of terrorism. *Public Choice, 138*, 317–346.

Hanestad, B. R., & Albrektsen, G. (1992). The stability of quality of life experience in people with type 1 diabetes over a period of a year. *Journal of Advanced Nursing, 17*, 777–784.

Headey, B., & Wearing, A. (1989). Personality, life events, and subjective well-being: Toward a dynamic equilibrium model. *Journal of Personality and Social Psychology, 57*, 731–739.

Henderson, S. (1977). The social network, support and neurosis. The function of attachment in adult life. *The British Journal of Psychiatry, 131*, 185–191.

Hill, N. E., & Herman-Stahl, M. A. (2002). Neighborhood safety and social involvement: Associations with parenting behaviors and depressive symptoms among African American and Euro-American mothers. *Journal of Family Psychology, 16*, 209–219.

Hoffman, B. (1998). *Inside terrorism*. New York: Columbia University Press.

Huelsman, I. J., Nemanick, R. C., & Munz, D. C. (1998). Scales to measure four dimensions of dispositional mood: Positive energy, tiredness, negative activation, and relaxation. *Educational and Psychological Measurement, 58*, 804–819.

International Wellbeing Group. (2006). *Personal wellbeing index manual*. Melbourne: Deain University. Retrieved June 30, 2009, from http://www.deakin.edu.au/research/acqol/instruments/wellbeing_index.htm

Kitchen, P., & Williams, A. (2010). Quality of life and perceptions of crime in Saskatoon, Canada. *Social Indicators Research, 95*, 33–62.

Klasen, S. (2000). Measuring poverty and deprivation in South Africa. *Review of Income and Wealth, 46*, 33–58.

Kling, J. R., Liebman, J. B., & Katz, L. F. (2001). *Bullets don't got no name: Consequences of fear in the ghetto. Joint Center for Poverty Research, Working Paper 225*. Retrieved July 1, 2010, from http://www.northwestern.edu/ipr/jcpr/workingpapers/wpfiles/kling_liebman_katz.PDF

Lau, A. L. D., Cummins, R. A., & McPherson, W. (2005). An investigation into the cross-cultural equivalence of the personal wellbeing index. *Social Indicators Research, 72*, 403–430. doi:10.1007/s11205-004-0561-z.

Lau, A. L. D., Chi, I., Cummins, R. A., Lee, T. M. C., Chou, K. L., & Chung, L. W. M. (2008). The SARS (severe acute respiratory syndrome) pandemic in Hong Kong: Effects on the subjective wellbeing of elderly and younger people. *Aging & Mental Health, 12*, 746–760. doi:10.1080/13607860802380607.

Liska, A. E., & Baccaglini, W. (1990). Feeling safe by comparison: Crime in the newspapers. *Social Problems, 37*, 360–374.

Liska, A. E., Sanchirico, A., & Reed, M. D. (1988). Fear of crime and constrained behavior: Specifying and estimating a reciprocal effects model. *Social Forces, 66*, 827–837.

Lykken, D., & Tellegen, A. (1996). Happiness is a stochastic phenomenon. *Psychological Science, 7*, 186–189.

Macleans, C. A. (2008). *The most dangerous cities in Canada: Overall crime score—By rank. March 24, 38–46*. Retrieved July 9, 2010, from http://www2.macleans.ca/2009/03/04/the-most-dangerous-cities-in-canada-overall-crime-score%E2%80%94by-rank/

Mattes, R., Bratton, M., & Davids, Y. D. (2003). *Poverty, survival and democracy in Southern Africa. Afrobarometer Paper No. 23*. Cape Town/Accra/East Lansing: Afrobarometer.

McDonell, J. R. (2007). Neighborhood characteristics, parenting, and children's safety. *Social Indicators Research, 83*, 177–199.

Merriam-Webster Online. (2011). Retrieved January 17, 2011, from http://www.merriam-webster.com

Michalos, A. C., & Zumbo, B. D. (2000). Criminal victimization and the quality of life. *Social Indicators Research, 50*, 245–295.

Moller, V. (2005). Resilient or resigned? Criminal victimization and quality of life in South Africa. *Social Indicators Research, 72*, 263–317.

NationMaster. (2011). Retrieved January 19, 2011, from http://www.nationmaster.com/index.php

Patmore, G. (2010). *Happiness as an objective of labour law.* Working Paper No. 48 Centre for Employment and Labour Relations Law. Retrieved July 13, 2010 from http://www.apo.org.au/node/20821.

Rothbaum, F., Weisz, J. R., & Snyder, S. S. (1982). Changing the world and changing the self: A two-process model of perceived control. *Journal of Personality and Social Psychology, 42*, 5–37.

Russell, J. A. (2003). Core affect and the psychological construction of emotion. *Psychological Review, 110*, 145–172.

Sarason, I. G., Sarason, B. R., & Pierce, G. R. (1990). Social support: The search for theory. *Journal of Social and Clinical Psychology, 9*, 137–147.

Schwarz, N., & Strack, F. (1991). Evaluating one's life: A judgement model of subjective well-being. In F. Strack, M. Argyle, & N. Schwarz (Eds.), *Subjective well-being* (pp. 27–47). Oxford: Pergamon Press.

Schwarz, N., & Strack, F. (1999). Reports of subjective well-being: Judgmental processes and their methodological limitations. In D. Kahneman, E. Diener, & N. Schwarz (Eds.), *The foundation of hedonic happiness* (pp. 61–84). New York: Russell Sage.

Shek, D. T. L. (2010). Using students' weekly diaries to evaluate positive youth development programs: Are findings based on multiple studies consistent. *Social Indicators Research, 95*, 475–487.

Smyth, R., Nielsen, I., & Zhai, Q. G. (2010). Personal well-being in urban China. *Social Indicators Research, 95*, 231–252.

Tiliouine, H., Cummins, R. A., & Davern, M. (2006). Measuring wellbeing in developing countries: The case of Algeria. *Social Indicators Research, 75*, 1–30. doi:10.1007/s11205-004-2012-2.

Wei, H.-S., & Chen, J.-K. (2010). School attachment among Taiwanese adolescents: The roles of individual characteristics, peer relationships, and teacher well-being. *Social Indicators Research, 95*, 421–436.

Wilkinson, P. (2000). *Terrorism versus democracy: The liberal state response.* London/Portland: Frank Cass.

Yik, M. S. M., Russell, J. A., & Barrett, L. F. (1999). Structure of self-reported current affect: Integration and beyond. *Journal of Personality and Social Psychology, 77*, 600–619.

Chapter 3
Terror, Fear and Individual and Community Well-Being

1 Introduction

> In March 2002, with much pomp, the Bush administration's new Department of Homeland Security introduced its color-coded terror alert system: green, "low"; blue, "guarded"; yellow, "elevated"; orange, "high"; red, "severe." The nation has danced ever since between yellow and orange. Life has restlessly settled, to all appearances permanently, on the redward end of the spectrum, the blue-greens of tranquillity a thing of the past. "Safe" doesn't even merit a hue. Safe, it would seem, has fallen off the spectrum of perception. Insecurity, the spectrum says, is the new normal.
>
> (Massumi 2005, p. 31)

On a typical Monday in March 2007, shoppers and workers in the Central Business District of the West Australian capital went about their daily business as usual. By midday, the heart of the city was in the grip of an emergency as police and security personnel evacuated one of Perth's busiest precincts. A 'suspicious' package had been sent to three inner city travel agencies. The panic sparked by the packages had little to do with their contents or appearance or even the circumstances under which they happened to arrive at the doorsteps of their intended recipients. Rather it was the name of the sender – Osama – emblazoned across the packages that caused the frenzied commotion. Osama, as it turned out, is the rather inopportune name of the employee at the printing company that had put together the packages of brochures. Ironically, the packages included safety information for travellers.

In that same year 2007, 40-year-old school teacher Michael Chalk walked into a pub in the Queensland city of Cairns. Chalk headed towards the dance floor, but not before laying the book he was reading face up on a nearby ledge. Moments later, he was approached by a security guard and escorted out of the pub. Chalk

A. Aly (✉)
School of Social Sciences and Asian Languages, Curtin University, Bentley, Australia
e-mail: anne.aly@curtin.edu.au

D. Webb and E. Wills-Herrera (eds.), *Subjective Well-Being and Security*,
Social Indicators Research Series 46, DOI 10.1007/978-94-007-2278-1_3,
© Springer Science+Business Media B.V. 2012

was asked to leave the pub after several other patrons complained that the book he was reading made them nervous. The title of that book was *The Unknown Terrorist*, by Australian novelist Richard Flanagan. The book is the fictional story of a Sydney dancer who becomes Australia's most wanted terrorist after spending a night with a stranger. Ironically, it is a cynical assessment of public panic about terrorism and the role of the media and politicians in creating and manipulating the fear of terrorism. The incident with Michael Chalk reinforced the message about moral panic and the fear of terrorism that Flanagan was trying to get across: 'Far from being far-fetched, my novel correctly predicted the future of Australia' (Marks 2007).

The terrorist attacks on the United States in September 2001, we were told, changed the world forever. The attacks heralded a new era of ideological conflict – the 'clash of civilisations' (Huntington 1993). In his Address to Congress and the American people on 20 September 2001, the then US President George W. Bush defined the attacks as a 'new' kind of war: one that extended beyond previously established margins of combat to the unchartered battlefields of ideological warfare:

> Americans have known wars – but for the past 136 years, they have been wars on foreign soil, except for one Sunday in 1941. Americans have known the casualties of war – but not at the center of a great city on a peaceful morning. Americans have known surprise attacks – but never before on thousands of civilians. All of this was brought upon us in a single day – and night fell on a different world, a world where freedom itself is under attack. (Bush 2001a, b)

Five years later, on the anniversary of the 2001 terrorist attacks, Bush reaffirmed the 'new' boundaries of the 'war on terror', stating, 'The war against this enemy is more than a military conflict. It is the decisive ideological struggle of the twenty-first century, and the calling of our generation' (Bush 2006).

In Australia, we were told to 'be alert but not alarmed'. In June 2002, the then Prime Minister, John Howard, invoked Australia's cultural kinship with the United States to position Australia (along with the rest of the 'free' world) as a target for terrorists: 'The horrifying events in the United States last September drew Australia, and the rest of the world, into a new and largely unpredictable security environment' (Attorney-General's Department 2002).

In a 'Post 9/11' world, 'Insecurity is the new normal' (Massumi 2005, p. 31). In this 'new normal', insecurity is transformed from a situational emotional response (Cameron and McCormick 1954) to a perpetual state of alertness, and terrorism is imagined as an unknown, but impending, doom. Everyday situations (travelling to and from work) and objects (a backpack, a credit card, a mobile phone, a book) become subliminally associated with the threat of terrorism. The terrorist threat, articulated through images of the ordinary and banal, is situated in the everyday: normalising threat and re-constructing what would otherwise be considered exceptional measures as rational, prudent, even necessary (Huysmans 2004). The increased security presence at airports, the persistent salience of the *National Security Information Campaign* urging Australians to report 'possible signs of terrorism to the National Security Hotline' over 6 years after it was first launched (2002) and the progressive introduction of over 30 legislative amendments in the interests of national security invoke the spectre of security and amplify threat in the public imagination. In public usage, 'terrorism' is expanded to refer as much to an *act of terrorism* as a *state of terror*. Terrorism (what we fear) is re-inscribed as terror (the state of intense fear), and the 'war on terror' is a referent for the 'war on terrorism'.

Insecurity is linked to threat (Cameron and McCormick 1954) and threat to anxiety and fear (Huddy et al. 2005). Fear motivates people to take action against the perceived threat. This action is moralised as a justified response to suffering. The state of insecurity belies community anxiety and fear that finds expression in increased aggression towards the perceived source of threat, greater in-group solidarity and support for extraordinary measures directed at members of the threatening group (Davis and Silver 2004; Huddy et al. 2005, p. 594). Through fear, society can reaffirm its commitment to a set of common political values that are threatened by an identified enemy. At an individual or group level, this reaffirmation may be expressed through a renewal of nationalist ideologies and patriotic behaviours. As Falk (2002) states, '…when a society is threatened by an external enemy there is a strong tendency to express patriotic feelings through tribal and ultra-nationalist displays of unconditional support' (p. 331).

Originally constructed as an attack on the United States, September 11 symbolised the threat of Islam to the entire Western world, of which Australia was a part. The evolving discourse on terrorism in the Australian media objectified and personified the threat of terrorism, constructing it in terms of an irreconcilable, dangerous and ominous 'other' that could not be appeased through reason or rationality. The 'other' implicated in this Australian discourse is Islam and, by implication, Muslims around the globe (including Australia). Muslims in Australia were positioned by the media and political discourses as potential terrorists. Insecurity thus precipitated community anxiety, and communal fear translated into acts of aggression, vilification and abuse against those who most saliently represented the threat of terrorism (HREOC 2004).

2 Fear, Anxiety and Well-Being

Economic and social indicators of community well-being tend to monitor phenomena such as economic performance, health, educational achievement and human development. Indicators of subjective well-being (SWB), on the other hand, focus on individuals' self judgements about themselves and the society in which they live. Subjective indicators of well-being draw attention to people's experiences in relation to the social environment in which these experiences occur. Importantly, these experiences and the perceptions, attitudes and values which they shape influence patterns of behaviour. Jowell (2009) makes this point when discussing the fear of crime. He argues that crime statistics (an objective measure of well-being) may not necessarily be as revealing as measures of the fear of crime (a subjective measure of well-being). Fear of crime is more likely to motivate patterns of behaviour that impact on quality of life and well-being. Jowell (2009) argues that subjective indicators of well-being should extend beyond people's affective feelings of happiness and life satisfaction to include underlying value structures and personal perceptions of tolerance, safety and fairness.

Perceptions of safety and personal security are included in the Personal Wellbeing Index which measures personal satisfaction in eight domains: standard of living, personal health, life achievement, personal relationships, personal safety, community-connectedness, future security and spirituality/religion (Chen 2009). These indicators establish a link between subjective well-being and perceptions of fear, security and safety. Further evidence of this link is found in research that proposes that avoidance of worst fears is negatively related to SWB. King's (1998) survey of the literature cites research into defensive pessimism which demonstrates that individuals who focus on dread rather than success forego the affective benefits of goal attainment. King concludes that there is sufficient evidence in the literature to suggest that fear avoidance is likely to correlate with poorer SWB.

3 The Fear of Terrorism

The next section of this chapter reports on the findings of a national study on the fear of terrorism. The study investigated how Australians constructed the media discourse on terrorism, their perceptions of threat and their behavioural responses to the fear of terrorism. In order to draw conclusions about the variant impact of fear on different communities, the research explored these themes with two different groups: Australian Muslims and (non-Muslim) members of the broader community.

3.1 Method

The methodology for the study was essentially interpretive using techniques borrowed from qualitative research traditions: grounded theory and phenomenological research. Phenomenological research focuses on individual experiences of a phenomenon to develop multiple perspectives as a means of understanding lived experience (Osborne 1994). In the first stage of the research, 10 focus groups were conducted with 86 participants of various backgrounds in terms of age, gender, religion and ethnicity. Of the ten focus groups, 4 were held with Australian Muslims, while 6 groups involved participants from the broader community. A combination of snowballing, purposive, quota and chain referral sampling was used to ensure that no group of participants with similar characteristics (age, gender, ethnicity) was omitted, under-represented or over-represented in the focus groups. Muslim participants were primarily recruited through the researcher's community links while participants from the broader community were recruited through a circulated Call for

Participants notice. Some focus groups were held at Edith Cowan University while others were held in community venues nominated by the group participants.

The focus group sessions were audio recorded and transcribed. Phenomenological analysis was applied to the focus group data set using NVivo, a qualitative analysis software package, to identify and extract salient themes and constructs for further investigation. The insights revealed through this analysis informed the subsequent focussed interviews with a further 60 research participants. The focussed interview, as described by Merton and Kendall's (2003) seminal paper originally published in 1946, uses an interview guide based on a prerequisite analysis of the situation under investigation. This allows the interviewer to use her foreknowledge of the situation (derived from analysis of the focus groups data) to determine the parameters and nature of participant accounts generated in the interview. The individual interviews were conducted with 30 Muslim respondents (15 males and 15 females) and 30 respondents from the broader community (15 males and 15 females). The interviews were audio taped and transcribed to produce a second data set. The combined focus group and individual interview transcripts yielded over 300 pages of qualitative data that was again analysed using NVivo to extract participants' understandings of terrorism, their experiences of the fear of terrorism and their behavioural responses to that fear.

The qualitative techniques used allowed the researcher to examine the range of issues that directed public discussion about terrorism and the fear of terrorism as well as the range of language used to express the psychological, behavioural and emotional responses to the perceived threat of terrorism. The results are reported in the next section using quotations from both the focus groups (reported as focus group, gender, target group) and the individual interviews (reported as gender, age range, target group).

3.2 Results

The extant literature on the fear of terrorism and the fear of crime makes some distinction between anxiety and fear. Studies that utilise the definition of anxiety established in the fields of neuroscience and psychology give primacy to anxiety and regard fear and worry as sub-sets of anxiety. Others distinguish between anxiety and fear. Among the literature on the fear of crime, Garafolo (1981) distinguishes actual fear from anticipated fear and defines the fear of crime as 'an emotional reaction characterised by a sense of danger and anxiety about physical harm'. Importantly, both actual and anticipatory fears can produce behavioural responses.

In short, the available literature offers a variety of approaches – sometimes conflicting – to understanding fear and anxiety in relation to terrorism or crime. Rather than adopt a pre-constructed definition of fear from the literature, the approach taken in this study was to allow the respondents to define the fear of terrorism through self-reported expressions of anxiety, distress, worry or concern.

The language used by participants in the study to express fear of terrorism ranged from candid expressions of psychological distress such as 'afraid', 'scared' and 'fearful of' to more subtle expressions of concern, anxiety or worry. The fear of terrorism, as constructed and conceptualised by the respondents in this study, refers broadly to an intense emotional and/or physical response as well as latent feelings of anxiety, concern or worry.

The analysis of the data collected in the focus groups and individual interviews revealed patterns in how both groups of respondents (Australian Muslims and the broader community) conceptualised and expressed their fear of terrorism. Four distinct but related thematic categories emerged from the data to describe the range of fears, anxieties and concerns around the perceived threat of terrorism:

Fear of physical harm
Political fear
Fear of losing civil liberties
Feeling insecure

These four thematic categories of fear were expressed by both groups in the study but were conceptualised in very different ways. Australian Muslims construct the fear of losing civil liberties, for example, in terms of their own fears of being targeted and implicated as a possible 'person of interest' by authorities. In contrast, members of the broader community construct this kind of fear in terms of the depreciation of the core values of liberal democracy. Thus, each type or category of the fear of terrorism was constructed in accordance with the real, lived experiences of the respondents and reflected their subjective positioning in the media and official discourses on terrorism. Australian Muslims who were positioned as potential threats and the objects of fear in the popular discourse on terrorism adopted behavioural and cognitive responses that reflect this positioning – they construct their fears of terrorism from the position of 'threatening other'. Members of the broader Australian community who were positioned as potential targets of a terrorist attack and likely victims of 'Islamic' terrorism construct their fears of terrorism in relation to this position.

3.2.1   Fear of Physical Harm

The fear of physical harm from a terrorist attack is an emotional and (sometimes) physical response that is aroused in the presence of certain stimuli in the proximate environment. Respondents expressed their fear of physical harm from a terrorist attack explicitly—

> When September 11 happened for me I was terrified! I wouldn't leave the house. I was freaking out over it (female, age 18–24, broader community)

—and implicitly through their recollections about experiences in which they described behavioural responses in certain threat situations. Drawing on their schematic knowledge of terrorist attacks developed through interaction with media images of actual attacks, the respondents constructed situations of threat salience. These were situations in which a combination of elements in the environment resonated with media images of the terrorist attacks in New York (2001), Bali (2002) or London (2005): a crowded train, a backpack or a suspicious package or person.

Often, these situations prompted behavioural responses to the fear of terrorism. In one focus group, a female participant who had lost a close family member in the Bali bombings did not believe that this experience had made her more fearful of a terrorist attack. However, she did recall a recent incident in Perth in which authorities closed off the city centre in response to a bomb threat. Stuck in a bus for 2 hours, this participant began to feel more and more anxious about a terrorist attack:

> … and so it just went through my head…is this real? Can this happen again?

Participants in the study related stories about being fearful on public transport, on aeroplanes, in airports and when viewing media reports of terrorist attacks. The fear of being harmed in a terrorist attack is reported as being felt at certain times and in response to particular stimuli through which danger becomes objectified and seems imminent and unavoidable. As such, this kind of fear appears to be fleeting – one that enters and exits and re-enters the conscious in response to particular stimuli and in certain situations of threat salience. In reference to this kind of modulated fear, Aly and Balnaves (2005) state: 'In the Australian context, after more than 4 years of collected traces of experiences of images of threat, responses to terrorism have become almost reflexive – even automated'.

For Muslim respondents, the fear of physical harm did not express fear of actually being harmed in a terrorist attack. Rather, and in accordance with their personal experiences of harm in the aftermath of the September 11 terrorist attacks, Muslim Australians fear the community backlash to a terrorist attack. The fear of physical harm from a possibly violent retaliation to a terrorist attack in Australia and its implications for Australian Muslims were the most prevalent fear expressed by the Muslim research participants. Participants used terminology such as 'afraid', 'scared' and 'terrified' to express their fears of retaliation from the broader community: their fear was specifically the fear of harm to self, family and community – both physical and psychological – from a retaliation:

> I'm utterly terrified. What frightens me is that my family are Muslim people, are living in this sea of hate and I have never felt that in my life before. (female, age 40–54, Muslim)

The fear of physical harm expressed by Muslim participants is based on the *real, lived* experiences of vilification – either directly or indirectly. A report released by the Human Rights and Equal Opportunity Commission (HREOC 2004) revealed heightened levels of discrimination, vilification and violence against Muslims in the aftermath of the 2001 terrorist attacks. In contrast, fear among members of the broader community is rarely based on *actual* personal experience of a terrorist attack. Rather, it centres on *imagined or anticipatory* experience.

3.2.2 Political Fear

Political fear refers to the promotion and manipulation of fear in order to consolidate and maintain control. Political fear hinges on chimera – the ability of the government to instil the population with a sense of dread of an unknown, but impending, collective harm. Focus group participants and individual respondents expressed anxiety about the manipulation of fear of terrorism in Australia to serve a political agenda:

> When John Howard [former Australian Prime Minister] used to tell us that we had to pre-pare for terrorist attacks, I was frightened to go to large shopping centres because I was becoming over conscious of it and I was thinking 'my goodness, you know if a bomb went off here you wouldn't be able to find the way out.' And I started getting very anxious about everything and then I thought, 'no this is silly' because I've probably got more of a chance of being skittled by a car if I step out the front of it or a plane falling out the sky. (female, age 55–70, broader community)

In particular, the research participants expressed anxiety about the possible social consequences of communal fear that defines a particular section of the community as the object of fear. Of most concern was the impact that political fear would have on social harmony and the fracturing of Australia's multicultural society.

Participants who were particularly aware of the political dimensions of terrorism were likely to express fearfulness or anxiety about the political motivations for ter-rorism and counterterrorism. The political and military responses to terrorism (the war on terror and interventions in Iraq and Afghanistan) were a source of fear and anxiety among some participants:

> There is also you know a sense for me, feeling that in a way we're creating it just as much… Western civilisation. (male, age 25–39, broader community)

Muslim participants were acutely aware of political fear and constructed the fear of terrorism among the broader community as a politically modulated fear that implicated Muslims as a threat in order to gain public support for contentious poli-cies. Thus, while the political fear experienced by Australian Muslims differs from that experienced by members of the broader community, the two manifestations of fear share a locus in the social repercussions of communal fear that is manipulated and sustained for a political agenda.

3.2.3   Fear of Losing Civil Liberties

The most commonly expressed fear of terrorism related to the threat of the loss of civil liberties and in particular the loss of freedom of speech. Participants from the broader community expressed concern about losing the right to oppose or question the official discourse on terrorism as demonstrated in the following quote:

> It's pretty kind of disillusioning that … worrying that… unless you fall in line, or you choose an alternative path that however you may have come to it, even if you have come to it by perfectly logical and you know, well researched reasoning you're still going to fall in, or fall as being one of the bad guys; for being one of the you know, lunatic terrorists. (male, age 18–24, broader community)

For Australian Muslim participants in the study, the fear of losing civil liberties was a pervasive fear in response to perceived increased security measures specifi-cally targeting Muslims and the possibility of being falsely implicated as a terrorist. The behavioural response to this fear among Australian Muslims is silence and an unwillingness to discuss issues of terrorism for fear of being marked a security risk. This was particularly observable in the off-record comments by some Muslim participants who alluded to reports about fellow Muslims being detained and questioned by authorities for articulating certain opinions.

3.2.4 Feeling Insecure

Feeling insecure was expressed as a feeling of reduced safety in their everyday lives. One of the most salient themes discussed in the focus groups was the loss of a sense of security and a heightened sense of insecurity since the September 11 terrorist attacks in the United States. Individual interviewees also expressed that the September 11 attacks had 'shattered' their sense of security. The Bali bombings in October 2002 had a significant impact in signalling that Australia was no longer viewed as a passive partner in the 'war on terror' and impacting the threat of a terrorist attack on Australian soil:

> I had this feeling that Australia was this remote country that nobody much knew about so we'd be safe…And so I didn't feel in any way threatened until Bali. (focus group, females, broader community)

The bombings on London's public transport system in 2005 reinvigorated feelings of insecurity and introduced the 'new' threat of 'home-grown' terrorists. In a focus group with females from the broader community, one participant expressed the impact of the London 2005 terrorist attacks in the following way:

> I think at times I did start to feel concerned about riding on the trains and things like that. So somewhere in my subconscious I've obviously taken on that feeling of fear that it's going to happen within my own country. Definitely at times I started to think about where would be safe for me to live instead of in a city. (focus group, females, broader community)

Increased security measures and the heightened salience of security were either a source of security and reassurance or constructed as symptomatic of a security culture and inspired fear about the related loss of freedoms. In the following excerpt, a female participant describes how the salience of security inspired her fear of terrorism related not to an actual terrorist attack but to the implications of a security culture:

> I just recently went overseas and when I got to the airport the thing that sent chills down my spine, that our society has progressed to the stage where there was such high level security, and I was travelling at the time where you couldn't have any cosmetics or anything like that. That sent chills down my spine, and when I got onto the plane, where typically you might start to feel those types of threats of terrorism, I wasn't, I wasn't concerned in any way, shape or form. It was the shock and sadness that I felt about how far our society has progressed in terms of giving up all this freedom and living our lives in fear that scared me more than any threat of terrorism. (female, age 25–39, broader community)

For Muslim participants, feelings of insecurity were strongly related to their perceptions of anti-Muslim sentiment among some sections of the community and in the media and political discourses. Muslim respondents expressed a noticeable shift in public opinion and attitudes towards Australian Muslims since the 2001 terrorist attacks and ensuing war on terror. This shift created feelings of anxiety, worry and fear expressed as a loss of safety and heightened insecurity among Australian Muslims. In the following excerpt from an interview with a female Muslim, the participant expresses how her sense of insecurity is closely tied to her Muslim identity and to feelings of 'othering':

> I think it [a terrorist attack] would have a very great impact. I think it might be quite severe as well – not just normal depression or stress. I think it's going to be really severe. I lived as a refugee Muslim all my life and being discriminated against. And when you know it's not your fault it's even harder and when you try to scream out and clear things out and get people to understand when it's happening and you don't seem to be making any difference or any impact – you are no-one. It hurts. (female, age 25–39, Muslim)

Perhaps the most significant finding of the research reported in this chapter is that the fear of terrorism is not limited to the fear of terrorists per se but is more broadly associated with a perceived state of terror in which insecurity, suspicion and the manipulation of fear for political purposes are the norm. Considering that one of the aims of terrorists, as defined by the Australian Defence Force, is to put 'the public or any section of the public in fear' (Hancock 2002), the findings regarding the nature of fear pervading the populace implicate the political and social responses to terrorism as significant factors in propagating community fear and anxiety. The ramifications of this fear on well-being are discussed in the next section.

4   Discussion

The study reported here demonstrates that the fear of terrorism is multi-dimensional and, unlike the fear of crime, is not focussed specifically on the fear of victimisation (physical harm). Nonetheless, there is some value to be gained from exploring the relationship between the fear of crime and well-being in the literature as it pertains to terrorism as a violent criminal offence.

Studies that explore the impact of the fear of crime on well-being conclude that the fear of crime has a negative impact on individual and community well-being. A study undertaken to inform crime prevention strategies in South Africa, a country with one of the highest crime rates by international standards, measured the fear of crime in terms of perceived likelihood of victimisation (Moller 2005). This study found that concern about personal safety, as opposed to actual victimisation, had a greater negative impact on life satisfaction – the fear of being a victim of a criminal act actually had a greater impact than the actual crime experience. Significantly, the study on the fear of terrorism reported in this chapter found that the fear of terrorism elicited protective and assertive responses from people who had not directly experienced a terrorist attack.

The live broadcasting and extended coverage of mass casualty terrorist attacks in New York, London and Bali positioned the global audience as witnesses. As such, the global audience who watched the demise of the Twin Towers and the carnage in Bali and London participated in the emotional responses to the terrorist attacks.

The claim that witnessing a terrorist attack by proxy (through mediated channels of communication) produces a fear effect that impacts on the broader population is supported by clinical studies that confirm that mass terrorist attacks psychiatrically impact on a broader population than the immediate victims. In one study by Galea et al. (2006) on residents of Manhattan (the borough in which the September 11 terrorist attacks occurred), the researchers found that residents who watched the most television coverage of the attacks had the highest likelihood of posttraumatic stress disorder. Many people in Galea's study described symptoms such as difficulty sleeping or concentrating. According to Galea, mass casualty terrorist attacks prompt behaviour changes that are damaging to health and quality of life: cigarette smoking, alcohol consumption and marijuana use rose among New Yorkers after September 11 for up to 9 months after the terrorist attacks. Two years after the attacks, the fear of flying had also increased (Lamberg 2005).

Apart from clinical symptoms of fear and their impact on well-being and health, individuals also adopt behavioural responses to fear that impact on well-being. The study reported in this chapter was used to inform the development of a metric of fear that was administered to a national sample of Australians (Aly et al. 2007; Aly and Balnaves 2007; Balnaves and Aly 2007). The results of this national survey pointed to the fear of terrorism as affecting two patterns of behavioural responses to fear: restrictive behaviours which assume that people constrain their behaviour to avoid circumstances considered unsafe and assertive behaviours which involve people adopting protective behaviours in circumstances perceived to be risky or unsafe (Liska et al. 1988). Restrictive behaviours included avoiding public transport or crowded shopping centres while protective behaviours included increased awareness of surroundings and behaviours described by participants as 'paranoia' or 'suspicion of others'. Such behaviours impact negatively on individual and community well-being. At the individual level, sustained high levels of anxiety and fear about a terrorist attack produce adverse health effects such as stress and depression. At the community level, risk assessments are based on popular discourses of terrorism which position the broader community as potential victims of terrorism and the Muslim 'other' as the object of fear. Behavioural responses are prompted by the salience of elements that are deemed to present risk. In the case of terrorism, the media and political framing of the terrorist threat as almost exclusively 'Muslim' effects behavioural responses in the presence of 'suspicious' persons – those who visually represent the terrorist threat. Ultimately, the impact has been a fracturing of social harmony and a marked increase in vilification and discrimination of Australian Muslims who are marked as the object of fear.

Muslim participants in the study expressed the most acute behavioural responses to global terrorist events. In several cases, female Muslims who wear the hijab (the traditional Islamic dress which covers the hair) expressed anxiety about venturing into public spaces for fear of being vilified or attacked. Often this anxiety was not based on personal experiences or relationships with individual members of the broader community, which were often described as positive, but on a perception of the Muslim community at risk of hostile and often violent responses from some members of the broader community. One woman stated that after the

September 11 attacks, she did not leave her home for 2 weeks. Reports about attacks on Muslim women wearing hijab in public circulated among the Muslim communities – promulgating fear, heightening anxiety and precipitating behavioural responses. Such extreme restrictive and protective behaviours have a significantly adverse impact on the social and economic health and well-being of the community, resulting in and contributing to community isolation and marginalisation.

5 Conclusion

Indicators of subjective well-being include feelings of safety, personal security and perceptions of tolerance and fairness (Chen 2009; Jowell 2009). The study reported here explored individual and group perceptions of fear and safety in relation to terrorism. Importantly, these perceptions are grounded in individual experiences of threat and, in the case of some of the Muslim respondents, actual experiences of vilification from some members of the broader community in response to terrorism. Perceptions of the terrorist threat may reveal more about community and individual well-being than statistical measures of threat or risk of a terrorist attack. The fear of terrorism is not necessarily a fear of being personally harmed in a terrorist attack. These feelings of fear not only are limited to the perceived risk of personal harm or injury in a terrorist incident but also encompass the fear of losing civil liberties, political fear and feelings of insecurity. In essence, the fear of terrorism can be described as a state of fear in which a terrorist attack impacts beyond the immediate victim and beyond the immediate event to a perpetual state of heightened anxiety.

Acknowledgements The research reported in this chapter was supported under Australian Research Council's Discovery Projects funding scheme (Project DP0559707), 'Australian responses to the images and discourses of terrorism and the other: Establishing a metric of fear', Edith Cowan University, Western Australia.

References

Aly, A., & Balnaves, M. (2005). The atmos*fear* of terror: Affective modulation and the war on terror. *MC Journal, 8*(6). http://journal.media-culture.org.au/0512/04-alybalnaves.php
Aly, A., & Balnaves, M. (2007). 'They want us to be afraid': Developing a metric for the fear of terrorism. *The International Journal of Diversity in Organisations, Communities and Nations, 6*(6), 113–122.
Aly, A., Balnaves, M., & Chalon, C. (2007). Behavioural responses to the terrorism threat: Applications of the metric of fear. In P. Mendis, J. Lai, E. Dawson, & H. Hussein Abbass (Eds.), *Recent advances in security technology: Proceedings of the 2007 RNSA security technology conference* (pp. 248–255). Melbourne: Australian Homeland Security Research Centre.

Attorney-General's Department. (2002). *Counter-Terrorism package*. Retrieved 4 October 2005 from http://www.attorneygeneralHome.nsf/Web+Pages/24C55CD617969BEA

Balnaves, M., & Aly, A. (2007). Media, 9/11, and fear: A national survey of Australian community responses to images of terror. *Australian Journal of Communication, 34*(3), 101–112.

Bush, G. W. (2001). President outlines war effort: Remarks by the President at the California Business Association Breakfast. Retrieved 11 June 2011 from http://www.whitehouse.gov/news/releases/2001/10/20011017–15.html

Bush, G. W. (2001). Statement by the president in his address to the nation. Retrieved 11 June 2011 from http://www.whitehouse.gov/news/releases/2001/09/20010911–16.html

Cameron, W. B., & McCormick, T. C. (1954). Concepts of security and insecurity. *The American Journal of Sociology, 59*(6), 556–564.

Chen, Z. (2009). 'Peace in a thatched hut—that is happiness': Subjective wellbeing among peasants in rural China. *Journal of Happiness Studies, 10*(2), 239–252.

Davis, D. W., & Silver, B. D. (2004). Civil liberties vs. security: Public opinion in the context of the terrorist attacks on America. *American Journal of Political Science, 48*(1), 28–46.

Falk, R. (2002). Testing patriotism and citizenship in the global terror war. In K. Booth & T. Dunne (Eds.), *Words in collision: Terror and the future of global order* (pp. 325–335). New York: Palgrave Macmillan.

Galea, S., Ahern, J., Resnick, H., & Vlahov, D. (2006). Post traumatic stress symptoms in the general population: Implications for public health. In Y. Neria, R. Gross, & R. Marshall (Eds.), *9/11 Mental health in the wake of terrorist attacks* (pp. 19–44). New York: Cambridge University Press.

Garofalo, J. (1981). The fear of crime: Causes and consequences. *The Journal of Criminal Law and Criminology, 72*(2), 843.

Hancock, N. (2002). Terrorism and the law in Australia: Supporting material. Canberra:Department of the Parliamentary Library.

Huddy, L. S., et al. (2005). Threat, anxiety and support of antiterrorism policies. *American Journal of Political Science, 49*(3), 593–608.

HREOC. (2004). *Ismaa- listen: National consultations on eliminating prejudice against Arab and Muslim Australians*. Sydney: Human Rights and Equal Opportunity Commission.

Huntington, S. P. (1993). The clash of civilizations? *Foreign Affairs, 72*(3).

Huysmans, J. (2004). Minding exceptions: The politics of insecurity and liberal democracy. *Contemporary Political Theory, 3*(3), 321–322.

Jowell, R. (2009). Happiness is not enough: Cognitive judgements as indicators of national well-being. *Social Indicators Research, 92*(1), 317.

King, L. A. (1998). Daily goals, life goals, and worst fears: Means, ends, and subjective well-being. *Journal of Personality, 66*(5), 713.

Lamberg, L. (2005). Terrorism assails nation's psyche. *Journal of the American Medical Association, 294*, 544–546.

Liska, A. E., Sanchirico, A., & Reed, M. D. (1988). Fear of crime and constrained behaviour: Specifying and estimating a reciprocal effects model. *Social Forces, 66*(3), 827–837.

Marks, K. (2007). Australian panic as 'unknown terrorist' sparks a pub ejection. The independent. Retrieved 7 June 2011 from http://www.independent.co.uk/news/world/australasia/australian-panic-as-unknown-terrorist-sparks-a-pub-ejection-400564.html

Massumi, B. (2005). Fear (The spectrum said). *Positions, 13*(1), 31–48.

Merton, R. K., & Kendall, P. L. (2003). The focused interview. In N. Fielding (Ed.), *Interviewing* (Vol. 1, pp. 232–260). London: Sage.

Moller, V. (2005). Resilient or resigned? Criminal victimisation and quality of life in South Africa. *Social Indicators Research, 72*(3), 263–317.

Osborne, J. W. (1994). Some similarities and differences among phenomenological and other methods of psychological qualitative research. *Canadian Psychology, 35*(2), 167–196.

Chapter 4
Personal Security and Fear of Crime as Predictors of Subjective Well-Being

Renata Franc, Zvjezdana Prizmic-Larsen, and Ljiljana Kaliterna Lipovčan

1 Introduction

1.1 Safety Needs

The modern age brings different types of threats which are becoming global and independent of the place where people live (Olsen et al. 2007; Christie 1997). However, in order to fulfill basic human safety needs, the security of someone's neighborhood, local area, city, or society is very important. Safety needs reflect order and predictability in the environment and the human desire for security and protection (Maslow 1943).

According to Maslow's needs hierarchy theory, only when lower-order needs (physiological, safety, belonging, and esteem) are gratified do people tend to satisfy their higher need for self-actualization (Maslow 1970). Lower-level needs appear to be more salient in extreme conditions such as natural disasters, wars, or poverty, but in modern functional societies, these are mostly met and fulfilled (McClinton 1990; Olsen et al. 2007). A number of researchers have used needs hierarchy theory to explain the relationships between subjective well-being and variables like income, food supply, nutrition, and shelter (Diener and Biswas-Diener 2002; Veenhoven 1991; Oishi et al. 1999; Rodríguez et al. 2008; Howell and Howell 2008). In general, findings suggest that people's life satisfaction depends on the extent to which their needs and values are fulfilled and satisfied. Oishi and colleagues (1999) found different associations between needs and global life satisfaction for poorer and

R. Franc (✉) • L. Kaliterna Lipovčan
Institute of Social Sciences Ivo Pilar, Zagreb, Croatia
e-mail: renata.franc@pilar.hr

Z. Prizmic-Larsen
Washington University in St. Louis, St. Louis, MO, USA

D. Webb and E. Wills-Herrera (eds.), *Subjective Well-Being and Security*,
Social Indicators Research Series 46, DOI 10.1007/978-94-007-2278-1_4,
© Springer Science+Business Media B.V. 2012

wealthier nations. Satisfaction with safety needs was a stronger predictor of life satisfaction in poorer nations, while belonging and esteem needs tended to be stronger predictors of life satisfaction in wealthy nations, the latter being also dependent on cultural values. Although needs hierarchy theory cannot completely explain societal differences in subjective well-being, especially in cases where the basic needs in a society are fulfilled (Diener and Lucas 2000), the theory still has a prominent place in explaining some of the differences in well-being between developing and wealthy nations (Howell and Howell 2008).

1.2   Fear of Crime and Perception of Crime

In general, crime is considered as deviant behavior or offense against the person, public, or property which violates the law and norms of a society (Ferraro and LaGrange 1987; Ramchand et al. 2009). Threat to personal safety in modern societies can range from robbery to violent crime. Regardless of actual crime, people tend to experience fear beyond objective risk, thus many countries regularly monitor levels of fear of crime in their society. Many reports, such as The British Crime Surveys, European Social Survey, and International Crime Victim Survey, confirm that fear of crime is common and widespread in societies (Gray et al. 2008; Hale 1996). There are different definitions of fear of crime, but it is most often categorized as personal fear, referring to risk for self-victimization, and more general fear, referring to risk for others being victimized (Ferraro and LaGrange 1987). Most researchers agree that measures of fear of crime have an affective component since feelings of anxiety and worry are included in such assessments (Ferraro and LaGrange 1987; Adams and Serpe 2000). While fear of crime is viewed as an emotional response to potential victimization, the perception of crime is described as more of a cognitive judgment than an affective evaluation. As an affective measure, fear of crime was shown to be more sensitive to objective conditions than perception of crime (Adams and Serpe 2000). It was found that people living in high-crime areas report greater fear compared to people living in low-crime areas (Adams and Serpe 2000; Taub et al. 1984), while the perception of crime and objective frequency of crime were found to be only weakly related (Adams and Serpe 2000; Forgas 1980).

1.3   Well-Being and Safety

Well-being is conceptualized as having a cognitive component, such as life satisfaction, as well as affective components, such as positive and negative affect (Diener 2006; Kuppens et al. 2008). The cognitive component refers to people's subjective evaluation of their life circumstances, while the affective component refers to the balance of positive and negative affect states experienced over time. The predictors of well-being have been researched widely, as well as the factors associated with it (Oishi et al. 1999; Diener and Seligman 2004). The links between well-being measures and factors such as income, health, marital status, age, gender, job morale, education have been demonstrated (for a review, see Diener et al. 1999; Diener and Seligman 2004; Dolan et al. 2008).

Several studies have explored the relationships between crime and quality of life (Michalos and Zumbo 1999; 2000; Møller 2005). For instance, Michalos and Zumbo (1999) showed that crime reduction is important for improving the quality of life, but in a later study when crime was measured subjectively (i.e., fear of victimization, neighborhood worries, beliefs about increases in local crime, satisfaction with personal and family safety), the authors concluded that criminal victimization, worries about safety, or defensive behavior related to personal safety had relatively little impact on respondents' well-being (Michalos and Zumbo 2000). In extensive research on victimization and quality of life in South Africa, Møller (2005) reported that poverty and unemployment are considered greater threats to the quality of life than victimization. However, she also found that perceived likelihood of victimization and concern about personal safety had a greater negative influence on life satisfaction than actual victimization did (Møller 2005).

Some researchers have incorporated items about safety in their well-being measures (Cummins 2002). The International Wellbeing Index (IWI) consists of two parts: the Personal Wellbeing Index (PWI) measuring satisfaction in specific life domains and the National Wellbeing Index (NWI) measuring satisfaction with living conditions in the country, which include items on personal safety and national security, respectively (Cummins 2002; International Wellbeing Group 2006). Satisfaction with national security is usually rated very highly in western countries (Renn et al. 2009; Cummins et al. 2003), while in developing countries, satisfaction with both personal safety and national security were much lower (Tiliouine et al. 2006; Lau et al. 2005).

Frequently, NWI is employed in research as a measure of satisfaction with living conditions at the national level. However, some authors explored NWI as a measure of satisfaction with living conditions at the local or city level (Wills-Herrera et al. 2009). In a comparative study between three cities (i.e., Bogotá, Toronto, and Belo Horizonte), which displayed different levels of development, Wills-Herrera and colleagues (2009) investigated the relationships between satisfaction with personal life domains and living conditions in the cities. The results showed that among the significant predictors of personal well-being were satisfaction with economic conditions, social relationships, and security level in the city and the possibility of doing business (Wills-Herrera et al. 2009). The authors concluded that citizen's perceptions of the objective circumstances at the local level are important when exploring personal well-being. In an analysis of the data obtained in 22 European countries, it was also found that poor neighborhood conditions (e.g., living in dangerous areas) lower individuals' life satisfaction, even after controlling for other variables such as low income, unemployment, and fewer social contacts (Lelkes 2006). Some authors point out that people's perceptions of neighborhood conditions provide an alternative when objective measures are not available (Elo et al. 2009).

1.4   Research in Croatia

Systematic research on crime-related variables and well-being of citizens in Croatia has not yet been done, to the best knowledge of the authors. However, there are studies that explored well-being and its predictors, as well as those that explored crime-related variables and its predictors. Most of these studies were conducted with large, nationally-representative samples.

The Cummins measures, PWI and NWI (Cummins 2002; International Wellbeing Group 2006), have been administered in several surveys (Kaliterna Lipovcan and Prizmic-Larsen 2006a, b, 2007; Kaliterna Lipovcan et al. 2009). Generally, results of surveys of Croatian citizens showed that among PWI domains, satisfaction with personal safety was rated among the top three domains (together with satisfaction with family and community), and among the NWI domains, satisfaction with national security was rated the highest (Kaliterna Lipovcan and Prizmic-Larsen 2006b). When attempting to predict well-being with satisfaction with personal and national domains, personal safety was revealed as a weak but significant predictor of happiness ($\beta = .06$, $p < 0.05$) in 2003 and 2005 (Kaliterna Lipovcan and Prizmic-Larsen 2006a), while in a 2008 dataset, neither satisfaction with personal safety nor satisfaction with national security was found to predict life satisfaction (Kaliterna Lipovcan et al. 2009).

The data on fear of crime collected in several surveys show that Croatian citizens experience relatively high levels of safety. For example, data from International Crime Victimization Survey (ICVS) in 1996/1997 and 2000 show that Croatian citizens, in comparison to citizens of other countries, experienced only medium rates of fear of crime (Alvazzi del Frate and Van Kesteren 2004; Ivicic et al. 2004; Zvekic 1998). More recent surveys (conducted in 2003, 2005, 2007, and 2008) showed that around 25% of Croatian citizens feel unsafe when alone on the street at night, which is similar to the proportion in 25 other European countries (Jackson and Kuha 2010; Franc et al. 2007; Sakic et al. 2009). When attempting to predict fear of crime, demographic variables were found to be relatively weak predictors, while satisfaction with both personal safety and national security, as well as perceptions of crime and neighborhood incivilities, were revealed to be much better predictors (Ivicic et al. 2004; Sakic et al. 2009).

According to official crime statistics, Croatia is a relatively safe country. The homicide rate per 100,000 population in 2008 was 1.62, while homicide rates across other European countries in the same year ranged from 0.54 in Slovenia and 0.57 in Austria to over 2.48 in Finland and 2.94 in Turkey and to as high as 6.26 in Estonia and 8.61 in Lithuania (Malby 2010, p. 14). Based on the most recent analyses of international data, in which the countries were divided into four groups of equal size according to the recorded crime rates for specifics crimes (Heiskanen 2010), Croatia was among the top 25% of countries in the world with the lowest recorded crime rates for assault (and major assault), as well as kidnapping. It was placed in the second quartile for rape and robbery and in the third quartile for burglary and car theft. According to the ranking of countries on the basis of 1-year overall victimization rates based on results of ICVS surveys carried out in the period 1996–2000, Croatia was 1 of the 15 countries with the lowest victimization rates (van Dijk et al. 2007, p. 124).

1.5 Present Study

The aim of this study was to examine the relationship between crime-related variables and life satisfaction in Croatian society. For crime-related variables, we employed the fear of crime experienced in three situations that can occur in everyday life (i.e., being alone at home at night, being at street at night, and in public transportation at night) and perception of different types of crimes and substance abuse in the local area (i.e., corruption, minor crime, violent crime, delinquency, domestic abuse, alcoholism, and drug abuse). We tested the hypothesis that there was a relationship between the life satisfaction as the dependent variable and crime-related variables as predictors, after controlling for the effect of demographic variables (i.e., age, gender, income, and education) and objective conditions in the local area that could affect fear and perception of crime (i.e., urbanization level and crime rates).

The relationships between various demographic variables as well as objective crime rates with fear and perception of crime were also explored to determine if they were congruent with the findings from other studies. Most results of previous studies revealed that female, older, and less-educated individuals express greater fear than male, younger, and better-educated individuals (see Adams and Serpe 2000; Sakic et al. 2009). In the literature, different explanations for gender differences (i.e., female reporting higher fear of crime than men) have been offered: women are either more vulnerable or victimized than men are, men are less accurate in their risk assessment, or men tend to suppress their fear of crime (Sutton and Farrall 2005; Smith and Torstensson 1997). Previous research also shows that greater fear of crime was associated with a higher level of urbanization (Ivicic et al. 2004). One of the explanations is related to population density, where poverty and social problems are most evident in urban areas (Adams and Serpe 2000). Research on criminal activity shows that higher criminal activity in the local area is associated with greater residents' fear (Taub et al. 1984). We predicted similar relationships between demographic and crime-related variables in our sample.

Previous research on safety and/or subjective well-being in Croatia included measures at the national level; however, in this study, we included measures of perception of crime in the local area. Citizens' ratings at the local level might better reflect their everyday life experience. In addition, objective measures of crime rates in the local area were included to control for a possible effect on the relationship between crime-related and well-being measures. Understanding the correlates of subjective well-being will help to inform public policy to assess the needs for certain policies, which is one possible implication of this study.

2   Method

2.1   Subjects and Procedures

Participants made up a representative sample of Croatian citizens ($N=4,000$) aged 18 and above. They were chosen as a multistage probability-based sample of the Croatian population. To ensure statistically representative results for the defined target population, 200 sample points were drawn on the basis of the latest statistical data on regional, community, and town levels. Two-stage stratification was used, by region and size of residence, and addresses were randomly selected at each sampling point. Out of 7,964 contacted persons, 4,000 agreed to participate, so that participation rate was 50.2%. The representativeness of the sample was checked by comparisons to demographics according to the last census (2001). It differed only by education level, where there were about 10% less respondents with elementary school, and accordingly, the proportion of participants with higher education was higher in the sample than in the population.

The survey was conducted in November 2008 through "face-to-face" interviews in participants' homes. All interviewers attended training sessions to become familiar with the questionnaire and procedure for selecting survey participants within a household.[1] Ten percent of the total sample was subject to fieldwork control.

Demographic characteristics of the sample are presented in Table 4.1. The sample comprised 51% females and 49% males, with a mean age of 47.1 years (standard deviation$= 17.23$) and median age of 47 years (range 18–86 years). Income was defined as household monthly income divided by number of persons in the household. Education level was measured by three categories: elementary representing 1–8 years of schooling, secondary representing 9–12 years of schooling, and higher representing over 12 years of schooling. Additionally, the information about urbanization level was provided, since it was one of the criteria for sampling procedure. Urbanization level was divided in four categories, from the least urbanized area to the highest urbanized area, according to Vresk's urbanization typology (Vresk 1992), which is an index comprised of four indicators: the size of the area, the percentage of farmers, the percentage of households without farm land, and the percentage of inhabitants working in the area.

As an objective measure of crime, crime rates at the local areas (counties) were added to the set of demographic variables. The crime rates obtained for the 21 counties in Croatia were based on two sources of information provided by Central Bureau of Statistics (CB).[2] The first being the number of reported adult perpetrators of

---

[1] The contacted person was asked the number of adults and the number of women in the household and the interviewer selected a participant on the basis of 2×2 matrix that crosses sex with age (Troldahl and Carter 1964). This method is a widely accepted technique for systematically selecting respondents from households and ensures that the sample accurately represents the eligible population according to its age and sex structure (Gaziano 2005).

[2] The CBS is a state administrative organization of the official statistics system of the Republic of Croatia.

Table 4.1 Demographic[a] characteristics of the sample of Croatian citizens (*N*=4,000)

Demographic variables	*N* (%)
Age groups	
18–35 years	1,169 (29%)
36–50 years	1,111 (28%)
51–65 years	1,007 (25%)
66+ years	713 (18%)
Gender	
Female	2,028 (51%)
Male	1,972 (49%)
Education	
Elementary (1–8 years)	983 (25%)
High school (9–12 years)	2,128 (53%)
Graduate and higher (>12 years)	889 (22%)
Monthly income divided by number of persons in family (in Euro)[b]	
<70–139	426 (12%)
140–279	1,166 (29%)
280–558	1,595(40%)
559+	740 (19%)
Urbanization level	
The lowest urban	660 (17%)
Medium urban	560 (14%)
High urban	820 (20%)
The highest urban	1,960 (49%)
Crime rates in the local area[c]	
The lowest crime rate (.0087 to .0124)	1,100 (28%)
Medium crime rate (.0125 to .0169)	1,500 (37%)
The highest crime rate (.0170 to .0298)	1,400 (35%)

[a]Although objective measures of urbanization level and crime rates are not "demographic variables" in a precise definition of that phrase, since they do not reflect the characteristics of human population, we shall use it in the text in that sense as they were included in the set of other demographic variables for the purpose of some analyses

[b]The income was recalculated in Euros based on the exchange rate as of November 2008 (1 Euro=7.18 Croatian Kuna)

[c]The crime rate was calculated as the number of reported criminal offenses in a local area divided by the residential population estimates of the area for 2008

criminal offences for each county for the year 2008 (Statistical Information 2009), and the second being the population estimates for the year 2008[3] by counties (Statistical Information 2010). We calculated crime rates for each county as a ratio between reported number of criminal offences and estimates of population for each county. For easier interpretation, we divided them into three categories according to

---

[3]The latest census in Croatia was in the year 2001, so population numbers were based on estimates.

the level of crime in each county, i.e., local areas with the lowest crime rates (from .0087 to .0124), medium crime rates (from .0125 to .0169), and highest crime rates (from .0170 to .0298). This was used as an objective measure of crime in further analyses. In Table 4.1, the frequency of each category of crime rates is presented. Additionally in Table 4.6 of the Appendix, we reported the number of adult perpetrators of criminal offences for 2008, population estimates for 2008, and calculated crime rates for the 21 counties.

2.2   Measures

2.2.1   Life Satisfaction

Assessment of life satisfaction, namely how a respondent evaluates his or her life as a whole, was used as a measure of subjective well-being (Diener 2006). The subjects were asked "All things considered, how satisfied are you with your life as a whole nowadays?." They rated their satisfaction with life using an 11-point scale where 0 represents "extremely dissatisfied" and 10 represents "extremely satisfied." The one-item measure was acquired from European Social Survey Well-Being module (Huppert et al. 2009), which was originally adapted from Diener et al. (1985) Life Satisfaction Scale.

2.2.2   Fear of Crime

Fear of crime was assessed by means of the most commonly asked question in determining fear of crime in large-scale national or cross-national surveys such as the British Crime Survey, International Crime Victim Survey, and the European Social Survey or Eurobarometer (Jansson 2007; Gray et al. 2008). The measure for fear of crime consisted of three items asking participants how physically safe they feel being alone on the streets at their neighborhood at night, being alone at their home at night, and being in the public transport at night. They rated their feelings of safety using a four-point scale ranging from 1 as "very safe" to 4 as "very unsafe."

2.2.3   Perception of Crime and Substance Abuse

Participants' perceptions of crime and substance abuse were based on responses to questions regarding the prevalence of various problems in their neighborhood. The participants rated how much they perceived a particular crime and substance abuse as problems in their local area using the four-point scale ranging from 1 as "not at all the problem" to 4 as "serious problem." The option to answer "I cannot judge" was also offered, but responses in such cases were excluded from subsequent analyses. The types of crime and substance abuse rated were: corruption, minor crime (i.e., burglary, theft), violent crime (i.e., assault, rape, and murder), delinquency, domestic abuse, alcoholism, and drug abuse.

2.3   Data Analysis

The analyses[4] consisted of two steps. First, descriptive statistics, including means, standard deviations, and Pearson's correlation coefficients, were obtained for test variables. T-tests for paired sample were performed to test the mean differences among fear of crime variables, as well as among perceptions of crime variables. Analyses of variance (ANOVAs), with Bonferroni post hoc test, were performed in testing the mean scores of fear of crime and perception of crime and substance abuse variables across various demographic variables. The demographic variables considered were as follows: age group (18–35, 36–50, 51–65, 66+ years), gender (female, male), monthly income (four categories from <70 Euros to 559+ Euros), education (elementary, high school, graduate, and higher), urbanization level (the lowest urbanized, medium, high, the highest urbanized area), and level of crime rates (the lowest crime rate, medium crime rate, the highest crime rate).

Second, hierarchical multiple regression was employed to evaluate the relationship between life satisfaction, as the dependent variable, and fear and perception of crime and substance abuse, as independent variables, while controlling for the impact of demographic variables and crime rates. The analysis measured the percentage of variation in dependent variables that could be explained by the set of independent variables (i.e., measuring impact of all variables together), as well as each variable individually (measuring the impact of each variable while controlling for influence of all other variables). The analysis added terms to the regression model in stages by entering the variables in blocks. In the first block, the demographic control variables were entered. In the second block, the three fear of crime items and seven perceptions of crime and substance abuse items were entered. The analysis calculated the regression weights and significance level for each stage.

Since the sample size in all analyses was relatively large, significance levels were set at $p < 0.01$ for all statistical tests.

3   Results

3.1   Relationships Between Demographic Variables, Fear of Crime, Perception of Crime and Substance Abuse, and Life Satisfaction

Descriptive statistics of fear of crime, perception of crime and substance abuse, and life satisfaction are presented in Table 4.2. Croatian citizens reported to be the most physically unsafe while using public transportations at night and the least unsafe while being alone at home at night ($M = 2.10$ and $M = 1.59$, respectively; $t = 40.36$,

---

[4] In analyses, treatment of missing values was set on "pairwise" which sometimes resulted in different N of cases per analyses.

Table 4.2 Mean (M) and standard deviations (SD) for fear of crime, perception of crime and substance abuse, and life satisfaction

Variables (theoretical range)	M (SD)	N
Fear of crime (1–4)		
Alone at streets at night	2.04 (0.94)	3,988
Alone at home at night	1.59 (0.75)	3,987
In public transp. at night	2.10 (0.93)	3,968
Perception of crime and substance abuse (1–4)		
Corruption	3.28 (0.91)	3,552
Minor crime	2.84 (0.95)	3,714
Violent crime	2.59 (1.10)	3,637
Delinquency	3.01 (0.97)	3,633
Domestic abuse	2.78 (0.95)	3,421
Alcoholism	3.04 (0.89)	3,774
Drug abuse	3.17 (0.95)	3,588
Life satisfaction (0–10)	6.58 (2.16)	3,975

Table 4.3 Zero-order correlations coefficients between fear of crime, perception of crime and substance abuse, and life satisfaction with demographic variables and objective crime rates

Variables	Age	Gender	Income	Education	Urban. level	Crime rate
Fear of crime						
Alone at streets at night	.05**	.17**	.01	.01	.19**	.11**
Alone at home at night	.09**	.13**	−.10**	−.06**	.05**	−.02
In public transp. at night	.02	.17**	.01	.03	.13**	.07**
Perception of crime and substance abuse						
Corruption	−.06**	.01	.10**	.10**	.38**	.22**
Minor crime	−.06**	.03	.10**	.10**	.38**	.17**
Violent crime	−.06**	.02	.10**	.11**	.41**	.26**
Delinquency	−.09**	.02	.12**	.13**	.36**	.10**
Domestic abuse	−.11**	.06**	.12**	.12**	.34**	.13**
Alcoholism	−.01	.08**	.03	.04**	.15**	.04
Drug abuse	−.05**	.01	.15**	.13**	.37**	.24**
Life satisfaction	−.19**	−.01	.25**	.17**	.03	.02

Age groups: 4 categories; Gender: Male = 1, Female = 2; Income: 4 categories; Education: 3 categories; Urbanization level: 4 categories; Crime rate: 3 categories
**$p<.01$

$df=3963$, $p<.001$). The perception of prevalence of different crimes in their local area was the highest for corruption and lowest for violent crime ($M=3.27$ and $M=2.59$, respectively; $t=37.76$, $df=p<.01$).

The associations between demographic variables with fear of crime, perception of crime and substance abuse, and life satisfaction are presented in Table 4.3, and interrelationships between independent and dependent variables (i.e., fear of crime, perception of crime and substance abuse, and life satisfaction) in Table 4.4.

Demographic characteristics (age, gender, income, and education) were significantly but weakly correlated with crime variables (fear and perception), with

Table 4.4 Zero-order correlations coefficients among fear of crime, perception of crime and substance abuse, and life satisfaction

	1	2	3	4	5	6	7	8	9	10
1. Alone at streets at night	–									
2. Alone at home at night	.61**	–								
3. In public transp. at night	.74**	.56**	–							
4. Corruption	.28**	.16**	.27**	–						
5. Minor crime	.37**	.26**	.31**	.58**	–					
6. Violent crime	.42**	.26**	.35**	.54**	.68**	–				
7. Delinquency	.29**	.19**	.24**	.49**	.61**	.57**	–			
8. Domestic abuse	.33**	.21**	.29**	.53**	.63**	.64**	.59**	–		
9. Alcoholism	.22**	.17**	.21**	.44**	.41**	.32**	.44**	.46**	–	
10. Drug abuse	.25**	.16**	.22**	.54**	.55**	.54**	.68**	.54**	.43**	–
11. Life satisfaction	−.13**	−.18**	−.13**	−.03	−.05**	−.03	−.01	−.02	.01	.01

$**p < .01$

correlation coefficients varying between $r=.05$ and $r=.17$ (Table 4.3). The associations of urbanization level and crime rates with different measures of fear and perception of crime and substance abuse were higher, ranging from $r=.05$ to $r=.41$. In general, results showed that living in a highly urbanized area with a higher crime rate was associated with higher fear and perception of all types of crime and substance abuse. Perceptions of crime and substance abuse as being a problem in the neighborhood showed stronger relationships with objective measures (urbanization level and crime rates) than fear of crime in different situations. It should be mentioned that urbanization level was positively associated with the crime rate in the local area (zero-order correlation between these two variables was $r=.36$, $p<.01$).

To get a more detailed picture of the associations between demographic character-istics, objective measures (urbanization level and crime rates), and perceptions and fear of crime, separate ANOVAs were performed to test the mean differences in sub-jective crime variables by demographics and objective crime measures. The results with F-ratio and corresponding level of significance are presented in Table 4.7 in the Appendix. Age was positively associated with fear of crime (Table 4.3). Also, the oldest age group (65+ years) reported more insecurity being alone at home ($F_{3,3984}=13.4$), at streets ($F_{3,3983}=13.4$), and in public transportation at night ($F_{3,3964}=6.2$) than all other age groups (posthoc comparisons all significant at $p<.01$). However, the associations between age and perception of crime and substance abuse were in different direction. Higher perceptions of different crimes and substance abuse were associated with younger age groups, with the exception of alcoholism (n.s.). The youngest group of respondents perceived more problems with corruption ($F_{3,3548}=8.0$), minor crime ($F_{3,3710}=5.9$), domestic abuse ($F_{3,3417}=14.8$), violent crime ($F_{3,3633}=9.6$), drug abuse ($F_{3,3584}=4.7$), and delinquency ($F_{3,3629}=11.8$) than other age groups (Table 4.7 in the Appendix). Women were feeling more unsafe in all three rated circumstances than men: being alone at streets ($F_{1,3986}=113.4$), at home ($F_{1,3985}=63.6$), and in public transportation ($F_{1,3966}=117.9$) at night. Also, women perceived alcoholism ($F_{1,3772}=26.4$) and domestic abuse ($F_{1,3419}=12.0$) as greater problems in their local area than men did, while other types of crime were not associ-ated with gender (Table 4.3; Table 4.7 in the Appendix). People with the highest incomes showed the least fear of being alone at home at night ($F_{1,3913}=13.1$) than other income groups. They perceived all types of crime and substance abuse: corrup-tion ($F_{3,3489}=13.7$), minor crime ($F_{3,3645}=15.2$), domestic abuse ($F_{3,3368}=19.6$), violent crime ($F_{3,3573}=13.4$), drug abuse ($F_{3,3522}=36.2$), and delinquency ($F_{3,3571}=21.6$) as greater problems in their local areas than other income groups did, except for alco-holism (Table 4.7 in the Appendix). People with the lowest level of education reported more fear of being alone at home at night ($F_{2,3984}=11.1$) than other groups did. However, the perception of crime and substance abuse in the local area was higher among people with higher education: corruption ($F_{2,3549}=16.8$), minor crime ($F_{2,3711}=19.5$), domestic abuse ($F_{2,3418}=25.8$), violent crime ($F_{2,3634}=30.5$), drug abuse ($F_{2,3585}=29.4$), and delinquency ($F_{2,3630}=34.8$) (Table 4.7 in the Appendix), with exception of alcoholism (n.s.). Compared to people living in all other areas, people living in highly urbanized and the most urbanized areas had significantly higher perception of all crimes: corruption ($F_{2,3549}=16.8$), minor crime ($F_{2,3711}=19.5$), domestic abuse ($F_{2,3418}=25.8$), violent crime ($F_{2,3634}=30.5$), drug abuse ($F_{2,3585}=29.4$), and delinquency ($F_{2,3630}=34.8$) (Table 4.7 in the Appendix). Fear of crime and perception of crimes and substance abuse, with exception of fear of being alone at home and alcoholism, were significantly different between the areas with different level of crime rates. People living in local areas with high crime rates had significantly higher perception of corruption ($F_{2,3551}=91.71$), minor crime ($F_{2,3713}=61.13$), domestic abuse ($F_{2,3420}=40.99$), violent crime ($F_{2,3636}=139.46$), drug abuse ($F_{2,3587}=86.14$), and delinquency ($F_{2,3632}=17.98$) than people living in the local areas with the lowest or medium levels of crime rates (Table 4.7 in the Appendix). [5]

Intercorrelations between fear and perception of crime and substance abuse variables, as well as correlations of these variables with life satisfaction, are presented in Table 4.4. Different fears of crime, as well as perception of crime and substance abuse items, were relatively largely positively intercorrelated (fear of crime items ranging from $r=.56$ to $r=.74$; perception of crime items from $r=.32$ to $r=.68$). The correlations between different aspects of fear and perception of crime and substance abuse were positive and moderate (from $r=.16$ to $r=42$), the highest associations were found for fear of being alone at streets at night and perceptions of violent crime ($r=.42$) or minor crime ($r=.37$). The correlations between life satisfaction and fear of crime showed significant but relatively low negative associations (in range from $r=-.13$ to $r=-.18$), while the associations between life satisfaction and perception of crime and substance abuse were not statistically significant, with exception of corruption, where the perception that it was a problem in the area had a significant but weak association with life satisfaction ($r = -.05$, $p<.01$; Table 4.4).

3.2 Fear of Crime and Perception of Crime and Substance Abuse as Predictors of Life Satisfaction

Hierarchical regression was used to test the hypothesis that there was a relationship between the dependent variable life satisfaction and the predictor variables, fear of crime and perception of crime and substance abuse, after controlling for the effect of demographic variables. This analysis allows us to measure the percentage of variation in life satisfaction that is explained by fear of crime and perception of crime and substance abuse variables taken together (i.e., total impact on life satisfaction) and individually (i.e., impact of one variable at a time), while controlling for the impact of demographic variables. In the first block, demographic variables (i.e., age, gender, income, education, urbanization level, and crime rates) were entered. In the second block, the ratings of fear of crime and perception of crime and substance abuse were entered. The results of the hierarchical regression analysis are presented in Table 4.5 which contains unstandardized coefficients (B), standard

---

[5] Post hoc comparison results are available from the authors upon request.

Table 4.5 Hierarchical regression analysis summary predicting life satisfaction from fear of crime and perception of crime and substance abuse while controlling for age, gender, income, education, urbanization level, and crime rates

Life satisfaction

Predictors	B	SEB	ß	T
Step 1:				
Age	−.26	.04	−.13	−7.29**
Gender[a]	.07	.07	.02	0.92
Income	.50	.05	.21	11.04**
Education	.21	.06	.07	3.44 **
Urbanization	−.06	.04	−.03	−1.45
Crime rates	−.04	.05	−.02	−.87
R^2 change	.09**			
Adjusted R^2	.09**			
Step 2:				
Age	−.24	.04	−.12	−6.77**
Gender[a]	.19	.07	.04	2.50
Income	.48	.05	.20	10.69**
Education	.20	.06	.07	3.45**
Urbanization	−.01	.04	−.01	−0.19
Crime rates	−.04	.05	−.01	−0.71
Alone at streets	−.06	.06	−.03	−0.89
Alone at home	−.31	.06	−.11	−4.90**
In public transp.	−.14	.06	−.06	−2.45**
Corruption	−.17	.05	−.07	−3.08**
Minor crime	.03	.06	.01	0.55
Violent crime	.06	.06	.03	1.21
Delinquency	.05	.06	.02	0.81
Domestic abuse	−.04	.06	−.02	−0.69
Alcoholism	.02	.05	−.07	0.31
Drug abuse	.01	.06	.01	0.16
R^2 change	.03**			
Adjusted R^2	.12**			
Total R	.34**			

**p<.01
[a]Gender variable was coded as 1=male and 2=female; B=unstandardized coefficients; SEB= standard error of B; β=standardized coefficients (beta); t=t-test value; R^2 change and Adjusted R^2 for each block

error of B (*SEB*), standardized coefficients beta (*β*), corresponding *t*-test value as test of significance of coefficients (*t*), *R* square changes associated with each of the steps (*R*² changes), and adjusted *R*² for each step.

The hierarchical regression analysis with life satisfaction as a dependent variable showed that multiple R for the final model was 0.34 (*p*<.01). Overall, all variables in the model explained 12% of the variance in life satisfaction, which was significant but low. Based on *R* square change, which tell us whether or not the variables added after the controls have a relationship to the dependent variable, the fear and perception of crime and substance abuse variables predicted only 3% of the variance in life satisfaction over and above the set of demographic variables. Demographic variables alone accounted for 9% of the variance in life satisfaction (Table 4.5). In other words, the contribution to the explanation of the variance in the life satisfaction was larger for demographic variables than it was for fear and perception of crime variables.

After controlling for the relationship between demographic variables and life satisfaction, the unique impact of each fear and perception of crime and substance abuse variables could be seen. Two fear of crime variables (alone at home at night, $\beta = -.11$; in public transportation at night, $\beta = -.06$) and one perception of crime and substance abuse variable (perception of corruption as a problem, $\beta = -.07$) emerged as significant predictors of life satisfaction (Table 4.5). Persons who were less afraid being alone at home and in public transportation at night, as well as persons who perceived less corruption in the local area, reported to have better life satisfaction.

4 Discussion

The purpose of this study was to examine the relationships between subjective measures of crime (fear and perception of crime and substance abuse in the local area) and well-being in Croatian citizens. Additionally, the relationships between these variables and demographic characteristics (age, gender, income, and education), urbanization level, and the objective measure of crime (crime rates in the local area) were explored.

Subjective measures of crime-related issues included feelings of personal safety in different everyday situations which are potentially unsafe (being alone at night at streets, at home, and in public transport), as well as perceptions of various crimes and substance abuse (corruption, minor crime, violent crime, delinquency, domestic abuse, alcoholism, and drug abuse) in the neighborhood. Among three potentially unsafe situations, Croatian citizens were feeling the most safe being at home at night and the most unsafe being in public transportation at night. Indirectly, these results can reflect citizens' feelings of safety in their neighborhood, as they were least fearful at home at night than all other situations. It should be mentioned, however, that the citizens expressed relatively low fear of crime in all three situations, with mean rankings below the theoretical mean of 2.5 on the scale 1–4 (Table 4.2). Perceptions of various types of crimes or substance abuse as a problem at the level of local area showed that the most problematic crime perceived by the citizens was corruption, while the least problematic one was violent crime. Corruption was perceived as a serious problem by almost half of the participants (47%). This is consistent with findings from recent surveys conducted in Croatia in 2003, 2005, and 2006 (Franc et al. 2007). In those studies, Croatian citizens perceived corruption, together with unemployment, poverty, and low socioeconomic standard, as the most severe social problems afflicting the country (Franc et al. 2007). According to the Croatian Bureau of Statistics (CBS 2009), reports of corruption in Croatia rose from 2002 to 2007, but the number of accused and convicted did not follow suit. Only 30% of the persons who were reported for corruption were accused, while 10% of them were actually convicted. This discrepancy in the number of reported and convicted corruption offenses is maybe one of the reasons why citizens perceive corruption in the local area to be the most severe problem. According to Transparency International (2009), Croatia was ranked 66th among 180 countries on the Corruption Perception Index in 2009, which highlights at least the potential severity of the issue.

The relationships between various demographic variables and fear of crime in our sample were congruent with findings from other studies. Gender, urbanization level, and crime rates were the strongest correlates of fear of crime (Table 4.3). Women reported higher fear of crime than men did, which is consistent with other studies (Sutton and Farrall 2005; Smith and Torstensson 1997) as well as previous results using Croatian samples (Ivicic et al. 2004; Sakic et al. 2008; Kaliterna Lipovcan and Prizmic-Larsen 2007). Research on associations between age and fear of crime mostly shows that the elderly expressed greater fear than younger people did, although some studies reported that a weak relationship (Adam and Serpe 2000; Sutton and Farrall 2005). In our study, we found a significant but very low association between age and fear of crime. Older people felt more unsafe on the street and at home alone at night than younger people did. In another study, we found that satisfaction with physical safety was significantly lower among older people than among younger people (Kaliterna Lipovcan and Prizmic-Larsen 2007). Since there are no objective data showing elderly Croatian are more often victimized than younger ones, it seems that these results show at least that older people feel more fragile in potentially unsafe situations.

Concerning the level of urbanization, previous research indicates that the fear of crime increases with city size and is associated positively with urban residence (Hale 1996). These findings were confirmed in our study, as feeling unsafe being alone at streets and in public transportation at night were higher in participants who lived in more urbanized areas. The fear in the same situations was associated also with higher crime rates reported in the local area (Table 4.3). Similar results obtained with two different measures of objective circumstances can be partly explained by its correlation ($r=.36$), indicating highly urbanized areas are associated with greater reports of actual crime. However, the obtained association of fear of crime and objective data on potentially unsafe environments are surprisingly low ($r=.05$ to $r=.19$). One explanation for such results is that the objective measures of urbanization level and crime rates used in this study were too general and did not fully reflect actual situations in the participants' neighborhoods. Another explanation is that living in a relatively safe society as Croatia can make people unaware of potential risks, so they express less fear. Other studies on fear of crime which analyzed structural level predictors such as urbanization levels and criminal activity in the community found conflicting results. While some authors found that different structural characteristics of the neighborhood conditions have an impact on fear of crime (Hale 1996; Taub et al. 1984), others found that disorder or incivility also play a small role (LaGrange et al. 1992).

Perception of crime variables showed stronger relationships with demographics than fear of crime, with the exception of gender and age. Associations of the perception of crime and substance abuse with age and gender were also quite low (ranging from $r = -.05$ to $r = -.11$ for age and from $r = .06$ to $r = .08$ for gender; Table 4.3). It is interesting that the association between perception of different crimes and age is in the opposite direction of that between age and fear of crime. Older people perceived various types of crime as less problematic than younger ones, which could be the consequence of older people not being as much involved in everyday ongoings in the local area as younger people are; consequently, they may be not aware of potential problems. Significant correlations with gender showed that women perceived alcoholism and domestic abuse as more problematic than men did. Such associations could be expected, since women are more often victims of domestic violence, which sometimes occur as a consequence of alcohol abuse by their partners. Both income and education were confirmed as consistent, albeit poor correlates of perception of crime and substance abuse (Table 4.3). Those more educated and with higher incomes perceived higher levels of crimes in the local area. Similarly to associations of demographic variables and fear of crime, the strongest consistent associations with perception of crime and substance abuse were found with urbanization level and crime rates in the local area. Both the higher level of urbanization and higher crime rate were associated with greater perceptions of all crimes in the local area (except alcoholism).

Life satisfaction showed significant negative associations with each of three measures of fear of crime, with the strongest being the relationship with the fear of being home alone at night (Table 4.4). In general, the more satisfied respondents were with their life in general, the less fear of crime they reported. This is in line with research showing inverse associations between fear of crime and mental health, physical, and cognitive functioning (Stafford et al. 2007). The only significant association with perception of crime and substance abuse was between life satisfaction and perception of corruption as a problem (Table 4.4). Perceiving higher corruption in the area was associated with lower life satisfaction.

More detailed analyses of the relationships between crime-related variables and life satisfaction showed that three fear of crime items and perception of various crimes in the local area together only explained 3% of variation in life satisfaction, when controlling for demographic variables. However, demographic variables alone accounted for 9% in life satisfaction variance, with the best predictors of life satisfaction being income, age, and education. Respondents with higher income, higher level of education, as well as younger respondents reported higher life satisfaction, which is in line with previous research on well-being correlates (Diener and Seligman 2004; Dolan et al. 2008).

One of the explanations for why crime-related issues did not appear as strong predictors of life satisfaction for Croatian citizens is that residents live in a relatively safe environment, where crime issues are of low priority in their everyday life. In such conditions, crime-related issues might not be personally important and have a little impact on person's quality of life, as some authors point out (Møller 2005).

When we analyzed the unique impact of each crime-related variable on life satisfaction, the impact of fear of being alone at home and in public transportation at night were significant but weak, with fear of being alone at home as the strongest predictor among the two. It could be speculated that citizens who feel unsafe at home have had some negative experience in the past that affected their life satisfaction. Among the perception of various crimes, only the perception of corruption as a problem in the local area had a significant impact on citizens' life satisfaction. Residents perceiving corruption to be a problem reported lower life satisfaction. It is interesting that from all types of perceived crimes, only corruption emerged as a significant predictor. There are two possible explanations: The first is connected with objective increase in corruption activity in Croatia in recent years, while the second is connected to increased media coverage on this issue.

The problem of corruption, which includes a range of activities from bribery of public officials to abuse of position or power at work and business to get personal advantage, is at the moment one of the central issues in Croatia. As previously described, corruption in Croatia has risen from 2002 to 2007 (CBS 2009). During that time, the Croatian government has tried to stamp it out by launching several anti-corruption campaigns in the country. Corruption in Croatia is recognized as a harmful social phenomenon. In 2008, the Croatian parliament defined the anti-corruption strategy, which was a revision of the National Anti-Corruption Programme planned for 2006 to 2008 to stamp out corruption. By launching the anti-corruption campaign to raise the general awareness about the harmfulness of corruption, it became one of the most frequently reported problems in the media. Media coverage, which emphasized particular crimes over others, can influence citizens' perception of crime. According to some authors, media coverage contributes to heightened fear among residents even in situations where they have not been personally exposed (Kitchen and Williams 2010). Other research shows that exposure to news reports in the media is associated with higher judgments of crime severity (Gebotys et al. 1988). Corruption is reported daily in the media in Croatia, thus emphasizing this problem over others, in turn affecting citizens' judgment of seriousness of this criminal activity.

It would be interesting for future research to explore the personal experience of respondents regarding different types of crime, which is lacking in this study. It is possible that in everyday life, people are confronted with some kinds of corruption (bribery of public officials, nepotism at work, etc.) more often than other crimes explored in this study, which is why corruption affects subjective well-being more than other crimes.

In conclusion, it should be stressed that the presented findings about fear of crime and especially perception of crime and substance abuse as weak predictors of well-being are based on a cross-sectional study, in which all variables were operationalized as subjective evaluations. As the objective measure of crime, we included crime rates in counties, but this measure was quite general and did not tap into various crime activities at local level. More sensitive measures of objective conditions regarding crime activities and neighborhood circumstances, together with actual victimization episodes among respondents, should be taken into consideration in future studies as these factors could also have negative impact on perception of crime and subjective well-being. Also, well-being measures should include more aspects, for example satisfaction with different life domains, instead of being limited to only one aspect of life satisfaction, which is the case in the present study. Finally, exploring the role of the mass media coverage of crime and how it affects people's perception of crime could help explain variations between actual crime activities and perceptions of crime.

In spite of some shortcomings of the present study, it showed several interesting results that could inform policy makers. First, it is obvious that corruption is a problem that Croatian citizens perceive it to be the most pronounced criminal activity in their neighborhood, and more importantly, such a perception is associated with lower levels of well-being. Second, although fear of crime is not very high in Croatian citizens, those who are fearful being at home or in public transportation at night also showed lower levels of well-being. And third, higher objective crime rates, as well as subjective perceptions of different crime activities and fear of crime, were associated with higher urbanization level. These are the points that should be taken into consideration when developing policy interventions to fight crime and increase the well-being of society. Research on crime-related issues and its impact on well-being of citizens should be taken as inputs into the political process, under the assumption that public policy is designed to improve well-being.

Appendix

Tables 4.6 and 4.7.

Table 4.6 Review by counties: number of reported adult perpetrators of criminal offenses in 2008, natural change of population for 2008, and crime rate for each county in 2008

Counties	Criminal offenses in 2008	Estimated population in 2008	Crime rate[a] (rank order of counties[b])
Zagrebacka	3,639	326,880	.0111 (6)
Krapinsko-zagorska	1,313	137,001	.0096 (5)
Sisacko-moslovacka	2,825	174,301	.0162 (14)
Karlovacka	2,281	133,405	.0171 (16)
Varazdinska	1,638	180,781	.0091 (2)
Koprivnicko-krizevacka	1,135	120,106	.0094 (3)
Bjelovarsko-bilogorska	1,573	125,652	.0125 (9)
Primorsko-goranska	4,123	304,750	.0135 (11)
Licko-senjska	1,200	50,576	.0237 (20)
Viroviticko-podravska	1,037	88,299	.0117 (7)
Pozesko-slavonska	722	82,548	.0087 (1)
Brodsko-posavska	2,075	173,628	.0120 (8)
Zadarska	3,092	174,595	.0177 (17)
Osjecko-baranjska	4,154	320,617	.0130 (10)
Sibensko-kninska	2,190	114,283	.0192 (18)

(continued)

Table 4.6 (continued)

Counties	Criminal offenses in 2008	Estimated population in 2008	Crime rate[a] (rank order of counties[b])
Vukovarsko-srijemska	3,044	198,289	.0154 (13)
Spiltsko-dalmatinska	7,812	481,872	.0162 (15)
Istarska	6,385	214,156	.0298 (21)
Dubrovacko-neretvanska	1,819	126,751	.0144 (12)
Medimurska	1,127	117,923	.0096 (4)
Grad Zagreb	18,037	788,095	.0229 (19)

[a]Crime rate is calculated as the number of reported criminal offenses in a local area divided by the residential population estimates of the area for 2008
[b]1 = lowest crime rate, 21 = highest crime rate

Table 4.7 One-way ANOVAs results for each predictor variables separately performed by age, gender, income, education, urbanization level, and crime rate

	Age	Gender	Income	Education	Urbanization level	Crime rate
Fear of crime						
Alone at streets at night	$F_{3,3984}=13.4$	$F_{1,3986}=113.4$	n.s.	n.s.	$F_{3,3984}=53.5$	$F_{2,3987}=26.8$
Alone at home at night	$F_{3,3983}=13.4$	$F_{1,3985}=63.6$	$F_{3,3913}=13.1$	$F_{2,3984}=11.1$	n.s.	n.s.
In public transp. at night	$F_{3,3964}=6.2$	$F_{1,3966}=117.9$	n.s.	n.s.	$F_{3,3964}=23.6$	$F_{2,3967}=24.5$
Perception of crime and substance abuse						
Corruption	$F_{3,3548}=8.0$	n.s.	$F_{3,3489}=13.7$	$F_{2,3549}=20.5$	$F_{3,3548}=207.6$	$F_{2,3551}=27.3$
Minor crime	$F_{3,3710}=5.9$	n.s.	$F_{3,3645}=15.1$	$F_{2,3711}=21.8$	$F_{3,3710}=216.7$	$F_{2,3713}=30.2$
Violent crime	$F_{3,3633}=9.6$	n.s.	$F_{3,3573}=13.4$	$F_{2,3634}=25.4$	$F_{3,3633}=295.3$	$F_{2,3636}=51.2$
Delinquency	$F_{3,3629}=11.8$	n.s.	$F_{3,3571}=21.6$	$F_{2,3630}=37.7$	$F_{3,3629}=196.7$	$F_{2,3632}=23.8$
Domestic abuse	$F_{3,3417}=14.8$	$F_{1,3419}=12.0$	$F_{3,3368}=19.6$	$F_{2,3418}=28.8$	$F_{3,3417}=171.7$	$F_{2,3420}=23.5$
Alcoholism	n.s.	$F_{1,3772}=26.3$	n.s.	n.s.	$F_{3,3770}=33.9$	n.s.
Drug abuse	$F_{3,3584}=4.7$	n.s.	$F_{3,3522}=36.2$	$F_{2,3585}=33.2$	$F_{3,3584}=203.8$	$F_{2,3587}=37.5$

F = F-values with corresponding degree of freedom; all F significant at $p<.01$
n.s. = not significant

References

Adams, R., & Serpe, R. (2000). Social integration, fear of crime, and life satisfaction. *Sociological Perspectives, 43*(4), 605–629. 6/14/2010.
Alvazzi del Frate, A., & Van Kesteren, J. N. (2004). *Criminal victimisation in urban Europe. Key findings of the 2000 International Crime Victims Survey.* UNICRI, Turin. http://rechten.uvt.nl/icvs/pdffiles/CriminalVictimisationUrbanEurope.pdf. Accessed June 20, 2010.
Christie, D. (1997). Reducing direct and structural violence: The human needs theory. *Peace and Conflict: Journal of Peace Psychology, 3*(4), 315–332.

Croatian bureau of statistics. (2009). *Koruptivna kaznena djela 2002–2007.* Zagreb. http://www.dzs.hr/Hrv/publication/korupcija/koruptivna_kaznena_djela_2009.pd

Cummins, R. A. (2002). *International wellbeing index*, Version 2 (Web document: http://acqol.deakin.edu.au/inter_wellbeing/Index-CoreItemsDraft2.doc). Accessed June 20, 2010.

Cummins, R. A., Eckersley, R., Pallant, J., van Vugt, J., & Misajon, R. (2003). Developing a national index of subjective wellbeing: The Australian unity wellbeing index. *Social Indicators Research, 64*, 159–190.

Diener, E. (2006). Guidelines for national indicators of subjective well-being and ill-being. *Journal of Happiness Studies, 7*, 397–404.

Diener, E., & Biswas-Diener, R. (2002). Will money increase subjective well-being? *Social Indicators Research, 57*, 119–169.

Diener, E., & Lucas, R. (2000). Explaining differences in societal levels of happiness: Relative standards need fulfillment, culture and evaluation theory. *Journal of Happiness Studies, 1*(1), 41–78.

Diener, E., & Seligman, M. (2004). Beyond money: Toward an economy of well-being. *Psychological Science in the Public Interest, 5*, 1–31.

Diener, E., Emmons, R. A., Larsen, R. J., & Griffin, S. (1985). The satisfaction with life scale. *Journal of Personality Assessment, 49*, 71–75.

Diener, E., Suh, E., Lucas, R., & Smith, H. (1999). Subjective well-being: Three decades of progress. *Psychological Bulletin, 125*, 276–302.

Dolan, P., Peasgood, T., & White, M. (2008). Do we really know what makes us happy? A review of the economic literature on the factors associated with subjective well-being. *Journal of Economic Psychology, 29*, 94–122.

Elo, I., Mykyta, L., Margolis, R., & Culhane, J. (2009). Perceptions of neighborhood disorder: The role of individual and neighborhood characteristics. *Social Science Quarterly, 90*(5), 1298–1320.

Ferraro, K., & LaGrange, R. (1987). The measurement of fear of crime. *Sociological Inquiry, 57*(1), 70–101.

Forgas, J. (1980). Images of crime: A multidimensional analysis of individual differences in crime perception. *International Journal of Psychology, 15*(4), 287.

Franc, R., Ivicic, I., & Sakic, V. (2007). Kriminal i nasilje kao društveni problem (Crime and violence as a problem in our society – Public perception). In V. Kolesaric, (Ed.), Vladimir (ur.). *Psihologija i nasilje u suvremenom društvu Zbornik radova znanstveno-stručnog skupa Psihologija nasilja i zlostavljanja* (pp. 103–116). Osijek: Sveučilište Josipa Jurja Strossmayera u Osijeku, Filozofski fakultet.

Gaziano, C. (2005). Comparative analysis of within-household respondent selection techniques. *Public Opinion Quarterly, 69*(1), 125–157.

Gebotys, R., Roberts, J., & DasGupta, B. (1988). News media use and public perceptions of crime seriousness. *Canadian Journal of Criminology, 30*(1), 3–16.

Gray, E., Jackson, J., & Farrall, S. (2008). Reassessing the fear of crime. *European Journal of Criminology, 5*(3), 363–380.

Hale, C. (1996). Fear of crime: A review of the literature. *International Review of Victimology, 4*(2), 79–150.

Heiskanen, S. (2010). Trends in police recorded crime. In S. Harrendorf, M. Heiskanen, S. Malby (Eds.), *International statistics on crime and justice* (pp. 21–48). European Institute for Crime prevention and control Affiliated with the United Nations (HEUNI) (Publication Series No. 64). Helsinki.

Howell, R., & Howell, C. (2008). The relation of economic status to subjective well-being in developing countries: A meta-analysis. *Psychological Bulletin, 134*(4), 536–560.

Huppert, F., Marks, N., Clark, A., Siegrist, J., Stutzer, A., Vittersø, J., et al. (2009). Measuring well-being across Europe: Description of the ESS well-being module and preliminary findings. *Social Indicators Research, 91*(3), 301–315.

International Wellbeing Group. (2006). *Personal wellbeing index* (4th ed.). Melbourne: Australian Centre on Quality of Life, Deakin University. http://www.deakin.edu.au/research/acqol/instruments/wellbeing_index.htm. Accessed June 20, 2010.

Ivicic, I., Sakic, V., & Franc, R. (2004). Fear of crime in Croatia: Its extent and predictors. In *4th Annual Conference of the European Society of Criminology, Global similarities, local differences, Programme & Abstracts* (p. 186). Amsterdam: European Society of Criminology.

Jackson, J., & Kuha, J. (2010, May 9). *Worry about crime among European citizens: A latent class analysis of cross-national data*. Available at SSRN: http://ssrn.com/abstract=1603465. Accessed June 20, 2010.

Jansson, K. (2007). *British crime survey: Measuring crime for 25 years*. London: Home Office. Available at http://www.homeoffice.gov.uk/rds/pdfs07/bcs25.pdf. Accessed October 20, 2010.

Kaliterna Lipovcan, Lj, & Prizmic-Larsen, Z. (2006a). What makes Croats happy? Predictors of happiness in representative sample. In A. Delle Fave (Ed.), *Dimensions of well-being. Research and intervention* (pp. 53–59). Milano: Franco Angeli.

Kaliterna Lipovcan, Lj., & Prizmic-Larsen, Z. (2006b), Quality of life, life satisfaction and happiness in Croatia in comparison to European countries. In: K. Ott (Ed.), *Croatia's Accession to the European Union. The Challenges of Participation* (pp. 189–208). Institute for Public Finances, Zagreb (also in Croatian edition (pp. 181–198)).

Kaliterna Lipovcan, Lj, & Prizmic-Larsen, Z. (2007). Importance and satisfaction with life domains in Croatia: Representative sample. In R. J. Estes (Ed.), *Advancing quality of life in a turbulent world* (pp. 41–51). Dordrecht: Springer.

Kaliterna Lipovcan, Lj., Prizmic, Z., & Brkljacic, T. (2009). International well-being index – The case of Croatia//IX ISQOLS Conference. Book of Abstracts/Ruviglioni, Elena; Trapani, Marco (ur.). Florence: Centro Editoriale Toscano (p. 266).

Kitchen, P., & Williams, A. (2010). Quality of life and perceptions of crime in Saskatoon, Canada. *Social Indicators Research, 95*(1), 33–61.

Kuppens, P., Realo, A., & Diener, E. (2008). The role of positive and negative emotions in life satisfaction judgment across nations. *Journal of Personality and Social Psychology, 95*, 66–75.

LaGrange, R. L., Ferraro, K. F., & Supancic, M. M. (1992). Perceived risk and fear of crime: role of social and physical incivilities. *Journal of Research in Crime and Delinquency, 29*, 311–334.

Lau, A., Cummins, R., & McPherson, W. (2005). An investigation into the cross-cultural equivalence of the personal wellbeing index. *Social Indicators Research, 72*(3), 403–430.

Lelkes, O. (2006). Knowing what is good for you: Empirical analysis of personal preferences and the 'objective good'. *The Journal of Socio-Economics, 35*(2), 285–307.

Malby, S. (2010). Homicide. In S. Harrendorf, M. Heiskanen, & S. Malby (Eds.), *International statistics on crime and justice* (pp. 7–20). European Institute for Crime prevention and control Affiliated with the United Nations (HEUNI) (Publication Series No. 64). Helsinki.

Maslow, A. (1943). A theory of human motivation. *Psychological Review, 50*(4), 370–396.

Maslow, A. H. (1970). *Motivation and personality*. New York: Harper & Row.

McClinton, J. (1990). Expecting the unexpected: The lessons of hurricane Hugo. *Police Chief, 57*(9), 34–38.

Michalos, A. C., & Zumbo, B. D. (1999). Public services and the quality of life. *Social Indicators Research, 48*(2), 125–156.

Michalos, A., & Zumbo, B. (2000). Criminal victimization and the quality of life. *Social Indicators Research, 50*(3), 245–295.

Møller, V. (2005). Resilient or resigned? Criminal victimisation and quality of life in South Africa. *Social Indicators Research, 72*(3), 263–317.

Oishi, S., Diener, E., Lucas, R., & Suh, E. (1999). Cross-cultural variations in predictors of life satisfaction: Perspectives from needs and values. *Personality and Social Psychology Bulletin, 25*(8), 980–990.

Olsen, O., Kruke, B., & Hovden, J. (2007). Societal safety: Concept, borders and dilemmas. *Journal of Contingencies and Crisis Management, 15*, 69–79.

Ramchand, R., MacDonald, J., Haviland, A., & Morral, A. (2009). A developmental approach for measuring the severity of crimes. *Journal of Quantitative Criminology, 25*(2), 129–153.

Renn, D., Pfaffenberger, N., Platter, M., Mitmansgruber, H., Cummins, R., & Höfer, S. (2009). International well-being index: The Austrian version. *Social Indicators Research, 90*(2), 243–256.

Rodríguez, A., Látková, P., & Sun, Y. (2008). The relationship between leisure and life satisfaction: Application of activity and need theory. *Social Indicators Research, 86*(1), 163–175.

Sakic, I., Franc, R., & Ivicic, I. (2008). Extent of fear of crime in Croatia and effects of television viewing on fear of crime. In A. Marcelo (Ed.), *Abstracts of the 8th annual conference on criminology in the public sphere* (pp. 147–147). Edinburgh: European Society of Criminology.

Sakic, I., Franc, R., & Sakic., V. (2009). Fear of crime and quality of life. In E. Ruviglioni, & M. Trapani (Eds.), *Quality of life studies: Measures and goals for the progress of societies. IX ISQOLS Conference – Book of Abstracts* (p. 189). Florence: Centro Editoriale Toscano.

Smith, W., & Torstensson, M. (1997). Gender differences in risk perception and neutralizing fear of crime. *British Journal of Criminology, 37*(4), 608.

Stafford, M., Chandola, T., & Marmot, M. (2007). Association between fear of crime and mental health and physical functioning. *American Journal of Public Health, 97*(11), 2076–2081.

Statistical Information 2009. (2009). *Central Bureau of Statistics of Republic of Croatia.* Zagreb. http://www.dzs.hr/default_e.htm

Statistical Information 2010. (2010). *Central Bureau of Statistics of Republic of Croatia.* Zagreb. http://www.dzs.hr/default_e.htm. Accessed October 30, 2010.

Sutton, R., & Farrall, S. (2005). Gender, socially desirable responding and the fear of crime: Are women really more anxious about crime? *British Journal of Criminology, 45*(2), 212–224.

Taub, R. P., Taylor, D. G., & Dunham, J. D. (1984). *Paths of neighborhood change.* Chicago: University of Chicago Press.

Tiliouine, H., Cummins, R., & Davern, M. (2006). Measuring wellbeing in developing countries: The case of Algeria. *Social Indicators Research, 75*(1), 1–30.

Transparency International. (2009). http://www.transparency.org/policy_research/surveys_indices/cpi/2009/cpi_2009_table. Accessed October 30, 2010.

Troldahl, V. C., & Carter, R. E., Jr. (1964). Random selection of respondents within households in phone surveys. *Journal of Marketing Research, 1*, 71–76.

Van Dijk, J., van Kesteren, J., & Smit, P. (2007). *Criminal victimization in international perspective.* The Hague: United Nations Office on Drug and Crime.

Veenhoven, R. (1991). Is happiness relative? *Social Indicators Research, 24*, 1–34.

Vresk, M. (1992). Urbanizacija Hrvatske 1981–1991. *Geografski glasnik, 54*, 99–116.

Wills-Herrera, E., Islam, G., & Hamilton, M. (2009). Subjective well-being in cities: A multidimensional concept of individual, social and cultural variables. *Applied Research in Quality of Life, 4*(2), 201–221.

Zvekic, U. (1998). *Criminal victimisation in countries in transition* (UNICRI Publication No. 61). Rome. http://rechten.uvt.nl/icvs/pdffiles/c01_61.PDF. Accessed June 20, 2010.

Chapter 5
The Impact of Objective and Subjective Measures of Security on Subjective Well Being: Evidence from Portugal

Patrícia Jardim da Palma, Miguel Pereira Lopes, and Ana Sofia Monteiro

1 Introduction

Since the 1960s, the social indicators movement has grown around the world. The movement monitors features of life and society beyond traditional economic indicators and seeks to analyze current determinants of change in living conditions and in the quality of life (Noll 2002), providing systematic data for political debate and social planning.

Measuring quality of life enables social agents to understand the extent to which individuals are really achieving their goals and choosing their ideal lifestyle (EFILWC 2003). As such, the quality-of-life concept goes beyond the living conditions approach, which often tends to focus only on the material resources available to individuals. As stated by Veenhoven (2002, p. 40), "objective indicators alone do not provide sufficient information" and are not enough to understand how people live and feel about their life conditions. Quality of life encompasses both the objective features – the actual living conditions – as well as the overall satisfaction of the individual citizens (Argyle 1996). Subjective indicators allow comprehensive and meaningful assessments of an individual's quality of life.

Several studies have been conducted to measure the quality of life of citizens, using indicators related to the most important domains to describe a person's life, such as employment, education, health care, and security (e.g., EFILWC 2007). Beyond a traditional perspective, the human security framing approach is more centered on people, aiming to protect individuals from sources of threats in order to maintain their well-being (UNDP 1994). Although the concept of human security has already

P.J. da Palma (✉) • M.P. Lopes • A.S. Monteiro
Instituto Superior de Ciências Sociais e Políticas, Universidade Técnica de Lisboa,
Rua Almerindo Lessa, 1300-633 Lisboa, Portugal
e-mail: ppalma@iscsp.utl.pt; mplopes@iscsp.utl.pt; ana.monteiro@iscsp.utl.pt

D. Webb and E. Wills-Herrera (eds.), *Subjective Well-Being and Security*,
Social Indicators Research Series 46, DOI 10.1007/978-94-007-2278-1_5,
© Springer Science+Business Media B.V. 2012

gained legitimacy within the academic community and with policy agents, there is no universally accepted approach to its assessment (Djuric 2009).

Human security has long been focused on violent threats (e.g., Krause 1998) or on a wider range of issues (e.g., poverty, disease, and environmental disasters) (e.g., Owen 2008) but considered mostly at a global level. Although we may consider several threats to human security, their significance varies across regions in the same country, as noted by Owen (2004) and Reiss (1983). Moreover, it is at the local and regional, rather than the national, level a more comprehensive and accurate understanding of security assessment is provided (Djuric 2009). Despite the fact that many cities, such as Ontario, Seattle, and Washington D.C., are already measuring their quality of life (Hardi and Pintér 2006), a clear approach to human security at a regional or a municipal level (i.e., subnational) is still missing.

Different measures of human security (i.e., objective and subjective indicators) are used in the literature, depending on the level of analysis researchers wish to investigate, neighborhood *vs.* country, for instance. An attempt to build a comprehensive framework to study citizen security at a municipal level, which includes the measurement of its multiple dimensions and impact on citizens, remains to be undertaken. This study seeks to shed some light on this state of the discussion by analyzing the impacts of both objective and subjective measures of citizen security at the municipal level[1] on subjective well-being (SWB).

The chapter is organized as follows: We begin by discussing the human security issue within cities and local communities, emphasizing the impact of security on SWB. Then we present our study, how we collected data on the 20 municipalities that we examined, and the measures we used. We continue by exploring and explaining the effects of both objective and subjective measures of citizen security at the municipal level on the SWB of citizens and conclude with the implications of our study for planners and policymakers.

2   Security in Cities and Local Communities

Since the end of the Cold War, the dominant traditional security paradigm has changed considerably (Owen 2004). The current belief is that despite macrolevel stability, such as that which existed in the East–West military balance during the Cold War, citizens are not necessarily safe. They may suffer from poverty, disease, hunger, or attacks of violence. With this notion at its root, several authors argue that the security concept must be broadened to include the individual's condition (e.g., Rothschild 1995) and the spectrum of threat and injury be expanded to embrace

---

[1] Based on Johnson et al. (2009) concept of neighborhood security, we will use the expression "citizen security at the municipal level," referring to security of individuals within the municipality that is based on the geographic boundaries and the administrative structure defined by the National Statistics.

economic security, health security, and regional or local security, just to name a few. With the individualization of security, the focus changes from the state to a narrower level: the regional or local community. Indeed, it is the regional or local community level that mostly affects the citizens' quality of life (Djuric 2009).

Increased urbanization has led to a substantial and parallel increase in violence. As a result of the uncontrolled growth of cities, solutions to social, economic, and cultural problems and effective responses to the needs of those living in the cities are often delayed (Senlier et al. 2009). The modern city is today a site of class and ethnic warfare, conflict that has produced the contemporary city of walls, realized architecturally, discursively, economically, and normatively (Shapiro 2009). Urban crimes include those against property (e.g., theft, burglary, and vandalism) and violent crimes, which include any act that causes a physical or psychological injury or damage (e.g., murder, infanticide, assault, rape, sexual abuse, and acts of intimidation and terror) (Vanderschueren 1996). Criminality occurs in poor neighborhoods as well as in middle-class and wealthy ones.

In order to promote urban sustainability, the monitoring of security in cities and local communities is a priority today. Subjective well-being is mostly influenced by proximal situational factors, which are presented at the level of the community or city rather than the nation (Wills-Herrera et al. 2009). It is generally measured by life satisfaction and happiness, which refer to the individual's own assessment of their quality of life and their situation (e.g., EFILWC 2003), and can thus be used as a useful guide to promote a better life. Several studies have measured the perceptions of security in cities and local communities in Europe (e.g., Senlier et al. 2009), North America (e.g., Gage 2006), and Latin America (e.g., Cáceres 2002).

3 Impact of Security on Subjective Well-Being

At a community level, security has been measured using both objective and subjective indicators. On a quantitative level, objective indices of crime, physical disorder (e.g., deviant behaviors, gang membership), or exposure to neighborhood crime have served as measures of security. Some studies (e.g., Powdthavee 2005; McLeer et al. 1988) have shown that mental health and psychological distress stem from the experience of these stressful life events. This research has evidenced that victims of crime suffer from a variety of significant and persistent psychological problems, such as depression, anxiety, fear, and posttraumatic stress disorder. Research indicates that these psychological symptoms are negatively associated with SWB and overall subjective quality of life (Michalos 1991).

Furthermore, using data from the OHS97 survey,[2] Powdthavee (2005) showed that crime victims reported significantly lower well-being than nonvictims, that

---

[2] This study used a data set from the October Household Survey of South Africa that was collected in 1997.

is, victims were less satisfied with life in general. In another study, McLeer and colleagues (1988) revealed that children and adolescents who were victims of physical and sexual abuse before adolescence have shown increased prevalence of anxiety, depression, and posttraumatic stress disorder. As evidenced, both late and early experiences of violence affect long-term psychological well-being.

Several studies (e.g., Clark et al. 2008; Kruger and Reisch 2007) have also focused on subjective measures of human security, such as perception of crime or perception of violence in the local community. Kruger and Reisch (2007) demonstrated that residents with higher perception of neighborhood crime and insecurity reported higher levels of stress and symptoms of depression. Also, using a sample of women receiving their health care at an urban community health center, Clark and colleagues (2008) demonstrated that women who witnessed violent acts in their neighborhood were twice as likely to experience symptoms of depression and anxiety as those who did not witness community violence. In another study, findings indicated that when parents of children aged 5–10 years expressed greater anxiety about neighborhood safety, the children engaged in less physical activity (Weir et al. 2006), reinforcing the importance of security perception in promoting physical activity and general health.

Although different measures of human security have been employed in the literature, their use depends heavily on the outcomes that the researchers wish to emphasize. While research analyzing mental health and SWB tends to focus on exposure to violence (i.e., victimization), studies comparing different communities generally use actual measures of crimes or disorders (Johnson et al. 2009). Moreover, perception of security is usually employed when authors examine general health or physical activity.

To date, the literature has not offered an integrated view of how crime rates and perception of security affect the SWB of citizens across different regions. As previous research has predominantly focused on either crime rates or perception of security, a clear and complete framework of community and municipal security is still missing in the literature. Indeed, this is important because community security has been found to be one of the most important predictors of the quality of life of individuals, determining their satisfaction with life (Sirgy and Cornwell 2002). Moreover, scholars have even reinforced the belief that the higher the crime rate, the more residents are willing to move away to a safer neighborhood (Reiss 1983).

As such, our goal is to analyze the impacts of both objective and subjective measures of citizen security at the municipal level on SWB. Specifically, we wish to examine the path of causality of both objective and subjective measures of citizen security at the municipal level on SWB in a single study, without separating the elements of the model, as in earlier research.

Given the many studies (e.g., Powdthavee 2005; McLeer et al. 1988) that have shown how exposure to crime, as an objective measure of security, impairs SWB of victims, we may postulate that:

H1: Objective measures of security at the municipal level (crime rates) have a negative impact on SWB of citizens.

Following Kruger and Reisch (2007) as well as Weir and colleagues (2006) who showed that perception of local insecurity, a subjective measure of security, has a positive influence on stress and depression as well as a negative one on general heath, we also postulate that:

> H2: Subjective measures of security at the municipal level (perception of security) have a positive impact on SWB of citizens.

4 Method

Twenty Portuguese municipalities were chosen for our research: Albufeira, Angra do Heroísmo, Beja, Bragança, Cartaxo, Covilhã, Estremoz, Figueira da Foz, Funchal, Grândola, Guarda, Leiria, Lisbon, Odivelas, Portalegre, Portimão, Porto, Santo Tirso, São João da Madeira, and Vila Real. All are autonomous administrative centers, and they are spread throughout the country from the North to the South, East, and West, and the islands. We used census tract data to select municipalities. Tracts provide a replicable sampling frame that facilitates geographic dispersion of municipalities across the country.

All regions of Portugal are geographically represented in our sample as the "municipality" was used as the unit of analysis. From a population of 308 Portuguese municipalities, 20 were assessed, in which 25% represent the North Region (Bragança, Porto, São João da Madeira, Santo Tirso, and Vila Real); 20%, the Center (Covilhã, Figueira da Foz, Guarda, and Leiria); 10%, the Lisbon metropolitan region (Lisboa and Odivelas); 25%, Alentejo (Beja, Cartaxo, Estremoz, Grândola, and Portalegre); 10%, Algarve (Albufeira and Portimão); and 10% localized in the Islands (Angra do Heroísmo and Funchal).

4.1 Participants

A random sample of 3,757 individuals from those 20 municipalities was used to analyze how residents perceive their community's security level. We relied on Statistics Portugal[3] to collect a random probabilistic sample in the 20 municipalities, based on age (18–65 years old), gender, literacy, and profession (INE 2008). If a selected household had more than one eligible member, one household member was again randomly selected. Samples from each municipality ranged between 150 and 250 residents according to the dimension of the municipality.

---

[3] Statistics Portugal is the official public institution which has legal personality, administrative autonomy, and technical independence in the exercise of its official statistical activity. The original name is INE (*Instituto Nacional de Estatística*) and represents the Portuguese official statistical database.

Table 5.1 Descriptive data of objective indicators of criminality

	Mean	S.D.
1. Absolute number of crimes		
N. of total crimes registered by authorities	3854.504	6685.57
N. of crimes against property	806.9954	1077.44
N. of physical crimes against the person	2177.871	4437.45
N. of crimes against peace, humanity, and life in society	418.4257	545.95
2. Number of crimes per 1,000 inhabitants		
N. of crimes registered by authorities per 1,000 inhabitants	51.22375	36.07
N. of crimes against property per 1,000 inhabitants	11.00918	4.47
N. of physical crimes against the person per 1,000 inhabitants	27.05685	21.81
N. of crimes against peace, humanity, and life in society per 1,000 inhabitants	6.686152	6.47
3. Crime rates		
Total crime rate	51.69083	37.37
Physical crime rate against the person	6.661889	2.54
Crime rate of pickpocketing/mugging in public streets	1.695181	2.11
Crime rate of car theft and carjacking	7.239985	5.32
Crime rate of drink-driving above 1.2 g/l of blood alcohol concentration	4.402263	5.13
Crime rate of driving without a license	3.899294	5.40

From a total of 3,757 individuals interviewed, 27.3% were between 15 and 34 years, 33.6% were between 35 and 54 years, and 39.1%, above 55 years old (mean age=47.7; SD=17.1). This sample included 53.7% males and a distribution of 71.9% residents in coastal communities. Regarding the regions, 39% of the individuals were in the North; 9.8%, in the Center; 11%, in the region of Lisbon; 18.3%, in Alentejo; 17.1%, in Algarve; and 4.9%, in the islands.

4.2 Measures

4.2.1 Objective Security

Data on security conditions across the 20 municipalities were obtained from the 2007 Statistics Portugal database. Objective indicators of criminality were reverse-coded items recognizing the lack of security in each municipality (see Table 5.1; INE 2008). We based our analysis on those indicators that best describe the security level in the community, on the one hand, and make comparisons possible among different municipalities, on the other. Fourteen indicators were collected from the Statistics Portugal database regarding three categories: absolute number of crimes, number of crimes per 1,000 inhabitants, and crime rates.

4.2.2   Subjective Security

The perception of security at the level of each municipality was measured by the amount of safety perceived in a potentially risky context: *"How safe are you when going for a walk alone at night?"* The subjective security dimension is measured in this study in a single-item approach, as this was the only possible approach because the data were retrieved from a previous and broader quality-of-life questionnaire, specified in the "Procedure." Although this construct is measured as a single item, its subjacent concept includes the individual's condition of security (e.g., Rothschild 1995). Consequently, this study focuses on a specific type of subjective security, as from a critical point of view, we suggest taking into account some more diverse and comprehensive security measures for future research (e.g., Senlier et al. 2009).

4.2.3   Subjective Well-Being

According to the literature, SWB was measured using four indicators (life satisfaction, overall happiness, optimism about the future, and meaningfulness of life) from the same scale published by Lopes et al. (2010). Life satisfaction and overall happiness were assessed by two items: *"All things considered, how satisfied are you with your life these days?"* and *"Taking all things together, how happy would you say you are?"* Optimism about the future and meaningfulness of life were assessed by two items: *"All things considered, how optimistic are you about your future?"* and *"Taking all things together, to what extent do you agree with the sentence 'life is meaningful'."* Responses range on a five-point scale from 1, "strongly disagree," to 5, "strongly agree."

This scale had a relatively low Cronbach's alpha of 0.64 because of the 4 different dimensions evaluated inside SWB. Although all the items contribute in a positive way to this result, removing any would lower the reliability of the subjective well-being scale. In this sense, it was decided to keep the advantages of a more inclusive scale, with all the items.

The descriptive data of the measures in this study are presented in Appendix.

4.3   Procedure

Subjective data were based on the 2009 "Great Place to Live" in Portugal project, an initiative run yearly by INTEC, a not-for-profit institute whose main results were published in a major Portuguese weekly newspaper.[4] The survey was designed to monitor the general quality of life as well as the SWB of the Portuguese citizens in

---

[4]The results were published in five editions of the national newspaper *SOL* (The Sun), distributed for mainstream population, in February and March of 2009.

all of the 20 municipalities. This quality-of-life questionnaire included 51 items, all with a response range on a five-point scale from 1, "strongly disagree," to 5, "strongly agree." This broader questionnaire, from which the subjective data were retrieved to the present study, was measured across 10 domains: Mobility; Economy and Employment; Education and Training; Diversity Tolerance and Safety; Happiness and Well-being; Health; Urbanism and Housing; Tourism; Culture and Leisure; and Environment.

We based our study on how citizens measured the security of their cities as well as their SWB. We operationalized municipalities based on the geographic boundaries and the administrative structure defined by Statistics Portugal (INE 2008). Consistent with Sampson et al. (2002), this delimitation is a larger community, that is, it is a collection of individuals and institutions occupying a spatially defined area, which is influenced by ecological, cultural, and political forces.

The survey was made by phone to a representative sample of citizens from each municipality between October and December of 2008. Residents were invited to participate in a 25-min survey conducted by trained interviewers. From around 5,000 phone calls, 3,757 respondents completed the survey. The survey was conducted in Portuguese, the native language of respondents.

5 Results

Primarily, both objective and subjective measures of citizen security at the municipal level were assessed for their impact on SWB through hierarchical linear modeling (HLM). The results demonstrate that the theoretical model was generally supported, indicating the impact of a secure environment on the well-being of different regions' citizens. By running such a regression analysis, we assumed that there were no problems of multicollinearity. We assumed this for two main reasons. First, as can be seen in Table 5.1, the correlations between the variables are generally low, which do not point to the existence of such a problem. Second, the face validity of the objective indicators also points to the fact that we should be measuring different and not extremely related constructs. Also, to better characterize the behavior of these variables, we present the difference of means in people's SWB in different criminality contexts, evidencing the main predictors responsible for a higher difference in SWB.

The second part of this section is a comparative analysis, with Portuguese regions compared against four criteria for a better understanding of variations in security, crime levels, and SWB.

The descriptive information and correlation analysis results are presented in Table 5.2. All the objective measures of criminality are significantly correlated with each other ($p < 0.001$) and generally present values higher than $r > 0.5$, which should be explained by the measurement of multiple manifestations related to the same assembly – criminality. Also, the indicators evaluating the same specific crime types seem to have a stronger correlation with each other (e.g., number of total crimes per

1,000 inhabitants and total crime rate, with .99 correlation; number of physical crimes against the person and physical crime rate against the person, with .97 correlation). The subjective security construct relates negatively to the general criminality indicators, which was as expected.

We also explain lower correlations between SWB and the objective measures of security, as they refer to different levels of analysis (individual and municipal). The only higher relation was with subjective security, as they were treated at the same level of analysis ($r=.16$; $p<.001$). In addition, significant relationships were found between SWB and total crime rate ($r=-.03$; $p<0.05$) and physical crime against the person ($r=-.06$; $p<0.001$), as well as relationships with the other crime indicators, drink-driving, and crimes against property and against society ($p<0.05$). SWB did not correlate with the indicators of criminality – pickpocketing/mugging ($r=.00$), car theft ($r=.02$), and driving without a license ($r=.02$) – nor with number of crimes ($r=.00$; $r=.01$). Finally, SWB is related to subjective security ($r=.16$; $p<0.001$).

5.1 Impact of Objective and Subjective Measures of Security on SWB

For a better understanding of the general direct impact of both objective and subjective security measures on subjective well-being, we used hierarchical linear modeling (HLM). HLM is a more advanced form of simple linear regression and multiple linear regression, which is more appropriate for use with nested data. It allows variance in outcome variables to be analyzed at multiple hierarchical levels, whereas in simple linear and multiple linear regression, all effects are modeled to occur at a single level (Raudenbush and Bryk 2002).

This study design refers to two kinds of predictors. First, the predictor at an individual level is the perception of security. Second, the predictors at a context level – nested data – are the criminal objective indicators for the 20 municipalities.

The results demonstrate that the theoretical model was generally supported for the total criminality indicators in regions, which were found to be negative predictors of the SWB ($b=-0.21$; $p<0.001$: Table 5.3), thus supporting H1. Similarly, the perception of being safe also revealed an impact on people's overall well-being ($b=0.09$; $p<0.001$). H2 was thus confirmed.

An interesting finding remains for the specific types of crime with a significant impact on SWB. The model shows that only the crimes against property are predictive of SWB levels ($b=-0.35$, $b=-0.34$; $p<0.05$). Also, the comparative information criteria indices (Table 5.3 – AIC, BIC) demonstrate a higher quality for Model 3, as they have lower indices when we add each variable on the model. This means that each variable included improved the quality of the model.

In fact, the SWB coefficient seems to rise 0.087 when the subjective security rises and fall when the objective criminality rises. A significant impact of the crimes against property in the SWB ($b=-0.35$; $p<0.05$) was also found, as SWB decreases when this indicator increases. Additionally, this model demonstrates that there are

Table 5.2 Descriptive information on objective security and individual-level measures

Measure	N	M	SD	1	1a	1b	1c	1d	1e
Context level									
1. Total crime rate	20	51.7	37.4						
1a. Physical crime against the person	20	6.7	2.5	.54***					
1b. Pickpocketing/ mugging	20	1.7	2.1	.59***	.43***				
1c. Car theft	20	7.2	5.3	.92***	.56***	.68***			
1d. Drink-driving	20	4.4	5.1	.84***	.23***	.29***	.60***		
1e. Driving without a license	20	3.9	5.4	.92***	.27***	.42***	.78***	.91***	
1 f. Against property	20	27.3	22.5	.98***	.51***	.67***	.97***	.75***	.88***
2. N total crimes	20	3854.5	6685.6	.29***	.24***	.84***	.33***	.07***	.13***
2a. Physical crime against the person	20	807.0	1077.4	.11***	.24***	.77***	.19***	−.11***	−.04**
2b. Against property	20	2177.9	4437.4	.28***	.23***	.84***	.33***	.05**	.11***
2c. Against society life and peace	20	418.4	545.9	.47***	.25***	.84***	.44***	.35***	.36***
3. N crimes per 1,000 inhabitants	20	51.2	36.1	.99***	.56***	.61***	.92***	.83***	.91***
3a. Physical crime against the person	20	11.0	4.5	.53***	.97***	.28***	.51***	.26***	.28***
3b. Against property	20	27.1	21.8	.98***	.53***	.68***	.97***	.74***	.87***
3c. Against society life and peace	20	6.7	6.5	.88***	.27***	.35***	.66***	.99***	.93***
Individual level									
4. Subjective security	3705	2.8	0.7	−.03	−.04*	−.20***	−.11***	.07	.00
5. SWB	3722	3.2	0.4	−.03*	−.06***	.00	−.02	−.04*	−.02

NOTE: *p<0.05; ***p<0.001

1f	2	2a	2b	2c	3	3a	3b	3c	4
.35***									
.18***	.96***								
.35***	1***	.95***							
.50***	.94***	.88***	.92***						
.98***	.31***	.13***	.30***	.48***					
.48***	.14***	.12***	.13***	.16***	.54***				
.99***	.37***	.20***	.37***	.51***	.98***	.49***			
.81***	.12***	−.06***	.10***	.39***	.88***	.30***	.80***		
−.06***	−.15***	−.17***	−.15***	−.12***	−.03***	.01	−.07***	−.06***	
−.03*	−.01	−.01	−.01	.00	−.03*	−.06***	−.03*	−.03*	.16***

Table 5.3 HLM of criminality indices and perceptions of security in respect to SWB ($N=3,757$)

	Model 1	Model 2	Model 3
Intercept	3.17(0.12)***	2.92(0.03)***	2.89(0.03)***
Level 1			
Subjective security		0.09(0.01)***	0.09(0.01)***
Level 2			
Total criminality rate			−0.21(0.09)*
N total crimes per inhabitant			−0.21(0.09)*
Crime rate against property			−0.35(0.16)*
N crimes against property			−0.34(0.16)*
Information criteria			
AIC[a]	3489.172	3431.826	3358.387
BIC[b]	3501.796	3444.425	3370.984

NOTE: *$p<0.05$; ***$p<0.001$
[a]Akaike information criterion
[b]Bayes information criterion

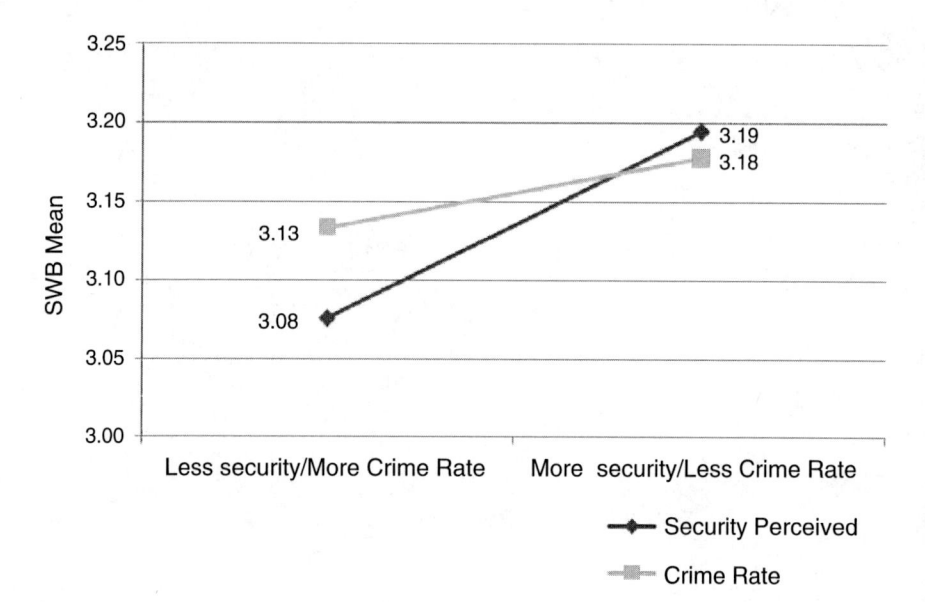

Fig. 5.1 Comparison of SWB between subjective security and crime rate means

significantly different levels of SWB between regions, explained by the different levels of security and criminality. When adding the criminality context predictor to the model, its quality criterion increases.

In the comparison between lower and higher crime and security (Fig. 5.1), a higher SWB in citizens living in regions with a generally lower crime rate ($F=-7.268$; $p=0.007$) was detected, as the same results were found regarding their perception to be safe walking down the streets at night ($Z=8.506$; $p<0.001$).

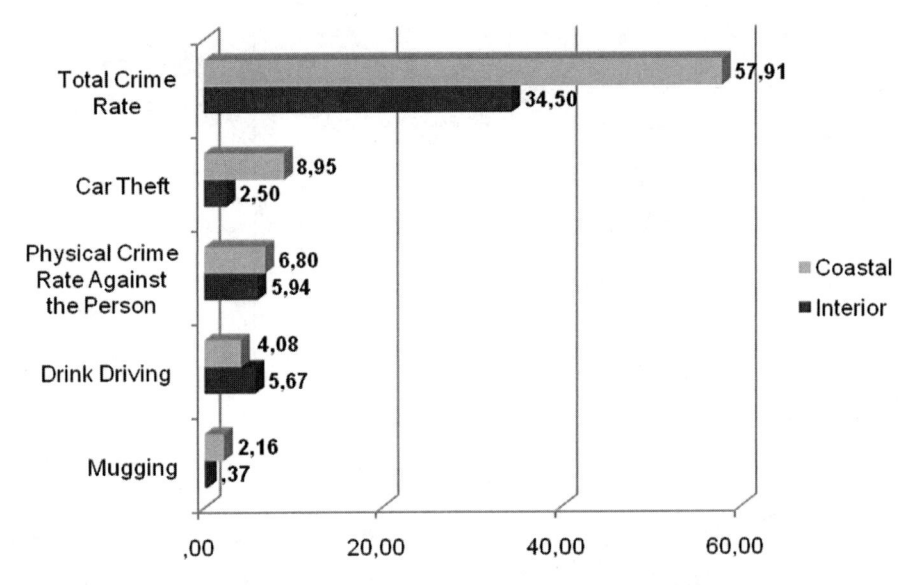

Fig. 5.2 Comparison of crime rate means between coastal and interior regions

The main objective indicators of crime associated with the differences observed in well-being are attributed to the physical crime rate against the person ($F=-4.160$; $p=0.041$) and against property ($F=-4.109$; $p=0.043$), drink-driving ($F=-3.390$; $p=0.001$), and driving without a license ($F=-9.460$; $p=0.002$). These indicators are shown to have an impact on the general well-being of Portuguese citizens, contrasting with the following crime rates where an equivalence of means between the groups was found. That was the case of crimes against society and peace ($F=-1.287$; $p=0.257$), car theft ($F=-1.770$; $p=0.184$), and pickpocketing, mugging, or purse-snatching ($F=-2.365$; $p=0.124$).

5.2   Differences Among Municipalities

Regarding the geographic characteristics of Portugal, the 20 regions were aggregated and compared in four domains: division of interior and coastal regions; continent and islands; division of the five regions; and comparison between metropolitan cities and the other remaining municipalities. These comparisons allow us to obtain a better understanding of the variations in the contribution of the security and crime levels to the SWB of its inhabitants.

At first, the comparison of the characteristics in the interior and coastal regions demonstrates that, besides the equivalence in respect to well-being ($F=0.151$; $p=0.698$), the interior seems to have a greater sense of security about walking through the streets ($F=-13.084$; $p<0.001$). This can be explained by the lower rates of criminality observed in the interior compared to the coastal regions ($F=-7.917$; $p<0.001$; Fig. 5.2). The only exception to the rule is the higher rate of drink-driving observed in the interior regions ($F=-25.979$; $p<0.001$).

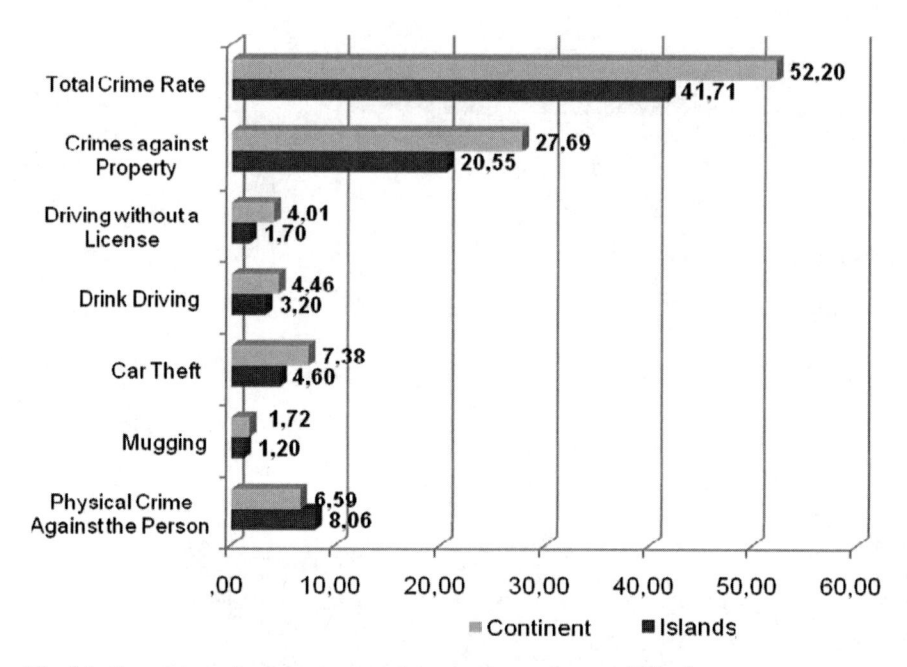

Fig. 5.3 Comparison of crime rate means between the continent and islands

Another comparison was between the Portuguese continent and the Madeira and Azores islands (Fig. 5.3). In this case, SWB is significantly higher in the islands than in the continent ($F=-4.875$; $p<0.001$), and the perception of insecurity is proportionally lower ($F=138.584$; $p<0.001$). These results are in line with the islands' crime rates ($F=-5.862$; $p<0.001$), which are lower for all types of crimes. The only exception is the higher number of physical crimes against the person in the islands, with a difference of 1.47 in the mean of the indicator ($F=-11.454$; $p<0.001$).

In the comparison among the main territories of Portugal (North, Center, Lisbon, Alentejo, Algarve, and Islands; Fig. 5.4), Lisbon demonstrates the lowest subjective security ($p<0.001$), as the Islands present the highest security, which is significantly higher than that in Lisbon and Algarve ($p<0.001$). In the SWB, the Islands also present the highest score ($p<0.001$) in relation to the rest of the statistically equivalent territories.

Contrary to the notion of higher crime rates in the metropolitan areas, Algarve seems to be the main target of criminality, significantly greater than all of the other territories ($p<0.001$; Fig. 5.5). The highest criminality is against peace and humanity, against property, driving without a license, drink-driving, and car theft ($p<0.001$).

Regarding the last comparison between the metropolitan areas and the remaining regions (Fig. 5.6), a perception of greater insecurity was found in these large cities (Lisbon and Oporto; $F=-13.927$; $p<0.001$) despite the equivalence in SWB ($F=-0.074$; $p=0.784$). This finding can be explained by some criminality indices

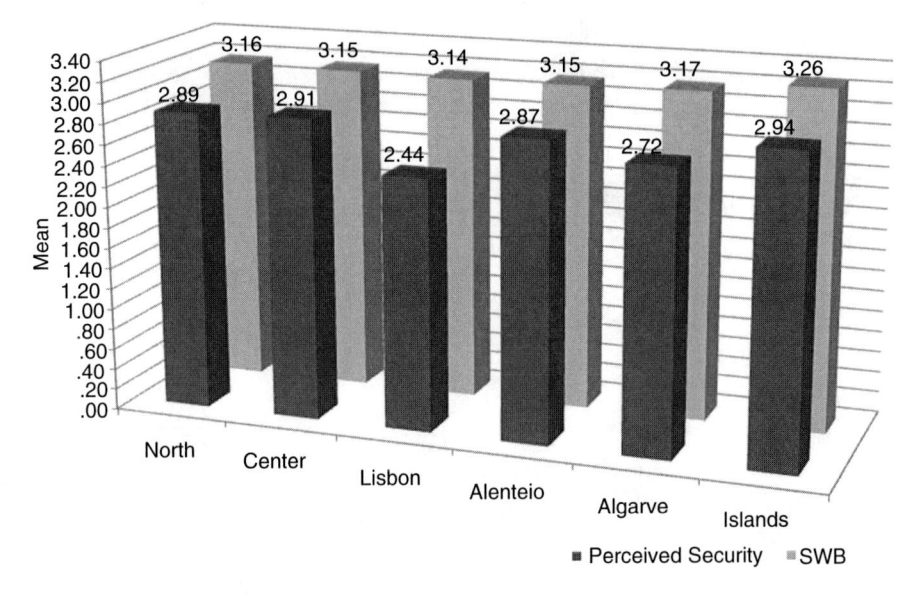

Fig. 5.4 Comparison of subjective security and SWB means between regions

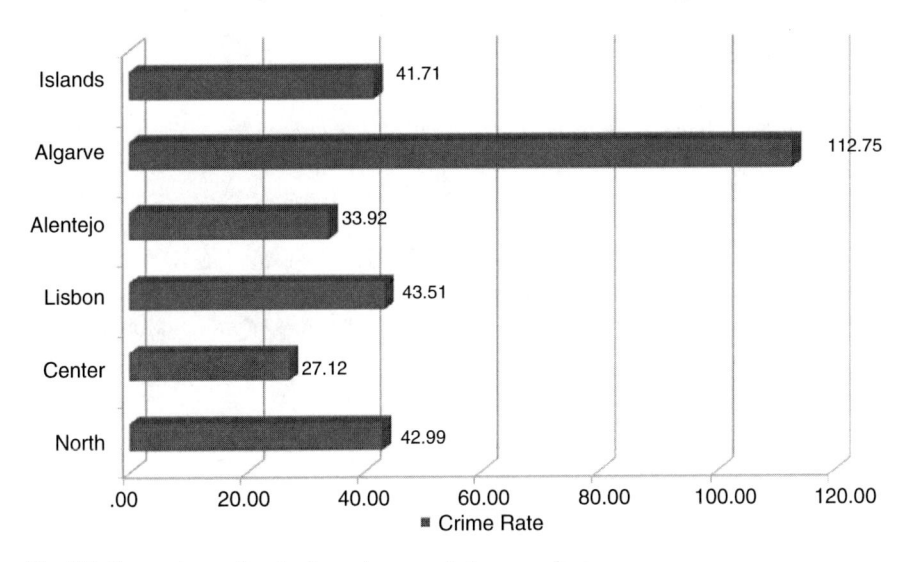

Fig. 5.5 Comparison of total crime rate means between regions

existing in these places, namely, crimes against property ($Z=-8.027$; $p<0.001$) and physical crimes against the person ($F=-10.392$; $p<0.001$), mugging attacks ($Z=-28.476$; $p<0.001$), and car theft ($Z=-15.485$; $p<0.001$). However, the remaining regions still present significantly higher crimes against peace and society ($Z=-11.906$; $p<0.001$), drink-driving ($Z=-9.724$; $p<0.001$), and driving without a license ($Z=-14.388$; $p<0.001$), as compared to Lisbon and Oporto.

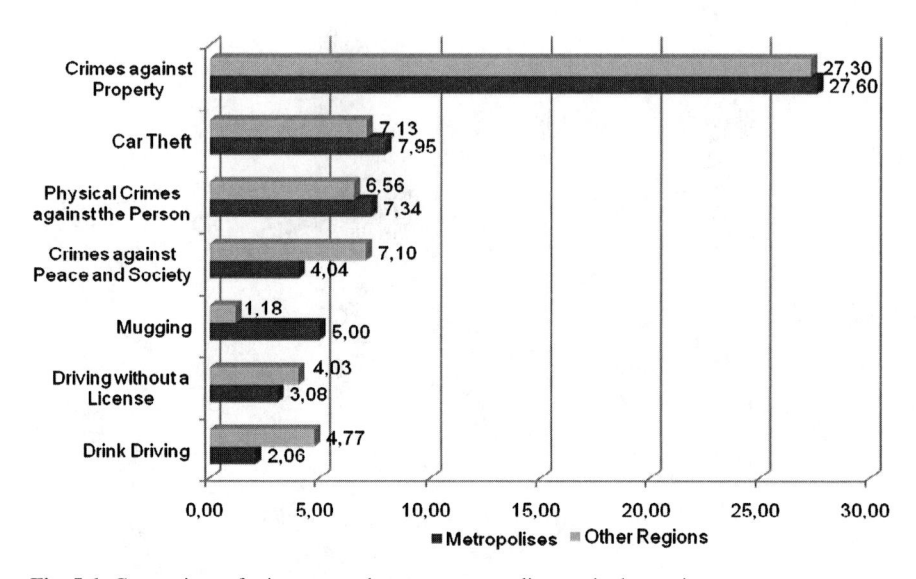

Fig. 5.6 Comparison of crime means between metropolises and other regions

6 Discussion

Past researchers have used different measures of human security, depending on the outcomes they wish to highlight. The analysis of SWB has tended to be based on victimization, whereas objective measures of security have been used mainly to compare different communities, while subjective ones were related to general health or physical activity (Johnson et al. 2009). An integrated understanding of how different security measures that vary across regions influence the SWB of citizens has not been made until now. Given this situation, we contribute to a more comprehensive and complete framework of citizen security at the municipal level by analyzing the impacts of both objective and subjective measures of security on SWB. To understand if both measures influence the quality of life of citizens, we explored in a single study the impact of both the objective measures of crime and the subjective perceptions of security on SWB across 20 Portuguese municipalities.

As expected, the model that best fit the data showed that the SWB of citizens was influenced by both objective and subjective indicators of security.

As predicted (H1), we found that objective measures of citizen security at the municipal level had an impact on the SWB of residents. In line with previous research (e.g., Powdthavee 2005; McLeer et al. 1988), our study showed that crime indices affect SWB of citizens. In the municipalities where the index crime was higher, residents were less happy and satisfied with their life in general. Indeed, some researchers have already emphasized that the gap between crime victims and nonvictims could be smaller, especially in higher crime-rate regions (e.g., Alesina et al. 2004; Powdthavee 2005). We demonstrated that the SWB of citizens was affected by crime rates, even though these citizens may not have been victims of crime.

Our study contributes to a more comprehensive understanding of security in municipalities. More than demonstrating that crime victims are less satisfied with their lives, as does much of the earlier literature, our study advances this line of research by showing that higher crime indices lead to lower SWB in citizens.

Specifically, our model reveals a significant impact of crimes against property on SWB, when compared to other crimes. Relying on Powdthavee (2005), a possible explanation for this impact is the fact that property crimes take place mainly inside the home, while pickpocketing, mugging, or purse-snatching happen elsewhere, away from one's home. Besides property crime, physical crimes against the person, drink-driving, and driving without a license also seemed to diminish SWB of citizens, revealing that those crimes are also crucial to quality of life. Although the literature does not explore these differences, one possible explanation rests on their frequency. Statistics indicate that property crime and physical crimes against the person are more frequent, which makes them more visible to citizens, thus affecting their SWB. According to Statistics Portugal, crime against property accounted for 53.2% of the total number of crimes in 2007, followed by physical crimes against the person, which represented 22.8% (INE 2008).

Moreover, our study indicates that SWB is higher in the interior municipalities where crime rates are lower. Consistent with Roh and Choo (2008), crime has been regarded as a major city problem due to the higher crime rates in major and coastal cities than in interior cities and municipalities. Since the 1960s, the major Portuguese cities (e.g., Lisbon, Oporto, and Aveiro) have grown quickly as rural workers moved to the coastal cities, seeking better life and work conditions (Antunes 1981). As those metropolitan areas have witnessed unemployment, social inequality, and diversity in socioeconomic conditions, they no longer remain immune to many social problems, such as crime and disorder.

Furthermore, our study reveals that the perception of violence has an impact on the SWB of citizens (H2). As earlier demonstrated (e.g., Kruger and Reisch 2007; Weir et al. 2006), residents with higher perceptions of neighborhood crime and insecurity reported higher levels of stress and symptoms of depression and were less engaged in physical activity. Our study emphasizes that in municipalities where residents perceive less security, happiness and satisfaction with life are lower. This effect is especially true with regard to walking on the streets at night. Consistent with Green et al. (2002), fear of walking on the streets at night is the best predictor of health status and reduced mental and social well-being.

Our study highlighted that, more than affecting physical and general health, perception of insecurity had a significant effect on the SWB of citizens.

Our study also reveals that the perception of security is greater among citizens from the interior municipalities, when compared with those based along the coast (e.g., Lisbon, Oporto). Given that crime rates are higher on the coast (as evidenced by our study), the citizens' fear of crime may also be higher. According to Powdthavee (2005), the greater the crime rate, the more the fear of crime becomes evident, thus reducing the SWB of citizens (Powdthavee 2005).

Perception of security is also greater in the islands, compared to the mainland municipalities. Several studies have already shown that both crime rates and perceptions of insecurity are lower in the islands (e.g., Briceño-León et al. 2008), although for different reasons. In their study, Briceño-León et al. (2008) revealed that the crime rate was lower in Cuba's and Costa Rica's islands, compared with Brazil, Mexico, and Venezuela, due mostly to an unfavorable social context (e.g., social inequalities, lack of employment opportunities, and urban segregation). Concerning Portugal and its social context, statistics for 2009[5] show that unemployment is significantly lower in the islands (8.3%) than in the continent (10.1%). This may help to explain why residents feel more secure in the islands.

In conclusion, our study contributes to a more complete framework of citizen security at the municipal level. More than demonstrating that crime victims are less satisfied with their lives or that perception of insecurity produces significant effects on physical and general health (Johnson et al. 2009), our study advances these lines of research by showing that SWB of citizens is affected by both higher crime index and perceptions of insecurity.

As emphasized by some authors (e.g., Veenhoven 1996, 2002), our study reinforces the belief that objective indicators alone are inadequate to understand the quality of life of citizens. Given that both objective and subjective measures of human security impact on SWB, both measures must be taken into account to obtain a more complete view of human security. Moreover, subjective measures are crucial for policymaking. Given that urban violence and security are of major concern for policymakers, planners, and development practitioners in cities around the world, measuring citizens' perceptions is very important in selecting policy goals and monitoring the outcomes of policy interventions (e.g., Diener 2006; Sirgy et al. 2010). In addition, when studying SWB, community planners are able to monitor community well-being over time and to check residents' satisfaction with the community, thus adjusting the policies and programs needed. Studying the impact of human security on SWB is also important for comparing municipalities. Understanding the sources of satisfaction/dissatisfaction with life allows community planners to propose programs and services to enhance residents' satisfaction, thus increasing the quality of life there.

Our study emphasizes the sources of security that promote SWB of citizens in their community. Future research could follow the longitudinal implementation of several programs to enhance SWB, thus exploring the efficacy of those programs. More studies are needed to better understand why the islands are perceived as more secure than the mainland and why the security indices have different impacts on SWB. Moreover, more studies analyzing both objective and subjective measures of citizen security at the local, municipal, and regional levels are needed to develop a more complete and comprehensive framework of citizen security.

---

[5]4th trimester (INE 2009).

Appendix: Descriptive Data and Quality Indices of Measuresss

Measures	Mean	S.D.
Subjective security (single-item)		
How safe are you when going for a walk alone at night?	2.81	0.67
Subjective well-being ($\alpha=0.64$)	3.16	0.37
All things considered, how satisfied are you with your life these days?	3.00	0.55
Taking all things together, how happy would you say you are?	3.13	0.50
All things considered, how optimistic are you about your future?	2.74	0.58
Taking all things together, to what extent do you agree with the sentence "life is meaningful"?	3.76	0.50

References

Alesina, A., Di Tella, R., & MacCulloch, R. (2004). Inequality and happiness: Are Europeans and Americans different? *Journal of Public Economics, 88*(9–10), 2009–2042.

Antunes, M. (1981). Migrações, mobilidade social e identidade cultural: Factos e hipóteses sobre o caso português. *Análise Social, XVII*(65), 17–27.

Argyle, M. (1996). Subjective well-being. In A. Offer (Ed.), *In pursuit of the quality of life* (pp. 18–45). Oxford: Oxford University Press.

Briceño-León, R., Villaveces, A., & Concha-Eastman, A. (2008). Understanding the uneven distribution of the incidence of homicide in Latin America. *International Journal of Epidemiology, 37*, 751–757.

Cáceres, M. (2002). More training, less security? Training and the quality of life at work in Argentina, Brazil and Chile. *International Labour Review, 141*(4), 359–384.

Clark, C., Ryan, L., Kawachi, I., Canner, M., Berkman, L., & Wright, R. (2008). Witnessing community violence in residential neighborhoods: A mental health hazard for urban women. *Journal of Urban Health, 85*(1), 22–38.

Diener, E. (2006). Guidelines for national indicators of subjective well-being and ill-being. *Journal of Happiness Studies, 7*(4), 397–404.

Djuric, S. (2009). Qualitative approach to the research into the parameters of human security in the community. *Policing: An International Journal of Police Strategies and Management, 32*(3), 541–559.

European Foundation for the Improvement of Living and Working Conditions (EFILWC). (2003). *Quality of life in Europe. First European quality of life survey 2003*. Luxembourg: Office for Official publications of the European Communities. Resource document. http://www.eurofound.europa.eu/pubdocs/2004/105/en/1/ef04105en.pdf.

European Foundation for the Improvement of Living and Working Conditions (EFILWC). (2007). *Second European quality of life survey overview*. Luxembourg: Office for official publications of the European Communities. Resource document http://www.eurofound.europa.eu.

Gage, L. (2006). Comparison of Census 2000 and American Community Survey 1999–2001 Estimates: San Francisco and Tulare Counties, California. *Population Research and Policy Review, 25*, 243–256.

Green, G., Gilbertson, J., & Grimsley, M. (2002). Fear of crime and health in residential tower blocks: A case study in Liverpool, UK. *European Journal of Public Health, 12*(1), 10–15.

Hardi, P., & Pintér, L. (2006). City of Winnipeg quality-of-life indicators. In J. Sirgy, D. Rahtz, & D. Swain (Eds.), *Community quality-of-life indicators: Best cases II* (pp. 127–176). Dordecht: Springer.

INE – Instituto Nacional de Estatística. (2008). *Statistical yearbook of Portugal. Resource document.* http://www.ine.pt/ngt_server/attachfileu.jsp?look_parentBoui=83354386&att_display=n&att_ download=y

INE – Instituto Nacional de Estatística. (2009). *Resource document.* http://www.ine.pt/xportal/ xmain?xpid=INE&xpgid=ine_unid_territorial&menuBOUI=13707095&contexto=ut&selTa b=tab3

Johnson, S., Solomon, B., Shields, W., McDonald, E., McKenzie, L., & Gielen, A. (2009). Neighborhood violence and its association with mothers' health: Assessing the relative importance of perceived safety and exposure to violence. *Journal of Urban Health: Bulletin of the New York Academy of Medicine, 86*(4), 538–550.

Krause, K. (1998). Critical theory and security studies: The research programme of "critical security studies". *Cooperation and Conflict: Nordic Journal of International Studies, 33*(3), 298–333.

Kruger, D., & Reisch, T. (2007). Neighborhood social conditions mediate the association between physical deterioration and mental health. *American Journal of Community Psychology, 40,* 261–271.

Lopes, M., Palma, P., & Cunha, M. (2010). Tolerance is not enough: The moderating role of optimism on perceptions of regional economic performance. *Social Indicators Research, 102*(2), 333–350.

McLeer, S., Deblinger, E., Atkins, M., Foa, E., & Ralphe, D. (1988). Post-traumatic stress disorder in sexually abused children. *Journal of the American Academy of Child and Adolescent Psychiatry, 27,* 650–654.

Michalos, A. (1991). *Global report on student well-being* (Life satisfaction and happiness, Vol. 1). New York: Springer.

Noll, H. (2002). Towards a European system of social indicators: Theoretical framework and system architecture. *Social Indicators Research, 58,* 47–87.

Owen, T. (2004). Are we really secure?: Challenges and opportunities for defining and measuring human security. *Disarmament Forum, 2,* 2–24.

Owen, T. (2008). In all but name: The uncertain future of human security in the UN. In *Rethinking human security.* Oxford: Blackell Press.

Powdthavee, N. (2005). Unhappiness and crime: Evidence from South Africa. *Economica, 72,* 531–547.

Raudenbush, S., & Bryk, A. (2002). *Hierarchical linear models* (2nd ed.). Thousand Oaks: Sage Publications.

Reiss, A. (1983). Crime control and the quality of life. *American Behavioral Scientist, 27*(1), 43–58.

Roh, S., & Choo, T. (2008). Looking inside Zone V: Testing social disorganization theory in suburban areas. *Western Criminology Review, 9,* 1–16.

Rothschild, E. (1995). What is security? *Daedalus, 124*(43), 53–90.

Sampson, R., Morenoff, J., & Gannon-Rowley, T. (2002). Assessing neighborhood effects: Social processes and new directions in research. *Annual Review of Sociology, 28,* 443–478.

Senlier, N., Yildiz, R., & Aktas, E. (2009). A perception survey for the evaluation of urban quality of life in Kocaeli and a comparison of the life satisfaction with the European Cities. *Social Indicators Research, 94,* 213–226.

Shapiro, M. (2009). Managing urban security: City walls and urban metis. *Security Dialogue, 40,* 443–461.

Sirgy, M., & Cornwell, T. (2002). How neighborhood features affect quality of life. *Social Indicators Research, 59,* 79–114.

Sirgy, M., Widgery, R., Lee, D., & Yu, G. (2010). Developing a measure of community well-being based on perceptions of impact in various life domains. *Social Indicators Research, 96*(2), 295–311.

United Nations Development Programme (UNDP). (1994). *Human development report.* New York: Oxford University Press.

Vanderschueren, F. (1996). From violence to justice and security in cities. *Environment and Urbanization, 8*(1), 93–112.

Veenhoven, R. (1996). Happy life-expectancy: A comprehensive measure of quality-of-life in nations. *Social Indicators Research, 39,* 1–58.

Veenhoven, R. (2002). Why social policy needs subjective indicators. *Social Indicators Research, 58,* 33–45.

Weir, L., Etelson, D., & Brand, D. (2006). Parents' perceptions of neighborhood safety and children's physical activity. *Preventive Medicine, 43*(3), 212–217.

Wills-Herrera, E., Islam, G., & Hamilton, M. (2009). Subjective well-being in cities: A multidimensional concept of individual, social and cultural variables. *Applied Research in Quality of Life, 4*(2), 201–221.

Chapter 6
An Assessment of How Urban Crime and Victimization Affects Life Satisfaction

Carlos Medina and Jorge Andrés Tamayo

1 Introduction

The rise in crime that has taken place since the Second World War has been quoted by Layard (2005) as "the clearest failure of community life" (Layard 2005, p. 80). As the author points out, the increase in crime in the United States and Britain goes beyond the usually argued poverty or inequality concerns, since as crime has increased, inequality and unemployment have decreased. In the case of Colombia, the key parties responsible for perpetuating its high crime rates have been the guerrilla groups and the drug dealers. Drug trafficking has strengthened organized crime in the last several decades. In Colombian urban cities, the influence of drug dealers is the most relevant force driving crime. They took over the domestic drug market and split it among them, with strict and enforceable boundaries within some neighborhoods of each of the main cities. Whenever there is disequilibrium in the forces among the groups controlling the market, a war among them takes place and crime rates abruptly increase, as has been the case in the last few years.[1]

In this chapter, we assess the effect that crime, households' perception of security in their respective neighborhoods, and individuals' victimization have on perceived quality of life which we also refer to as *life satisfaction*. This approach complements previous estimates of the costs of crime in urban areas obtained by other means, either accounting for their direct and indirect costs, or by means of empirical models like the hedonic model, which estimates the capitalization of crime on property values. By assessing whether these variables affect life satisfaction, we go beyond the market approach and are able to test whether each one of

---

[1] See Information System for Security and Coexistence (2009).

C. Medina (✉) • J.A. Tamayo
Banco de la República, Medellin, Colombia
e-mail: cmedindu@banrep.gov.co; jtamayca@banrep.gov.co

D. Webb and E. Wills-Herrera (eds.), *Subjective Well-Being and Security*,
Social Indicators Research Series 46, DOI 10.1007/978-94-007-2278-1_6,
© Springer Science+Business Media B.V. 2012

crime, neighborhood satisfaction, and victimization actually affects the much broader concept of perceived quality of life.

Identifying the effect of the variables of interest on crime is not an easy task since households sort endogenously across neighborhoods, accounting in that process for the levels of those variables in each of the potential neighborhoods they might move to, thus making it challenging to disentangle their actual effect. We exploit the large variation in the homicide rates between the different neighborhoods of Medellín. Using a large data set with the census of its homicides over several years, we build homicide rates at the block level, and split the sample, in a way that allows us to get reasonable estimates of the effect of the homicide rate, individual's perception of security in their neighborhood of residence, and the effect of their having been victimized, on life satisfaction. We control for a battery of socioeconomic variables at the household level, and fixed effects of the neighborhoods where the household currently and previously lived.

We find a negative effect of the homicide rate on life satisfaction for a subsample of individuals who have been living in their current houses for at least 10 years or more, and additionally, who had moved to their current house at some point in the past, as opposed to those who have lived in their current houses forever, or have moved to their house less than 10 years ago. On the contrary, the arrest rates, defined as the ratio of captures to homicides at the block level, significantly increase life satisfaction. We also find a positive and robust effect of the perception of security in the households' neighborhood for the whole sample and for each of the subsamples considered. Having been victim of an offense is also robustly negatively related to life satisfaction, and particularly so in the case where the offense was robbery.

We present in the following section a brief review of relevant literature before proceeding to describe our data and key empirical regularities. We finally present our identification strategy and results, and provide the conclusions.

2   Previous Work

As Di Tella et al. (2008) highlight that the relationship between criminal victimization and well-being has been studied by both psychologists and sociologists. In fact, psychologists and sociologists have studied the impact of different economic and social variables on life satisfaction. Sirgy and Cornwell (2002) present a complete review of studies that have analyzed the link between different neighborhood features and life satisfaction. They classify those features in three main aspects: physical, social, and economic features of the neighborhood and analyzed how neighborhood features affect the quality of life.[2] They conclude that their effect on quality of life can be explained through the mediating effects of community

---

[2] For these three features, they present a complete literature review of studies that analyzed the impact of this features on life satisfaction.

satisfaction, housing satisfaction, and home satisfaction. Specifically, satisfaction with the neighborhood social features contributes significantly to one's overall feelings about community satisfaction. "These overall feelings about the community, in turn, play a significant role in life satisfaction" (Sirgy and Cornwell 2002, p. 103).[3]

Particularly, Ross and Jang (2000) stress similar conclusions. From a representative sample of 2,482 Illinois residents collected by telephone in 1995, they conclude that "people who live in neighborhoods where they see a lot of disorder have significantly higher levels of both fear and mistrust than those who live in neighborhoods characterized by social control and order" (Ross and Jang 2000, p. 409). The stress of living in a place where the streets are dirty and dangerous takes its toll in feelings of depression and anxiety, and consequently in less well-being.[4] Latkin and Curry (2003) find a strong and positive association between perceived neighborhood characteristics and subsequent depressive symptoms. "The data also suggest that neighborhood and social disorganization is a powerful chronic stressor among inner-city population" (Latkin and Curry 2003, p. 40).[5]

Relevant issues on this topic are the possible predictors of perceived disorder in neighborhoods that at the end are connected with well-being perceptions. Franzini et al. (2008), in a neighborhood study conducted in Baltimore, conclude that perceptions of disorder are associated with aspects of observed physical disorder (overall conditions of buildings and public spaces rather than the presence of trash and graffiti) and neighborhood structural compositions (economic disadvantage and violence). Similarly, Latkin et al. (2009) conclude that perceptions of neighborhood disorder are based on objective factors, measured by police crime reports; individual's experiences, measured by the time spent on the streets; and the experience of others, measured by membership to specific networks.

On the other hand, Sampson and Raudenbush (2004) find that class and racial composition appears to be a strong predictor of perceived disorder. That is, perceptions of disorder are socially constructed and are shaped by much more than actual and observe levels of disorder. "Our larger point, however, is that the social and especially the racial composition of a local area, which is associated statistically with disorder, is highly salient in contemporary culture and deeply imbued with stereotypes" (Sampson and Raudenbush 2004, p. 323).

Recently, economists have revisited the concept of happiness and well-being. For example, Easterlin (1974 and 2003), Blanchflower and Oswald (2004), Clark and Oswald (1994), Graham and Pettinato (2002), and Layard (2005) are some of

---

[3] Diener et al. (1999) present a review for physiologist modern and past theories of subjective well-being.

[4] Geis and Ross (1998), Ross et al. (2000), Cutrona et al. (2000), among others obtain similar results. Scarbourough et al. (2010) studied the relationship between individual characteristic, neighborhood context, and fear of crime and find that relationship between demographic characteristics and fear of crime is conditions by neighborhood factors.

[5] This article mentioned a large literature that emphasizes social disorders in urban disadvantaged neighborhoods, illicit drug use, drug purchasing, and other criminal activities.

the key references in this literature.[6] Despite the extant literature in respect to life satisfaction and quality of life, only a few articles have analyzed the relationship between crime and life satisfaction.

Using Gallup World Poll, Di Tella et al. (2008) show that individuals who have experienced property crimes or have been mugged or assaulted within the last 12 months (victimized) have lower levels of well-being.[7] They use different specifications to define well-being based on "subjective well-being" (asked directly to individuals) and innovative questions such as "whether the individual smiled yesterday" or "if they would like more days like yesterday." They also show that individuals who have been mugged are "less likely to believe that effort pays."[8]

Cohen (2008) analyzed the U.S. General Social Survey which is administered to 2,800 individuals annually for the years with life satisfaction data available.[9] The question of interest in the GSS asks "Taken all together, how would you say things are these days?" (very happy, pretty happy, or not happy). Combining this information with county level data that include economic social variables and different measures of crime, they find that county level crime rates have little impact on overall life satisfaction. They also find that controlling for actual victimization reduces the significance level of impact to live in a perceived unsafe neighborhood. Cohen (2008) argues that one reason that might explain why county crime rates and perception of safety do not have an impact (or little) on life satisfaction is because "for those who live in unsafe neighborhoods these same individuals are already compensated for the higher risk of victimization through lower housing and rental prices. Thus, higher disposable income might offset the effect of less safety" (Cohen 2008, p. 23). On the other hand, the author finds a quite large effect of a home burglary on life satisfaction.

Michalos and Zumbo (2000) analyzed crime-related issues on happiness, satisfaction with life as whole in Prince George, British Columbia. They show that

---

[6] There are many articles that have tried to link life satisfaction with different themes. An example of those are the following: Helburn (1982), who analyzed the link between geography and quality of life; studies that analyzed unemployment and quality of life, Winkelmann and Winkelmann (1998), Frey and Stutzer (1999), and Blanchflower and Oswald (2003); relationship between absolute and relative income and quality of life, Clark and Oswald (1996), McBride (2000), Easterlin (2001), Deaton (2008), and Ferrer-i-Carbonell (2005); Di Tella et al. (2001, 2003) analyzed the impact of macroeconomics indicators on life satisfaction; Alesina et al. (2004) analyzed the relationship between inequality and quality of life.

[7] The Gallup World Poll is a survey covering more than 130 countries in all regions of the world which allows for comparison of patterns of victimization and safety perceptions. The poll asks if in the last 12 months interviewed individuals were victims of property crime or crime against the person (assaulted or mugged).

[8] They also presented interesting statistics about the patterns of victimization across groups, like "males are more often victimized than females," age is negatively correlated with victimization, etc. For more, see DiTella et al. (2008).

[9] Those are 1993, 1994, 1996, 1998, 2000, 2002, and 2004.

victims of crime reported lower measures of happiness and life satisfaction as a whole. They also point out that measures of fear correlate negatively with life satisfaction. However, they found that crime-related issues were displaced by other measures like satisfaction with family life, health, self-esteem among others, explaining the variation in overall happiness, life satisfaction, and satisfaction with overall quality of life scores.

Powdthavee (2005) analyzed the level of well-being of crime victims on post-apartheid South Africa (1995–nowadays), using subjective measures of well-being reported on October Household Survey of 1997 (OHS97). Data of 2,121 crime victims (violent and property offenses) are used to determine whether, ceteris paribus, crime episodes are negatively correlated with the well-being of households or not. Controlling for household expenditure, differences of race, sex, education, and other variables, Powdthavee (2005) finds that there are substantial differences in reported welfare of crime and noncrime victims, as well as a "fear of crime" effect on nonvictims' quality of life perception (felonies around the household or neighborhood increase the perceived probability of victimization). However, an interesting finding is that the negative correlation between well-being measures and crime experiences for females "is attenuated as crime on others rises" (he calls this a social norm effect: individuals may feel safer if a large percentage of the population in the neighborhood shares their experiences of criminal victimization). The effect is always negative for males.

3 Data and Empirical Regularities

In this section, we describe the evolution of crime in Medellin and present the main statistics of the variables employed in this study. Our main sources for the empirical exercises and variables described in this section are: at census sector level, 2005 Population Census, provided by the Administrative Department of National Statistics (DANE, by its acronym in Spanish); we also have data available at the household level with the survey *Encuesta de Calidad de Vida de Medellin* (ECVM) for 2008 collected by the Municipality of Medellin, which has detailed information about living conditions of households in Medellin, with more than 18,500 households interviewed across all the neighborhoods in the city.[10]

Finally, we use information of homicides and individuals captured in the act for different types of crime at spatial coordinates recorded by the Judicial Police Sectional of the National Police Department (SIJIN by its acronym in Spanish).

---

[10] See Map 6.4. There are a total of 242 census sectors (these are spatial units employed by Dane when surveying households) and 249 neighborhoods (these are the spatial administrative units in which the Municipality of Medellin splits the city) in Medellín. In the case of Medellin, these spatial units are very similar.

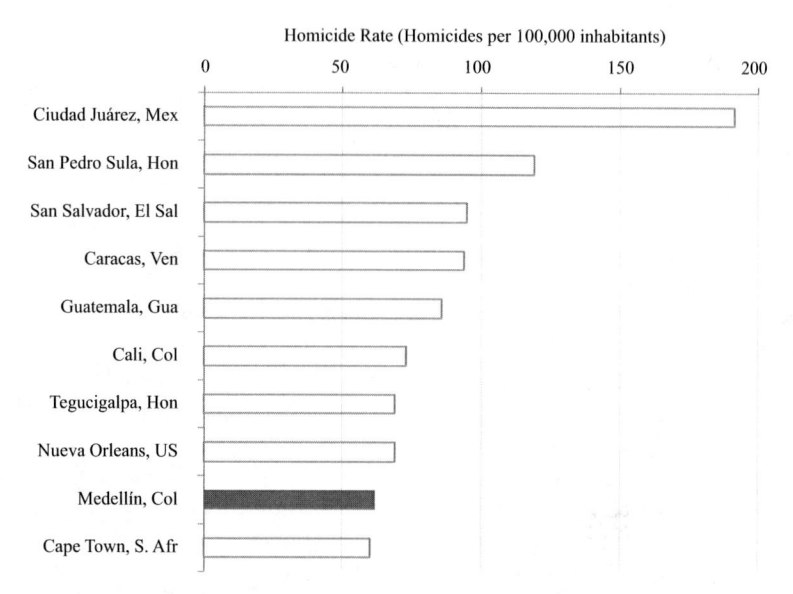

Fig. 6.1   Cities with the highest homicide rates of the world, 2009 (Source: *Consejo Ciudadano para la Seguridad Pública y la Justicia Penal* (CCSPJP) and *Movimiento Blanco*)

3.1   Empirical Regularities

Medellín has, over the last three decades, been one of the most violent cities in the world, and at times, it has had the highest homicide rate. Even though current homicide rates are much lower than the ones the city registered in the early 1990s, Medellín was still recently ranked among the ten most violent cities of the world, as it can be observed in Fig. 6.1, where it was ranked ninth by a study published by two Mexican non-governmental organizations.[11]

Medellín's violence has traditionally been high due to the existence of guerrilla groups. However, the drug business that took off in the late 1970s and early 1980s fueled initially the emergence of organized crime to support the business. This lead to the existence of the guerrilla groups who were hired to care for the drug crops, and finally, the emergence of paramilitary groups to care for both the entire business chain and any other armed group.[12] It also becomes apparent in Fig. 6.1 that the drug business is a driving force of violence not only in Medellín and Colombia, but also

[11] Patterns of crime by country in Latin America can be found in Soares and Naritomi (2010).

[12] Bullinton (1992) reports the huge share of cocaine and marijuana entering the US in the 1980s through Bahamas and Miami, and the role of Colombian drug dealers in sending it, as it is also described by Riley (1996). See also Gamarra (2003) who argues that most Colombian migrants to the US since the late 1970s and until the mid 1990s were linked to the growth of the international narcotics trade. See also Thoumi (1995) and Gugliotta and Leen (1989) on this. The relation between drug dealers, guerrillas, and paramilitary groups is described in Villamarin (1996).

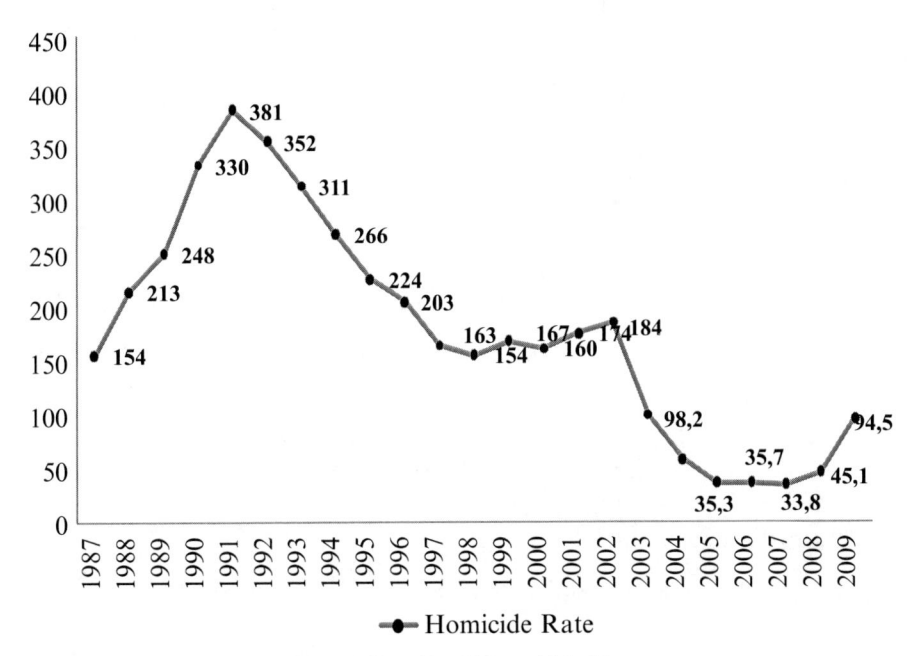

Source: Government Secretary's Office of Medellín, published inreport
of Civil Security from "Medellín Como Vamos"

Fig. 6.2 Homicide rate in Medellin (Source: Government Secretary's Office of Medellín, published in report of Civil Security from "Medellín Como Vamos")

in other countries of the world. In particular, it is the main cause for the recent increase in the homicide rate in Mexico, and for the presence of Ciudad Juárez as the most violent city of the world in Fig. 6.1.

Figure 6.2 shows the evolution of the homicide rate in Medellin over the period 1987–2009. There are three main aspects to highlight from this figure. First, the homicide rate began to rise in the mid 1980s and continued increasing until the early 1990s, when the homicide rate reached its highest level and began a persistent decline reaching levels not seen since the late 1970s. As stressed by Gaviria et al. (2010b), the observed peak of the homicide rate in the early 1990s was due to the "boom of the Medellin drug cartel, and its declaration of war to the government and other illegal groups" (Gaviria et al. 2010b, p. 10).

Secondly, the homicide rate presents a severe decline observed in October of 2002 due to the "hot-spot," called *Operación Orion*, perpetuated by military forces against the urban militias of the guerrillas (FARC and ELN by their acronyms in Spanish), which took place in the 13 commune, *San Javier*, located at the west zone of the city, and the *Cacique Nutibara*, paramilitary demobilization process that took place in November of 2003. These operations had a huge impact on the reduction in the number of homicides in the city.[13]

---

[13] Giraldo (2008) finds positive effects of the *Operación Orion* but questions the outcomes of the BCN demobilization (see also Palau and Llorente 2009 and the references therein).

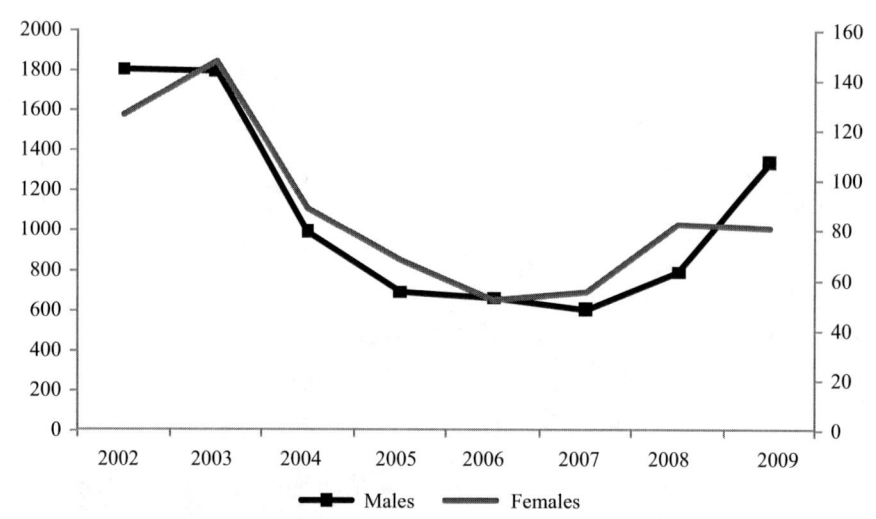

Source: National Police Department of Statistics

Fig. 6.3 Homicide rate, by gender (Source: National Police Department of Statistics)

Third, the renewed increase in the homicide rate beginning in 2008, the year in which key paramilitary leaders were extradited to the United States, and the capture of other leaders in April of 2009, has been interpreted as being caused by a fight among drug dealers to gain power within their organization and among the potential owners of the domestic urban drug market.

Figure 6.3 presents homicide rates for females and males over the period 2002–2009. Although they are highly correlated, the homicide rate is 12 times higher for males than for females. This is a very important feature of the violence in Medellin because this fact, coupled with the statistics presented in Fig. 6.4, gives us a better understanding of who the participants are and their motives for the violence in the city.[14]

Figure 6.4 shows that the average age of the victims and murderers (who were captured in the act) are around 17–25 years old.[15] This fact shows that victims and murderers have many characteristics in common. In fact, Giraldo et al. (2010) argued that victims and murderers have similar levels of education, age, sex (Fig. 6.3), neighborhood where they live, and activity, among others. This and other mentioned facts suggest that a great share of armed actors is not related to ordinary crime but rather to organized crime fighting for territory control.[16]

---

[14] Giraldo et al. (2010) present a complete characterization of the violent crime in Medellin.

[15] We present only statistics for murderers captured in the act. Later we are going to use that variable as a proxy for different types of criminal activity.

[16] For example, 75% of the victims murdered in Medellín in the first semester of 2009 were murdered in their neighborhood of residence, which is linked to the hiring of killers or to fight for territory control among gangs that belong to the organized crime. See Information System for Security and Coexistence (2009).

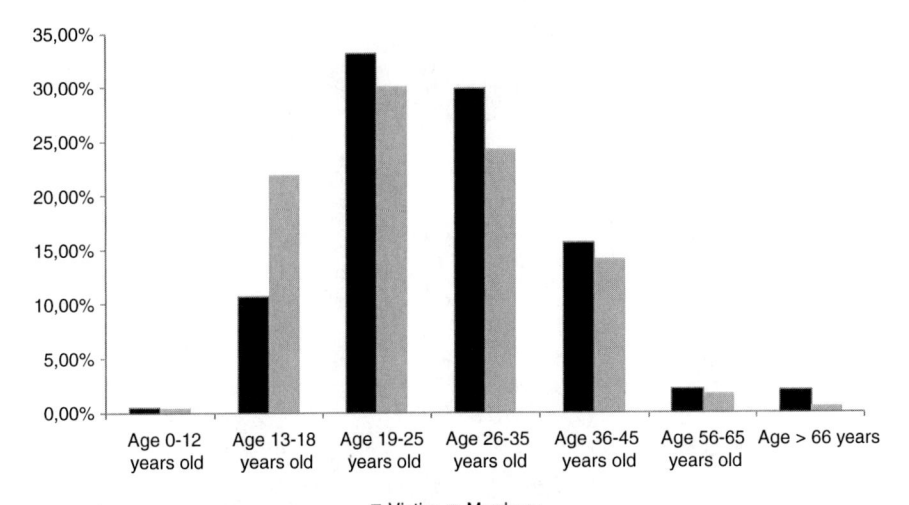

■ Victim ■ Murderer
Source:National Police Department, Sectional Judicial Police (SIJIN)

Fig. 6.4 Age of the victim and murder apprehended in the act (Source: National Police Department, Sectional Judicial Police (SIJIN))

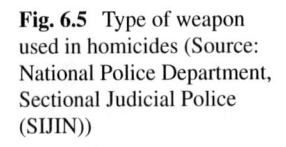

Fig. 6.5 Type of weapon used in homicides (Source: National Police Department, Sectional Judicial Police (SIJIN))

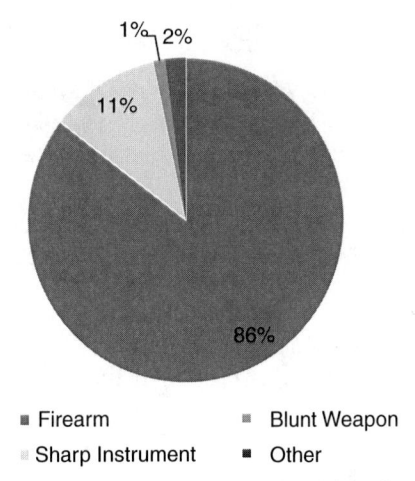

Source: National Police Department, Sectional Judicial Police (SIJIN)

The type of weapon used to commit homicides is presented in Fig. 6.5. The pie diagram shows that most of the homicides are committed with fire arms. Cohen and Rubio (2007), based on estimates of the World Health Organization (WHO), stress that the number of homicides committed with firearms in Latin America has reached three times the world average. This is a very important aspect since as stressed by Gaviria et al. (2010b), the easy access to firearms might be one of the main prob-

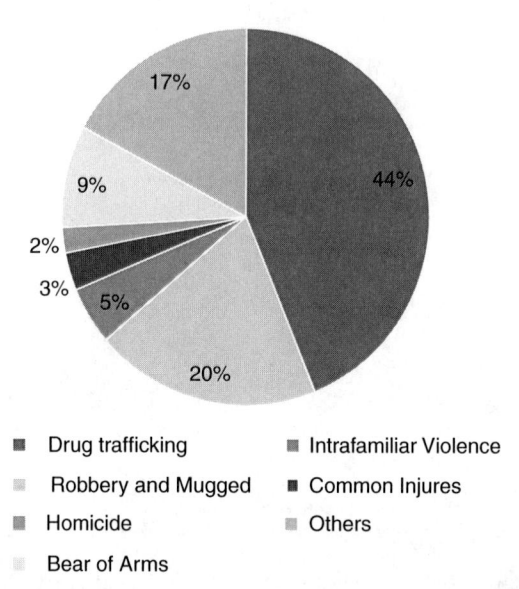

Source: National Police Department, Sectional Judicial Police (SIJIN)

Fig. 6.6 Captures by type of crime (Source: National Police Department, Sectional Judicial Police (SIJIN))

lems associated with the high incidence of crime. Krug et al. (2002) show that the increase in the homicide rate, experienced in the late 1990s in Colombia was associated with the increase in the use of guns as a method of attack: "youth homicides increased by 159%, from 36.7 per 100,000 to 95 per 100,000, with 80% of cases at the end of this period involving guns" (Krug et al. 2002, pp. 27). Cohen and Rubio (2007) also argue that the problem of young gangs and violence are also a matter of concern.

Figure 6.6 shows the shares of the different causes by which individuals were captured in Medellín. Drug trafficking and robbery are the main reasons why people were captured during the period 2002–2009, reflecting the nature of the conflict in Medellin.

We proceed to analyze the spatial distribution of some socio-economic characteristics in Medellin. Map 6.1 shows the spatial distribution of the school attendance rate in Medellin based on the Population Census of 2005. It can be seen that secondary school attendance has reached all socioeconomic strata of the city in a considerable spatially homogeneous way. A different situation happens with college attendance, since only at the southeast and center-west of the city can we observe rates above 50%. In addition, there is a clear pattern of higher college attendance in the better neighborhoods, as becomes clear when comparing Maps 6.1 and 6.2, which includes the location of households according to their income quintile.

Many studies have emphasized that dropping out of school seems to be a strong risk factor determining crime and gang membership. In fact, Gaviria et al. (2010b)

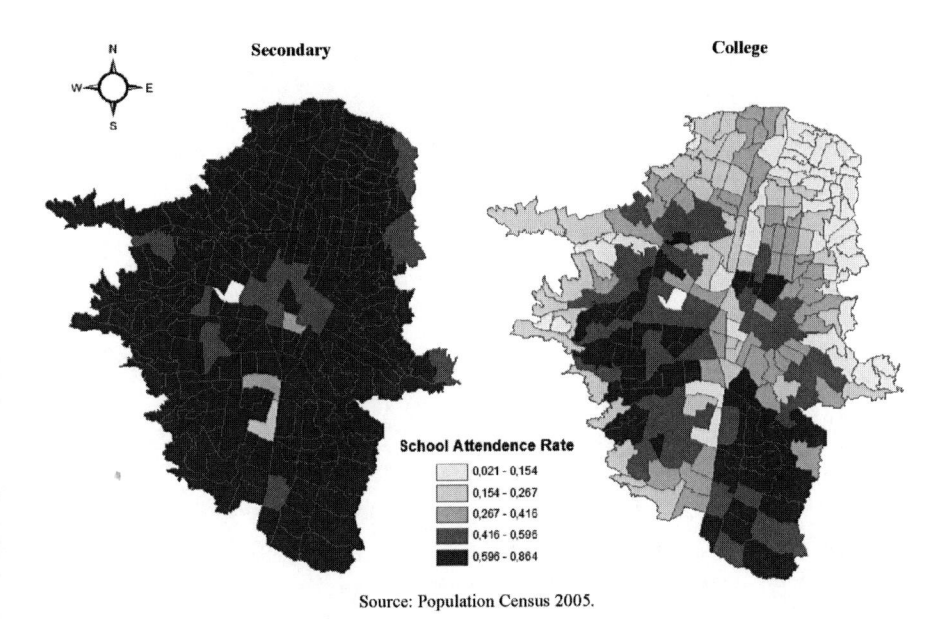

Map 6.1   School attendance rate, 2005 (Source: Population Census 2005)

found that "actually neighborhoods with (1) high effective adolescent fertility rates, (2) low secondary enrollment, and (3) high crime rates at the moment the children of their teen mothers become teenagers, are more likely to have higher homicide rates in the future, when those children reach their peak crime ages, estimated to be between 18 and 26 years old in violent cities of Colombia" (Gaviria 2010b, p. 39). Lochner and Moretti (2004) also find that education reduces crime and the probabilities of incarceration and arrests. Buvinic et al. (2005) stress that dropping out of high school and low school performance are reasons that explain high youth criminality in Latin America. Presenting a corresponding argument, Heckman and Masterov (2007) argue that education is a more cost-effective policy to reduce crime than increasing the number of police.

Map 6.2 also shows the areas with the highest unemployment rates, which are located mostly in the periphery of the west, north, and east of the city, matching the areas with the lowest levels of income and college attendance.

We now describe the most affected areas of the city by homicides. Map 6.3 shows homicide rates and the average distance to the homicides. Both figures were estimated at the block level using the kernel procedure described in Appendix 1. The figures have some features in common but are different because they have two different concepts behind them. The homicide rate indicates the (unconditional) probability of someone living in a specific block to be murdered. The distance indicates the average number of meters from the block in which someone lives to the location where victims have been killed, that is, we use the distance from the individual's residence to each of the places where people have been murdered and average

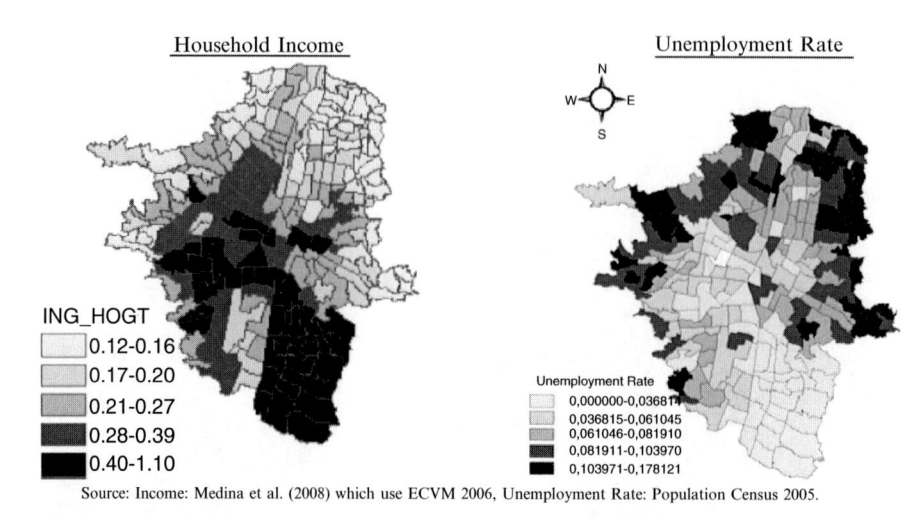

Source: Income: Medina et al. (2008) which use ECVM 2006, Unemployment Rate: Population Census 2005.

Map 6.2 Household income and the unemployment rate (Source: Income: Medina et al. (2008) which use ECVM 2006, unemployment rate: population census 2005)

all those.[17] The center of the map contains downtown Medellín (circled area), where we can observe both a high homicide rate and a short distance to crime, but although blocks in the northeast of the city does not seem to have a high homicide rate, they do have short distances to crime, which might be explained by the high population density of the sector, which allows to have both many people being killed nearby and still low homicide rates.

Map 6.4 shows the distribution of the households interviewed in the ECVM 2008 which we are using in our empirical work. While the units of observation in Map 6.3 are the blocks of the city, those of Map 6.4 are its neighborhoods. The random design of the sample implies the high population density existent at the north of the city, in the two dense subset of population separated by the river of the city and the highways that surround it. That is, Map 6.4 shows that from each neighborhood, households were selected randomly in a way that could include households in each of the six strata.[18]

Map 6.5 shows the location where criminals committing homicide, robbery, intra-family violence, or drug trafficking have been captured. Homicides and robbery are mostly located in downtown Medellín, and intra-family violence takes place mostly in the poorest neighborhoods. Finally, drug-related offenses demark a

---

[17] See Appendix 1 for more details on the way these variables were constructed.

[18] Urban areas in Colombia are split into six socioeconomic strata in which, the first one has the lowest QoL levels. The strata are used by authorities to target social spending like that in the supply of public services (water, electricity), housing, health insurance for the poor, etc.

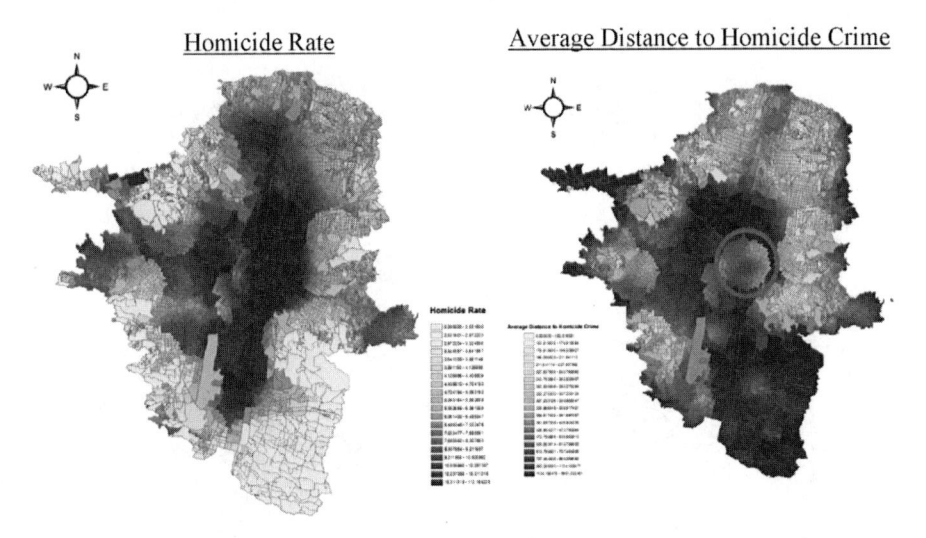

Homicide Rate   **Average Distance to Homicide Crime**

Map 6.3 Homicide rate and average distance to homicide crime, 2008

Map 6.4 Distribution of interviewed individuals, ECV, 2008

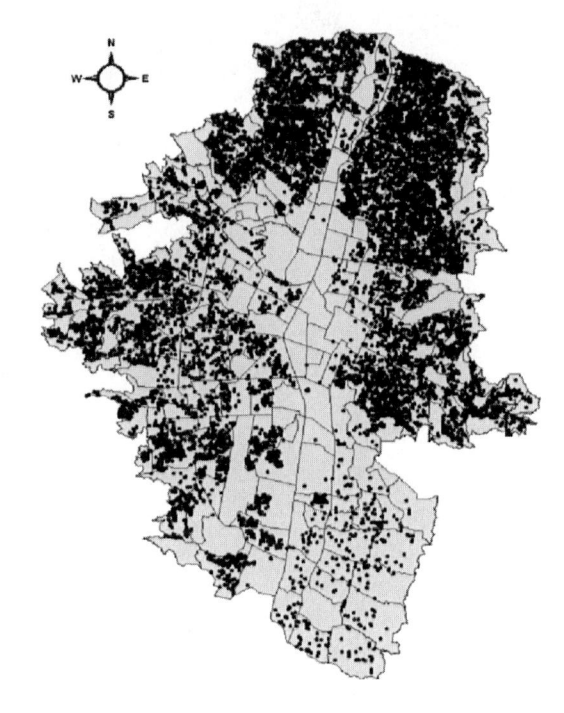

corridor that goes from the west through downtown up to the northeast of the city, which implies an asymmetry in that offense on that part of the city with respect to the northwest, an area with similar characteristics that could have been expected to have been as well affected as much by drugs.

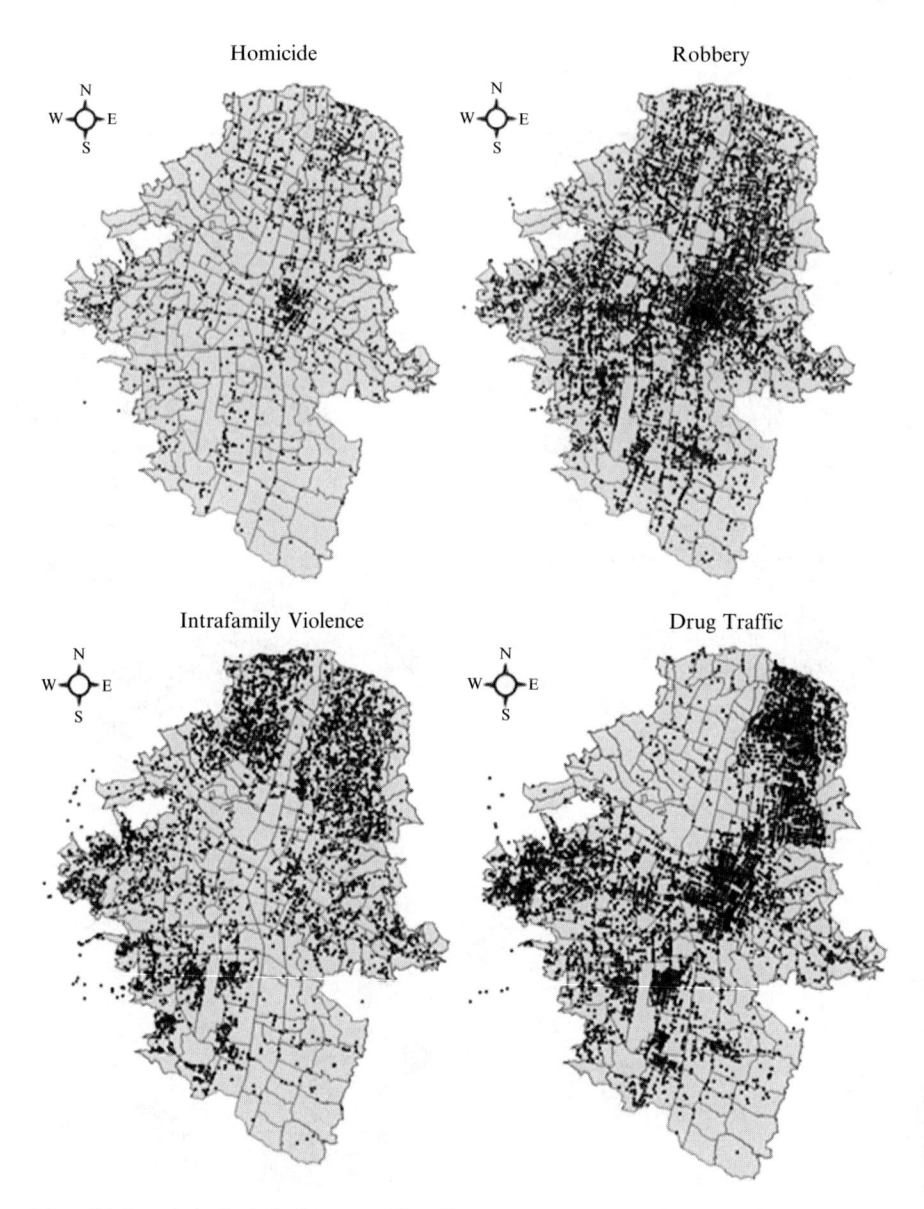

Map 6.5 Location of criminals captured by offense

3.2 *Patterns of Crime and Quality of Life*

The survey *Encuesta de Calidad de Vida de Medellin* (ECVM) for 2008, collected by the Municipality of Medellin, provides an opportunity to analyze the patterns of crime, victimization, and perceptions of safety with life satisfaction.

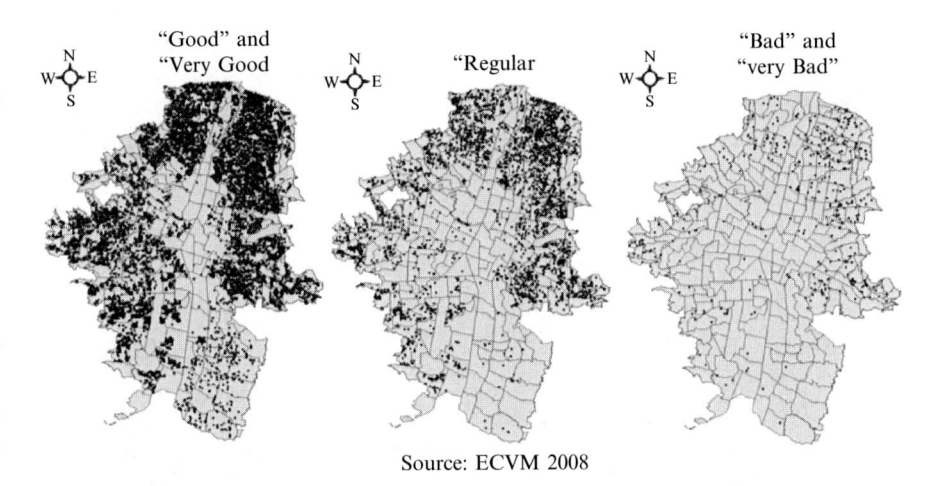

Source: ECVM 2008

Map 6.6 Quality of life perceptions (Source: ECVM 2008)

The survey asks the household head: "Currently, what are the quality of life conditions in your household?" It allows individuals to choose from among the following options: "very good," "good," "fair," "bad," and "very bad." We use the answer to this question to define that a household has "good quality life perceptions" if the household head answered "very good" or "good," as it is usually assumed in the quality of life literature (reference to back this statement up).

The survey also asks them: "How do you feel in the Neighborhood or district where you live?" In this case, individuals classify their safety perceptions of the neighborhood in four categories: "very safe," "safe," "insecure," and "very insecure."

Map 6.6 shows the residence location for individuals who answer "good and very good," "regular," or "bad and very bad" quality of life perceptions. Surprisingly, people who have "good and very good" perceptions of life satisfaction are spatially distributed across the city, while people with "regular" and "bad and very bad" perceptions of quality of life are concentrated among neighborhoods with low levels of income, in the periphery of the city at the west, north, and east.

Additionally, the ECVM explores victimization asking individuals if at least one member of their household was a victim of crimes against life, property, and personal security, among others: "During the last 12 months, have you or other member of your family been victim of a crime?"[19]

We analyzed reported patterns for these three questions taking into account stratum, age, and household income. A first look at reported patterns reveals that life satisfaction perceptions are positively correlated with the socioeconomic strata

---

[19]Interviewers asked interviewed individuals to specify which one of the 25 crime categories of the survey they were victim of.

Table 6.1 Key variable statistics by socioeconomic strata (%) (Source: ECVM 2008)

Socioeconomic stratum	Number of households	Good quality life perceptions	Good security neighborhood perceptions	Victimization
1	1,994	59.8	79.9	8.2
2	6,505	70.9	88.0	8.1
3	5,803	80.1	88.7	8.3
4	2,012	91.5	83.5	10.3
5	1,501	95.9	85.7	8.1
6	776	97.8	94.7	6.1
Total	18,591	78.0	87.0	8.3

(the correlation between these two variables is around 0.26).[20] Table 6.1 shows that at higher levels of socioeconomic strata, the quality of life perceptions are better. Regarding perceptions of security of neighborhoods, stratum 6 presents the highest "good perceptions," while stratum 1 the worst. This table presents an interesting fact, which is that strata 2 and 3 have better perceptions of neighborhood security than strata 4 and 5, which suggest that the better-off households residing in socioeconomic strata 4 and 5 might be more demanding in security standards. For households in stratum 6, the provision of security by own households' means might explain the difference with the answer provided by households in strata 4 and 5, which although still in a good socioeconomic situation might not have as many resources to fund their private security.[21] Finally, victimization seems to have high incidence in strata 3 and 4, while stratum 6 presents the lowest victimization rates.

Table 6.2 presents the rate of victimized households by age range. It shows that victimization is higher among the youngest individuals, while the best security perceptions of the neighborhood are among the oldest. These age patterns are similar to those reported in Di Tella et al. (2008) for Latin-American Countries and the rest of the world. On the other hand, good quality of life perceptions are higher among the people aged between 20 and 30 years old and the older than 50 years than for the other age groups.[22]

The ECVM also asks respondents to report their personal income in local currency, and also to report the income of the each individual at home. We construct household income adding the incomes of all household members, and then we determine the income quintile that each household is in. Table 6.3 shows the means of our key variables by income quintile. People with higher income are more likely to report having been a victim of crime, and having higher quality of life perceptions (except for quintile 1 which again presents on average better perception than quintiles 2 and 3). Good safety perceptions of the neighborhood are higher among people

---

[20] See also their spatial correlation in Maps 6.1, 6.2, and 6.6.

[21] See Di Tella et al. (2010) and Gaviria and Vélez (2001) for more on this.

[22] In our empirical estimations, we will find the standard U-shaped relationship between life satisfaction and age.

Table 6.2 Key variables statistics by age range[a] (%) (Source: ECVM 2008)

Age	Good quality life perceptions	Good security neighborhood perceptions	Victimization
20–30 years	80.4	86.0	9.3
30–40 years	77.2	85.5	9.1
40–50 years	77.4	85.6	9.5
50–60 years	78.1	87.1	9.0
60–70 years	78.2	87.5	7.0
More 70 years	77.4	88.7	6.0
Total	78.0	87.0	8.3

[a]Good quality of life perceptions is a dummy variable equal to one if individuals responded that current conditions in their household were "very good" or "good," and zero otherwise; good security neighborhood perceptions is a dummy variable equal to one if individuals reported to live in a "very safe" or "safe" neighborhood, and zero otherwise; victimization is a dummy variable equal to one if any member of the household was a victim of any offense (robbery, burglary, personal, and other), and zero otherwise

Table 6.3 Key variables statistics by income quintile (%) (Source: ECVM 2008)

Quintile	Good quality life perceptions	Good security neighborhood perceptions	Victimization
1	77.9	86.9	7.5
2	60.4	83.4	8.8
3	72.4	85.8	8.5
4	80.6	87.0	8.3
5	89.5	88.7	10.1
Total	78.0	87.0	8.3

with higher income except for quintile 1 whose perceptions are on average better than the perceptions of quintiles 2 and 3. Di Tella et al. (2008) report similar conclusions for Latin-American countries regarding quality of life perceptions; however, their conclusions do not apply to the perception of safety in the neighborhood since they reported that feelings of insecurity and lack of trust in the police in Latin America were increasing with income.

4 Identification and Estimation

Robust evidence of a statistical relationship between the homicide rate and life satisfaction is scarce in the literature. Previous work by Cohen (2008) does not find a significant effect of crime on life satisfaction, although Cohen (2008), Powdthavee (2005), and Michalos and Zumbo (2000) find a negative effect of victimization on

life satisfaction.[23] Previous work by Medina et al. (2010) using data for Bogotá and
Medellín evidenced the challenge to uncover the relationship between the homicide
rate and life satisfaction. They estimate both standard hedonic models using as
dependent variable property prices, and life satisfaction models, and although their
hedonic models captured a negative capitalization of the homicide rate on property
values in both Bogotá and Medellín, their life satisfaction models did not register
any statistically significant relationship between the homicide rate and life
satisfaction.[24]

Both the results of these authors and ours might just be lacking a correct identification strategy of the effect of the homicide rate on life satisfaction. However, due
to the complex nature of our dependent variable, which is very much related to
everything, it is implausible to come up with a variable that could allow us to implement a standard instrumental variable approach, and thus, any strategy would rely
more on accounting for as many observables as possible and determining on what
subsamples of the population it would actually be more likely to identify the relationship of interest.

An individual's decision to move to a specific neighborhood considers his or her
expectations regarding the characteristics of houses and amenities of all potential
places he or she might move to, including the homicide rate. To that extent, we could
expect endogeneity, due to household sorting across neighborhoods, to be larger;
the movement of households across neighborhoods and, in particular, the share of
households that had moved recently are also larger. It is possible that self-reported
life satisfaction of recent movers is more likely to have already discounted the cost
borne by the current homicide rate faced in his/her neighborhood than it would be
the case for individuals who have stayed in that neighborhood for several years,
since the latter might be facing constraints that prevent them or make them more
costly to move to another neighborhood, thus having to internalize the dissatisfaction caused by its homicide rate. Among the rigidities that might prevent people
from moving to another neighborhood include homeownership, the proximity to
their workplace or to their children's schools, etc.

The approach we follow is assessing the effect of the homicide on life satisfaction on three samples according to the length of time they have been living in their
current houses: (1) people living in their current house at least 10 years ago and that
have always lived there, (2) people living in their current house at least 10 years ago
and that moved there at some point in the past, and (3) people living in their current
houses less than 10 years ago.

We now analyze households' characteristics of those three groups. Table 6.4 contains descriptive statistics of these populations, splitting the sample of households
that have been living in their current neighborhoods for at least 10 years into those

---

[23] Powdthavee (2005) also includes in his estimation an interaction variable between his crime rate
and whether the individual had been a victim of crime, finding a positive coefficient on that interaction variable.

[24] Gaviria et al. (2010a) had as well found a negative capitalization of the homicide rate on property
values in the case of Bogotá.

Table 6.4 Descriptive statistics of *recent* and *previous movers*, and *settlers*

	In current neighborhood less than 10 years ago		In current neighborhood 10 or more years ago					
			Always in current neighborhood		Movers			
	Mean	Std. dev.	Mean	Std. dev.	Mean	Std. dev.	t-Statistic	
Variable	(i)	(ii)	(iii)	(iv)	(v)	(vi)	(i)–(iii)	(iii)–(v)
Life satisfaction	0.8003	0.3998	0.7885	0.4084	**0.7374**	0.4401	1.71	6.43*
Homicide rate	**7.32**	8.47	6.41	4.78	6.33	4.67	7.50*	0.98
Capture rate/homicide rate	**0.351**	0.181	0.339	0.179	0.339	0.179	3.79*	0.00
Homicide rate in previous neighborhood	**86.5**	163.6	139.8	153.5	146.2	152.9	−19.6*	−2.2*
Distance to crime	**466.0**	379.2	377.1	278.7	363.4	260.4	15.4*	2.7*
Years living in this place	3.7	2.6	38.8	18.4	25.8	13.0	−166*	46*
Safe neighborhood	0.8668	0.3398	0.8744	0.3314	0.8655	0.3412	−1.32	1.43
Victim of offense	**0.0918**	0.2888	0.0713	0.2573	0.0917	0.2886	4.37*	−3.97*
Household income	**933,132**	3,407,075	701,320	1,484,833	587,428	1,532,429	4.98*	4.06*
Number of persons in household	3.71	1.69	3.86	1.73	3.79	1.90	−4.89*	1.89
Age	**45.89**	14.76	52.49	15.47	58.44	14.76	−25.6*	−21.4*
Age^2	2,324	1,467	2,995	1,702	3,634	1,731	−24.9*	−20.0*
Socioeconomic stratum 1	0.1038	0.3050	0.0880	0.2834	0.1439	0.3510	3.13*	−9.22*
Socioeconomic stratum 2	0.2821	0.4501	0.3730	0.4836	0.4012	0.4902	−11.4*	−3.1*
Socioeconomic stratum 3	0.2875	0.4526	0.3513	0.4774	0.2799	0.4490	−8.1*	8.4*
Socioeconomic stratum 4	0.1471	0.3542	0.0900	0.2862	0.0876	0.2827	10.3*	0.5
Socioeconomic stratum 5 or 6	**0.1796**	0.3839	0.0977	0.2969	0.0874	0.2824	13.8*	1.9
Male	0.6609	0.4735	0.6063	0.4886	0.5656	0.4957	6.6*	4.5*
Household head with primary	0.2641	0.4409	0.3496	0.4769	0.3671	0.4821	−11.0*	−2.0*
Household head with secondary	0.3382	0.4731	0.3189	0.4661	0.2157	0.4113	2.4*	12.9*

(continued)

Table 6.4 Descriptive statistics of *recent* and *previous movers*, and *settlers* (continued)

Variable	In current neighborhood less than 10 years ago		In current neighborhood 10 or more years ago				t-Statistic	
			Always in current neighborhood		Movers			
	Mean	Std. dev.	Mean	Std. dev.	Mean	Std. dev.	(i)–(iii)	(iii)–(v)
	(i)	(ii)	(iii)	(iv)	(v)	(vi)		
House hold head with technique education	0.0739	0.2617	0.0514	0.2209	0.0360	0.1863	5.4*	4.2*
Household head single	0.1822	0.3860	0.1692	0.3750	0.1557	0.3626	1.98*	1.99*
Household head married	0.3913	0.4881	0.4249	0.4944	0.4097	0.4918	−4.0*	1.7
Household Head separated	0.1087	0.3113	0.1062	0.3081	0.1064	0.3084	0.47	−0.04
Household head lives with partner	0.2280	0.4196	0.1475	0.3546	0.1204	0.3254	12.0*	4.3*
Employed	**0.6924**	0.4615	0.5825	0.4932	0.4832	0.4998	13.5*	10.8*
Unemployed	0.0361	0.1865	0.0343	0.1820	0.0210	0.1434	0.57	4.51*
Household occupation rate	**0.4200**	0.2885	0.3857	0.2701	0.3619	0.2791	7.2*	4.6*
Household unemployment rate	0.0430	0.1282	0.0421	0.1243	0.0415	0.1207	0.42	0.28
Homeownership, house totally paid	**0.3513**	0.4774	0.6642	0.4723	0.6978	0.4593	−38.6*	−3.9*
Homeownership, house partially paid	0.0676	0.2511	0.0294	0.1689	0.0326	0.1775	10.2*	−1.0
Tenant	0.5413	0.4983	0.2349	0.4239	0.2037	0.4028	38.4*	4.1*
House with fixed phone line	0.8994	0.3008	0.9096	0.2867	0.9163	0.2770	−2.03*	−1.27
House with electricity	0.9612	0.1932	0.9704	0.1696	0.9694	0.1723	−2.94*	0.31
House with aqueduct	0.9483	0.2214	0.9546	0.2081	0.9537	0.2101	−1.71	0.23
House with sewerage	0.9573	0.2023	0.9640	0.1862	0.9621	0.1910	−2.03*	0.56
House with gas for cooking	0.4708	0.4992	0.4537	0.4979	0.4498	0.4975	2.00*	0.43
House with natural gas	0.4847	0.4998	0.4771	0.4995	0.4616	0.4986	0.90	1.68
House with internet	**0.3562**	0.4789	0.2824	0.4502	0.2388	0.4264	9.3*	5.4*

Table 6.4 Descriptive statistics of *recent* and *previous movers*, and *settlers* (continued)

Variable	In current neighborhood less than 10 years ago		In current neighborhood 10 or more years ago				t-Statistic	
			Always in current neighborhood		Movers			
	Mean	Std. dev.	Mean	Std. dev.	Mean	Std. dev.	(i)–(iii)	(iii)–(v)
	(i)	(ii)	(iii)	(iv)	(v)	(vi)		
House with cable TV	0.7124	0.4527	0.6854	0.4644	0.6592	0.4740	3.5*	3.0*
Number of rooms in household	0.3763	0.7192	0.3038	0.6969	0.4080	0.7922	6.0*	−7.4*
Enrolled in private health insurance	0.7275	0.4453	0.6968	0.4597	0.6815	0.4659	4.0*	1.8
Enrolled in public health insurance	0.1609	0.3674	0.2044	0.4033	0.2354	0.4243	−6.6*	−4.0*
Enrolled in pension fund	0.2694	0.4437	0.2212	0.4151	0.1656	0.3717	6.5*	7.7*
Good health	0.8721	0.3341	0.8485	0.3586	0.7377	0.4399	4.0*	14.5*
Educational attainment	8.95	5.12	7.72	4.85	6.06	5.01	14*	18*
Number of observations	6,154		7,747		4,669			

*Means difference of statistically significant

that have always lived there (columns (iii) and (iv)), and those that moved there at some point (columns (v) and (vi)). The last column of the table compares the mean of households living in their current neighborhoods less than 10 years ago (*recent movers*) with that of those who have always lived there (*settlers*, columns (i) minus (iii)), and the later with the mean of households who have been living in their current neighborhood for at least 10 years and that moved at some point there (*previous movers*, columns (iii) minus (v)). Characteristics with an asterisk in those columns mean that the difference is statistically different from zero.

The three samples of households (*recent movers, settlers,* and *previous movers*) are very different. We can say that *recent movers* have, on the whole, better quality of life than *settlers*, and *settlers* have better quality of life than *previous movers*. The order is supported by the monotone decreasing relation observed in household income, the share of household head employed, having good health, enrolled in private health insurance or a pension fund, and their educational attainment. Households also show a monotone decreasing relation in the probability to have internet or cable TV, their occupation rate, and the share in socioeconomic stratum 5 or 6.

Besides having most variables indicating that they have the lowest quality of life of the three groups, *previous movers* are also the less satisfied with their lives of the three groups. Although *settlers* currently live in the neighborhoods with the highest homicide rates, they used to live in neighborhoods with the lowest homicide rates, and additionally, they are the ones who live on average farther from the places where homicides take place. In addition, both *recent* and *previous movers* are more likely to have been victimized.

Finally, and not least important, *recent movers* are the households less likely to own their house, with just 35% of them owning their houses, as compared to 66% and 70% for *settlers* and *previous movers*, respectively. This gives support to our hypothesis claiming the existence of rigidities for households moving across neighborhoods, according to which home ownership would imply a form of rigidity.

To assess the effect of the homicide rate on life satisfaction, we estimate a standard life satisfaction model of the form:

$$LS = \alpha_0 + \alpha_1 Y + \alpha_2 \text{Crime} + \alpha_3 H + \alpha_4 A + u \qquad (6.1)$$

where Y is household income, *Crime* is a measure of the homicide rate in the vicinity of the individual, H is a vector of household and individual's variables, and A is a vector of amenities of the neighborhood.

4.1 Results on life Satisfaction

Table 6.5 presents the results of the estimating Eq. 6.1. The table contains two panels, one for the whole sample and the other includes only households living in their current house longer than 10 years (*settlers*). Column (i) is the simplest specification, controlling only for the variables, most arguably exogenous, that we had available from the LSMS survey, namely the basic household's head characteristics like gender, age, education, and years of living in current abode, and the key variables related to crime we are interested to assess, like the household's homicide rate, its average distance to crime, the household head's perception of how safe the neighborhood is, and whether he or she has been victim of any offense, which includes a wide variety of crimes like mugging, burglary, car theft, threats, etc.

As a first attempt to account for the endogeneity of the residential location of households, we control for predetermined characteristics, and actually, for characteristics predetermined even before the individual moved to their current neighborhood, by including in the estimation of column (ii) the fixed effects for the household's previous neighborhood of residence. Column (iii), in addition, controls for both past and current neighborhood fixed effects, and adds a few other housing covariates such as availability of a fixed phone line, electricity, aqueduct, and the number of rooms. Note that we can include both fixed effects and still identify the effect of the homicide rate since we estimated a different homicide rate figure by household, allowing us to have variation within neighborhoods.

Column (iv) drops the variable of the head of the household's perception of security in his/her neighborhood, while columns (v) and (vi) include each additional covariate to the previous columns, home ownership, and other housing characteristics in column (v), and individual's variables related to his/her labor market performance and enrollment in health insurance and pension funds.

First, note that the control variables included have the expected effects on life satisfaction. Life satisfaction decreases with age at a decreasing rate, decreases with the number of people in the household, and increases with income, the socioeconomic stratum and education, and it is higher for males and for the married household head than for single or divorced persons.[25]

Secondly, when we include in the estimation all household heads in our sample, we cannot identify any statistically significant effect of the homicide rate on life satisfaction (if something, a positive coefficient in column (ii)) or of the arrest rates or the distance to crime. Both the individual's perception of security in the neighborhood and them having been a victim of any offense result in significant and robust positive and negative effects on life satisfaction, respectively.

In order to attempt to attenuate the endogeneity problem previously described, we estimate model (1) only for the set of people who have been in their current neighborhood for at least 10 years (*settlers*).[26] The results are included in the second panel of Table 6.5 in columns (vii)–(xii). Here again, although the magnitude of the coefficients on the variables expressing whether the individual is feeling safe in the neighborhood and has been victimized turn, in general, smaller in their absolute values; their statistical significance is still robust. Nonetheless, for this sample,

---

[25] See Ferrer-i-Carbonell and Frijters (2004), Di Tella et al. (2008), and Medina et al. (2010), among others.

[26] We also got estimates of all regressions, splitting the sample with people living in their current neighborhood 9, 8, 7, 6, and 5 years ago, and we found similar results to the ones reported.

Table 6.5 Life satisfaction models. Dependent variable equal to one if satisfied or very satisfied

	All sample			
	coef	se	coef	se
Variable	(i)		(ii)	
Homicide rate	0.006*	0.004	0.007***	0.004
Capture rate/homicide rate	0.032	0.153	0.207	0.150
Distance to crime	**0.000***	**0.000**	0.000	0.000
Years living in this place	−0.000	0.001	0.001*	0.001
Safe neighborhood	**0.314***	**0.035**	**0.290***	**0.034**
Victim of offense	**−0.198***	**0.041**	**−0.231***	**0.045**
Household income	0.000***	0.000	0.000***	0.000
Number of persons in household	−0.067***	0.007	−0.069***	0.007
Age	−0.003	0.004	−0.005	0.004
Age2	0.000**	0.000	0.000	0.000
Male	0.093***	0.030	0.096***	0.032
Household head with primary	−0.105***	0.030	−0.065***	0.031
Household head with secondary	−0.084***	0.040	−0.036	0.040
Hhold head with technique education	0.010	0.073	0.048	0.075
Household head single	−0.243***	0.041	−0.232***	0.040
Household head married	0.050	0.041	0.058	0.043
Household head separated	−0.240***	0.043	−0.237***	0.046
Household head lives with partner	−0.199***	0.046	−0.141***	0.047
Educational attainment	0.071***	0.004	0.052***	0.004
House with fixed phone line				
House with electricity				
House with aqueduct				
House with sewerage				
Number of rooms in household				
Socioeconomic stratum 2				
Socioeconomic stratum 3				
Socioeconomic stratum 4				
Socioeconomic stratum 5 or 6				
Homeownership, house totally paid				
Homeownership, house partially paid				
Tenant				
House with gas for cooking				
House with natural gas				
House with internet				
House with cable TV				
Employed				
Unemployed				
Household occupation rate				
Household unemployment rate				
Enrolled in private health insurance				
Enrolled in public health insurance				
Enrolled in pension fund				
Good health				
Constant	0.114	0.145	0.362***	0.150
FE past neighborhood	No		Yes	
FE current neighborhood	No		No	
N	18,715		18,250	

*Significantly at 10%
**Significantly at 5%
***Significantly at 1%

Table 6.5 Life satisfaction models. Dependent variable equal to one if satisfied or very satisfied (continued)

All sample							
coef	se	coef	se	coef	se	coef	se
(iii)		(iv)		(v)		(vi)	
0.002	0.006	0.003	0.006	0.001	0.005	0.004	0.007
0.120	0.228	0.106	0.228	0.098	0.210	−0.170	0.242
−0.000	0.000	−0.000	0.000	−0.000	0.000	−0.000	0.000
0.001***	0.001	0.002***	0.001	0.002***	0.001	0.002***	0.001
0.272*	0.032**					**0.253***	0.037**
−0.213*	0.047**	**−0.270***	0.047**	**−0.305***	0.048**	**−0.238***	0.049**
0.000***	0.000	0.000***	0.000	0.000***	0.000	0.000***	0.000
−0.069***	0.007	−0.069***	0.007	−0.082***	0.007	−0.071***	0.008
−0.010***	0.005	−0.010***	0.005	−0.017***	0.005	−0.017***	0.005
0.000**	0.000	0.000**	0.000	0.000***	0.000	0.000***	0.000
0.118***	0.033	0.121***	0.033	0.131***	0.033	0.119***	0.036
−0.064**	0.033	−0.063**	0.033	−0.015	0.034	−0.042	0.037
−0.041	0.042	−0.037	0.042	0.035	0.046	−0.019	0.051
0.016	0.077	0.014	0.077	0.063	0.079	−0.026	0.092
−0.240***	0.042	−0.235***	0.041	−0.186***	0.043	−0.152***	0.047
0.031	0.044	0.029	0.044	−0.004	0.045	0.004	0.051
−0.252***	0.048	−0.252***	0.048	−0.232***	0.049	−0.185***	0.050
−0.137***	0.049	−0.137***	0.050	−0.109***	0.051	−0.067	0.055
0.044***	0.004	0.044***	0.004	0.027***	0.004	0.021***	0.005
0.397***	0.046	0.396***	0.046	0.293***	0.046	0.247***	0.051
−0.166	0.121	−0.178*	0.119	−0.183*	0.116	−0.202*	0.136
0.407***	0.074	0.418***	0.073	0.363***	0.075	0.324***	0.074
−0.048	0.107	−0.038	0.105	−0.045	0.104	−0.030	0.121
−0.044***	0.020	−0.047***	0.020	−0.052***	0.021	−0.042**	0.023
				0.037	0.068	−0.007	0.071
				0.163**	0.088	0.058	0.097
				0.568***	0.133	0.413***	0.146
				0.885***	0.156	0.681***	0.166
				0.296***	0.047	0.254***	0.051
				0.117*	0.073	0.063	0.080
				0.233***	0.056	0.202***	0.062
				−0.021	0.067	0.015	0.068
				0.200***	0.071	0.173***	0.074
				0.359***	0.034	0.310***	0.036
				0.328***	0.029	0.292***	0.031
						−0.181***	0.040
						−0.484***	0.086
						0.382***	0.067
						−0.420***	0.127
						0.251***	0.046
						−0.115***	0.046
						0.103***	0.040
						0.539***	0.035
−0.342	0.388	−0.130	0.396	−0.053	0.393	−0.421	0.449
Yes		Yes		Yes		Yes	
Yes		Yes		Yes		Yes	
17,936		17,936		17,936		15,228	

(continued)

Table 6.5 Life satisfaction models. Dependent variable equal to one if satisfied or very satisfied (continued)

	Living in current neighborhood 10 or more years ago			
	coef	se	coef	se
Variable	(vii)		(viii)	
Homicide rate	0.006	0.005	−0.006	0.005
Capture rate/homicide rate	−0.053	0.171	−0.058	0.283
Distance to crime	0.000*	0.000	−0.000	0.000
Years living in this place	0.000	0.001	0.001	0.001
Safe neighborhood	**0.288***	**0.043**	**0.256***	**0.041**
Victim of offense	**−0.139***	**0.052**	**−0.171***	**0.056**
Household income	0.000***	0.000	0.000***	0.000
Number of persons in household	−0.063***	0.009	−0.066***	0.009
Age	0.002	0.005	−0.002	0.005
Age2	0.000	0.000	0.000	0.000
Male	0.082***	0.035	0.090***	0.037
Household head with primary	−0.094***	0.038	−0.036	0.040
Household head with secondary	−0.077	0.055	−0.016	0.056
Hhold head with technique education	0.024	0.096	0.083	0.105
Household head single	−0.260***	0.046	−0.257***	0.046
Household head married	0.060	0.050	0.058	0.051
Household head separated	−0.291***	0.050	−0.305***	0.053
Household head lives with partner	−0.170***	0.058	−0.115**	0.060
Educational attainment	0.068***	0.005	0.045***	0.005
House with fixed phone line				
House with electricity				
House with aqueduct				
House with sewerage				
Number of rooms in household				
Socioeconomic stratum 2				
Socioeconomic stratum 3				
Socioeconomic stratum 4				
Socioeconomic stratum 5 or 6				
Homeownership, house totally paid				
Homeownership, house partially paid				
Tenant				
House with gas for cooking				
House with natural gas				
House with internet				
House with cable TV				
Employed				
Unemployed				
Household occupation rate				
Household unemployment rate				
Enrolled in private health insurance				
Enrolled in public health insurance				
Enrolled in pension fund				
Good health				
Constant	−0.012	0.183	−0.579***	0.218
FE past neighborhood	No		Yes	
FE current neighborhood	No		No	
N	12,521		11,894	

* Significantly at 10%
** Significantly at 5%
*** Significantly at 1%

Table 6.5 Life satisfaction models. Dependent variable equal to one if satisfied or very satisfied (continued)

Living in current neighborhood 10 or more years ago

coef	se	coef	se	coef	se	coef	se
(ix)		(x)		(xi)		(xii)	
−0.007	0.005	−0.007	0.006	−0.009*	0.006	−0.003	0.009
−0.073	0.283	−0.103	0.284	−0.069	0.269	−0.496**	0.296
0.000	0.000	0.000	0.000	−0.000	0.000	0.000	0.000
0.001	0.001	0.001	0.001	0.002***	0.001	0.002**	0.001
0.245*	**0.040**					**0.193***	**0.044**
−0.146*	**0.054**	**−0.200***	**0.054**	**−0.230***	**0.054**	**−0.160***	**0.061**
0.000***	0.000	0.000***	0.000	0.000***	0.000	0.000**	0.000
−0.062***	0.009	−0.062***	0.009	−0.079***	0.009	−0.069***	0.009
−0.004	0.006	−0.004	0.006	−0.012***	0.006	−0.011**	0.006
0.000	0.000	0.000	0.000	0.000**	0.000	0.000**	0.000
0.106***	0.037	0.108***	0.037	0.115***	0.036	0.105***	0.040
−0.037	0.040	−0.036	0.040	0.022	0.041	−0.005	0.042
−0.024	0.056	−0.020	0.056	0.072	0.058	−0.012	0.063
0.069	0.105	0.062	0.104	0.140	0.109	0.045	0.123
−0.253***	0.047	−0.249***	0.047	−0.195***	0.050	−0.153***	0.055
0.030	0.051	0.029	0.051	−0.005	0.052	0.005	0.057
−0.298***	0.052	−0.298***	0.052	−0.280***	0.054	−0.235***	0.057
−0.125***	0.058	−0.124***	0.058	−0.101**	0.060	−0.072	0.064
0.043***	0.005	0.043***	0.005	0.024***	0.005	0.019***	0.006
0.441***	0.061	0.439***	0.060	0.335***	0.059	0.285***	0.066
−0.143	0.140	−0.154	0.138	−0.168	0.133	−0.193	0.165
0.422***	0.092	0.435***	0.091	0.367***	0.095	0.333***	0.095
−0.079	0.126	−0.070	0.124	−0.091	0.122	−0.079	0.145
−0.030	0.023	−0.033	0.023	−0.042**	0.024	−0.022	0.027
				−0.010	0.087	−0.051	0.091
				0.104	0.106	0.010	0.111
				0.451***	0.165	0.289*	0.180
				0.897***	0.183	0.744***	0.196
				0.230***	0.050	0.172***	0.055
				0.030	0.098	−0.032	0.112
				0.196***	0.064	0.142***	0.068
				−0.088	0.086	−0.052	0.086
				0.274***	0.095	0.228***	0.095
				0.404***	0.041	0.330***	0.045
				0.343***	0.035	0.305***	0.038
						−0.182***	0.050
						−0.438***	0.103
						0.334***	0.082
						−0.500***	0.156
						0.260***	0.058
						−0.141***	0.060
						0.084**	0.049
						0.572***	0.041
−0.275	0.292	−0.838***	0.236	−0.245	0.326	−1.631***	0.755
Yes		Yes		Yes		Yes	
Yes		Yes		Yes		Yes	
11,894		11,894		11,894		9,875	

the coefficient on the homicide rate becomes negative although still not significant, and arrest rates actually become negative although not significant. Note also the importance of controlling for the households' past neighborhood fixed effects in allowing us to identify the negative effect of the homicide rate on life satisfaction, which becomes evident as we move from column (vii) to column (viii). Beyond the household's socioeconomic strata, an amenity that varies within each neighborhood which was already included in our estimation, the neighborhood fixed effects allow us to control for variation across neighborhoods on all other unobservable amenities.

As we showed previously, the subsample of households living in their current neighborhood for 10 or more years is comprised of two different sub populations, the *previous movers* and the *settlers*, with *settlers* having higher quality of life than *previous movers*.

As Parkes et al. (2002) claim, neighborhood characteristics are more likely to be more important for households living in the poorest areas than for those in the richest areas since the social life of the latter goes beyond the immediate possibilities provided by their neighborhoods. They also find that households living in the poorest areas are more sensitive to crime, being more likely to capitalize the costs of crime in their neighborhoods into lower levels of life satisfaction.

The previous argument suggests that it might be worth separately assessing the effect of the homicide rate on life satisfaction for the subsamples of *previous movers*, those registering the most unfavorable quality of life conditions and living in the poorest neighborhoods of our three groups and that of *settlers*. According to Parkes et al. (2002), we should be more likely to identify the effects of crime in the former group than in the latter. Although these authors use a measure of neighborhood satisfaction rather than our overall life satisfaction measure, both of these measures should help us to better understand the relationship of interest.

The results of estimating Eq. 6.1 for each of this two subsamples are presented in Table 6.6, which has the same structure of Table 6.5, but now the panel on the left is that for the *previous movers*, and the one on the right, that for the households which have always been in their current neighborhoods or *settlers*. There are almost two *settlers* per *previous mover*, and the homicide rate has negative coefficients for the subsample of *previous movers* once we control for the previous neighborhood fixed effects. In addition, the arrest rates now become positive and significantly related to life satisfaction for the subsample of *previous movers*. We still cannot identify any effect of the homicide rate on life satisfaction for the subsample of *settlers*. This result suggests that while *settlers* are more likely to have sunk the cost of the homicide rate levels of their neighborhoods, *previous movers* have a harder time to get used to it, and thus, are more likely to capitalize them into lower levels of overall life satisfaction, resembling in part the result found by Parkes et al. (2002).

It is also important to highlight that although feeling safe in the neighborhood is robustly linked to higher levels of life satisfaction for both subsamples, having been a victim of an offense only reduces life satisfaction in a statistically significant magnitude among the *settlers*. An interesting result (not reported here) is that having been victimized affects life satisfaction particularly of individuals living in places with high homicide rates.[27]

To have an idea of the magnitude of the effect of the homicide rate, the perception of security in the neighborhood, and the victimization, on life satisfaction, we reestimate a few of the previous specifications by OLS and get standardized coefficients (not reported here). We find that a standard deviation increase in each of the homicide rates, the share of households feeling safe in their neighborhoods, and the share of households reporting to have been victimized, implies a decrease of 5.3–4.7 (that is, an increase) and 1.8% of a standard deviation of life satisfaction, respectively.[28] The magnitudes are important since these effects are obtained once all other variables in our estimation are controlled for. To mention a couple of examples, a one standard deviation increase in household's income implies an increase of 4.4% of a standard deviation in life satisfaction, that is less than the effect a one standard deviation in the homicide rate would have on it. Education is the variable for which a one standard deviation increase affects the most life satisfaction: it would increase it in 10.7% of a standard deviation.

4.2   The Case of Very Happy Households

To assess whether the homicide rate affects not only whether individuals feel satisfied or very satisfied rather than unsatisfied, but also if it makes a difference in the likelihood of people feeling very satisfied with their lives, we estimate again equation (1) changing our definition of the dependent variable to be equal to one only for individuals who reported to be very satisfied, and zero for all the others. The results presented in Tables 6.5 and 6.6 with the previous definition are now repeated with the new definition in Tables 6.7 and 6.8.

First, we compare the results of Tables 6.5 and 6.7. As it was the case in Table 6.5 with the likelihood of individuals being satisfied, results in Table 6.7 do not show a significant relationship between the homicide rate and the likelihood of individuals feeling very happy. Distance to crime suggests impacts positively the likelihood of being very happy, nonetheless, the results are not robust with the inclusion of current neighborhood fixed effects. Feeling safe in the neighborhood also affects positively the likelihood of being very satisfied for both the total sample and the subsample of households living in their current neighborhood 10 or more years. Finally, having been victim of an offense does not affect the likelihood of individuals

---

[27] The result was obtained for the subsample of previous movers by estimating the model with an interaction of the homicide rate and the victimization variable. The coefficient on the interaction variable is negative and significant, while the victimization variable loses its significance. The homicide remains negative and significant.

[28] This result was found for the sample of previous movers with the specification in column (ii) in the tables, although other specification led to similar results.

Table 6.6 Life satisfaction models. Dependent variable equal to one if satisfied or very satisfied

| Variable | Living in current neighborhood 10 or more years ago, movers | | | |
	coef	se	coef	se
	(i)		(ii)	
Homicide rate	−0.004	0.005	**−0.027*****	**0.011**
Capture rate/homicide rate	−0.063	0.235	**0.987*****	**0.364**
Distance to crime	**0.000*****	**0.000**	−0.000	0.000
Years living in this place	−0.002	0.002	−0.000	0.002
Safe neighborhood	**0.218*****	**0.069**	**0.198*****	**0.070**
Victim of offense	**−0.098***	**0.066**	**−0.113***	**0.077**
Household income	0.000***	0.000	0.000***	0.000
Number of persons in household	−0.067***	0.014	−0.075***	0.014
Age	0.007	0.010	0.001	0.011
Age2	0.000	0.000	0.000	0.000
Male	0.047	0.058	0.089	0.065
Household head with primary	−0.106***	0.051	−0.039	0.061
Household head with secondary	−0.060	0.088	−0.029	0.107
Hhold head with technique education	−0.039	0.147	−0.024	0.179
Household head single	−0.149***	0.071	−0.192***	0.078
Household head married	0.123*	0.081	0.066	0.089
Household head separated	−0.309***	0.081	−0.367***	0.088
Household head lives with partner	−0.065	0.099	−0.049	0.108
Educational attainment	0.066***	0.008	0.041***	0.010
House with fixed phone line				
House with electricity				
House with aqueduct				
House with sewerage				
Number of rooms in household				
Socioeconomic stratum 2				
Socioeconomic stratum 3				
Socioeconomic stratum 4				
Socioeconomic stratum 5 or 6				
Homeownership, house totally paid				
Homeownership, house partially paid				
Tenant				
House with gas for cooking				
House with natural gas				
House with internet				
House with cable TV				
Employed				
Unemployed				
Household occupation rate				
Household unemployment rate				
Enrolled in private health insurance				
Enrolled in public health insurance				
Enrolled in pension fund				
Good health				
Constant	−0.155	0.339	−0.426	1.017
FE past neighborhood	No		Yes	
FE current neighborhood	No		No	
N	4,705		4,251	

* Significantly at 10%
** Significantly at 5%
*** Significantly at 1%

Table 6.6 Life satisfaction models. Dependent variable equal to one if satisfied or very satisfied (continued)

Living in current neighborhood 10 or more years ago, movers

coef	se	coef	se	coef	se	coef	se
(iii)		(iv)		(v)		(vi)	
−0.028***	0.011	−0.027***	0.011	−0.029***	0.011	−0.026**	0.014
0.919***	0.358	0.886***	0.358	0.906***	0.363	0.513	0.435
−0.000	0.000	−0.000	0.000	−0.000	0.000	0.000	0.000
−0.000	0.002	0.000	0.002	0.000	0.002	−0.001	0.002
0.196***	0.072					0.148**	0.077
−0.077	0.077	−0.112*	0.076	−0.117*	0.077	−0.086	0.092
0.000***	0.000	0.000***	0.000	0.000***	0.000	0.000***	0.000
−0.073***	0.014	−0.073***	0.014	−0.091***	0.014	−0.085***	0.014
−0.001	0.011	−0.002	0.011	−0.013	0.011	−0.011	0.012
0.000	0.000	0.000	0.000	0.000	0.000	0.000	0.000
0.115**	0.066	0.112**	0.066	0.125**	0.065	0.169***	0.072
−0.039	0.060	−0.042	0.060	0.012	0.062	−0.036	0.068
−0.031	0.107	−0.035	0.107	0.037	0.112	−0.047	0.119
−0.019	0.180	−0.035	0.176	0.022	0.188	−0.059	0.241
−0.195***	0.079	−0.193***	0.078	−0.119*	0.080	−0.129*	0.089
0.029	0.090	0.032	0.090	−0.017	0.089	−0.087	0.102
−0.359***	0.089	−0.353***	0.089	−0.323***	0.092	−0.327***	0.094
−0.066	0.106	−0.064	0.106	−0.056	0.109	−0.118	0.121
0.039***	0.010	0.039***	0.010	0.022***	0.010	0.017	0.012
0.447***	0.085	0.443***	0.084	0.302***	0.086	0.282***	0.099
−0.204	0.208	−0.213	0.207	−0.188	0.210	−0.337	0.291
0.391***	0.146	0.397***	0.147	0.345***	0.154	0.364***	0.165
−0.166	0.193	−0.147	0.192	−0.147	0.193	−0.100	0.224
−0.032	0.035	−0.033	0.035	−0.043	0.035	−0.032	0.039
				−0.010	0.092	−0.070	0.095
				−0.017	0.158	−0.130	0.167
				0.405**	0.243	0.231	0.262
				1.178***	0.295	1.194***	0.346
				0.273***	0.099	0.210***	0.104
				0.141	0.159	0.084	0.173
				0.198**	0.115	0.114	0.123
				−0.161	0.142	−0.181	0.158
				0.340***	0.156	0.390***	0.167
				0.366***	0.077	0.329***	0.092
				0.411***	0.055	0.373***	0.063
						−0.119*	0.078
						−0.224	0.191
						0.385***	0.117
						−0.652***	0.290
						0.185***	0.081
						−0.247***	0.096
						0.035	0.091
						0.627***	0.063
−0.802	1.023	−0.700	0.985	−0.757	0.992	−0.891	0.817
Yes		Yes		Yes		Yes	
Yes		Yes		Yes		Yes	
4,251		4,251		4,251		3,567	

(continued)

Table 6.6 Life satisfaction models. Dependent variable equal to one if satisfied or very satisfied (continued)

| Variable | Living in current neighborhood 10 or more years ago, always in current neighborhood | | | |
| | coef | se | coef | se |
	(vii)		(viii)	
Homicide rate	0.012*	0.007	−0.000	0.008
Capture rate/homicide rate	−0.035	0.165	−0.306	0.353
Distance to crime	0.000	0.000	−0.000	0.000
Years living in this place	−0.001	0.001	0.000	0.001
Safe neighborhood	**0.341***	**0.053**	**0.316***	**0.058**
Victim of offense	**−0.151***	**0.069**	**−0.202***	**0.077**
Household income	0.000***	0.000	0.000***	0.000
Number of persons in household	−0.063***	0.010	−0.062***	0.011
Age	0.001	0.007	−0.001	0.007
Age2	0.000	0.000	0.000	0.000
Male	0.104***	0.052	0.088**	0.052
Household head with primary	−0.097**	0.053	−0.026	0.057
Household head with secondary	−0.094*	0.065	−0.000	0.069
Hhold head with technique education	0.037	0.118	0.138	0.129
Household head single	−0.333***	0.065	−0.329***	0.071
Household head married	0.012	0.072	0.024	0.074
Household head separated	−0.284***	0.066	−0.287***	0.069
Household head lives with partner	−0.247***	0.077	−0.169***	0.080
Educational attainment	0.067***	0.006	0.049***	0.007
House with fixed phone line				
House with electricity				
House with aqueduct				
House with sewerage				
Number of rooms in household				
Socioeconomic stratum 2				
Socioeconomic stratum 3				
Socioeconomic stratum 4				
Socioeconomic stratum 5 or 6				
Homeownership, house totally paid				
Homeownership, house partially paid				
Tenant				
House with gas for cooking				
House with natural gas				
House with internet				
House with cable TV				
Employed				
Unemployed				
Household occupation rate				
Household unemployment rate				
Enrolled in private health insurance				
Enrolled in public health insurance				
Enrolled in pension fund				
Good health				
Constant	0.079	0.213	0.666***	0.220
FE past neighborhood	No		Yes	
FE current neighborhood	No		No	
N	7,811		7,181	

*Significantly at 10%
**Significantly at 5%
***Significantly at 1%

Table 6.6 Life satisfaction models. Dependent variable equal to one if satisfied or very satisfied (continued)

Living in current neighborhood 10 or more years ago, always in current neighborhood							
coef	se	coef	se	coef	se	coef	se
(ix)		(x)		(xi)		(xii)	
−0.002	0.008	−0.001	0.008	−0.005	0.009	−0.003	0.010
−0.301	0.348	−0.340	0.348	−0.334	0.361	**−0.814*****	**0.409**
0.000	0.000	−0.000	0.000	−0.000	0.000	−0.000	0.000
0.000	0.001	0.001	0.001	0.002*	0.001	0.002*	0.001
0.297***	**0.058**					**0.245*****	**0.070**
−0.185***	**0.075**	**−0.258*****	**0.073**	**−0.315*****	**0.073**	**−0.199*****	**0.085**
0.000***	0.000	0.000***	0.000	0.000***	0.000	0.000	0.000
−0.057***	0.011	−0.057***	0.011	−0.074***	0.011	−0.061***	0.013
−0.002	0.007	−0.002	0.007	−0.008	0.007	−0.008	0.008
0.000	0.000	0.000	0.000	0.000	0.000	0.000	0.000
0.096**	0.051	0.099***	0.050	0.105***	0.050	0.077	0.055
−0.029	0.058	−0.024	0.057	0.043	0.058	0.034	0.059
−0.017	0.067	−0.006	0.067	0.093	0.068	0.007	0.073
0.111	0.130	0.108	0.129	0.205*	0.133	0.106	0.146
−0.319***	0.072	−0.311***	0.072	−0.268***	0.076	−0.179***	0.083
0.005	0.075	0.003	0.074	−0.037	0.076	0.030	0.085
−0.276***	0.069	−0.282***	0.070	−0.274***	0.073	−0.176***	0.082
−0.173***	0.080	−0.173***	0.080	−0.151**	0.082	−0.064	0.088
0.047***	0.006	0.047***	0.006	0.027***	0.006	0.023***	0.007
0.456***	0.077	0.456***	0.076	0.360***	0.076	0.302***	0.085
−0.064	0.211	−0.076	0.208	−0.108	0.196	−0.117	0.220
0.441***	0.110	0.464***	0.108	0.398***	0.111	0.342***	0.112
−0.064	0.168	−0.064	0.165	−0.107	0.156	−0.105	0.180
−0.037	0.031	−0.041	0.031	−0.051*	0.032	−0.019	0.037
				−0.013	0.136	−0.051	0.144
				0.186	0.147	0.107	0.154
				0.534***	0.210	0.416**	0.236
				0.749***	0.232	0.560***	0.262
				0.199***	0.060	0.141***	0.068
				−0.053	0.128	−0.150	0.145
				0.201***	0.074	0.175***	0.082
				−0.066	0.103	0.005	0.109
				0.280***	0.110	0.191**	0.114
				0.449***	0.052	0.354***	0.059
				0.321***	0.051	0.279***	0.057
						−0.239***	0.063
						−0.552***	0.129
						0.308***	0.110
						−0.504***	0.197
						0.339***	0.074
						−0.078	0.074
						0.077	0.063
						0.557***	0.058
0.511***	0.224	0.604***	0.221	0.870***	0.258	−1.751***	0.790
Yes		Yes		Yes		Yes	
Yes		Yes		Yes		Yes	
7,181		7,181		7,181		5,897	

Table 6.7 Life satisfaction models. Dependent variable equal to one if very satisfied

Variable	All sample coef (i)	se	coef (ii)	se
Homicide rate	−0.008**	0.004	−0.006**	0.003
Capture rate/homicide rate	0.272**	0.158	0.374***	0.152
Distance to crime	0.000***	0.000	0.000***	0.000
Years living in this place	−0.002***	0.001	−0.002**	0.001
Safe neighborhood	0.113***	0.044	0.155***	0.048
Victim of offense	0.002	0.050	0.012	0.051
Household income	0.000**	0.000	0.000*	0.000
Number of persons in household	−0.051***	0.010	−0.046***	0.011
Age	−0.000	0.005	−0.006	0.005
Age2	0.000	0.000	0.000	0.000
Male	0.062*	0.038	0.063*	0.041
Household head with primary	−0.097***	0.041	−0.071*	0.043
Household head with secondary	−0.093***	0.040	−0.080***	0.040
Hhold head with technique education	−0.012	0.058	−0.009	0.057
Household head single	−0.142***	0.057	−0.143***	0.060
Household head married	0.049	0.054	0.070	0.060
Household head separated	−0.060	0.062	−0.032	0.066
Household head lives with partner	−0.228***	0.074	−0.181***	0.079
Educational attainment	0.054***	0.004	0.040***	0.004
House with fixed phone line				
House with electricity				
House with aqueduct				
House with sewerage				
Number of rooms in household				
Socioeconomic stratum 2				
Socioeconomic stratum 3				
Socioeconomic stratum 4				
Socioeconomic stratum 5 or 6				
Homeownership, house totally paid				
Homeownership, house partially paid				
Tenant				
House with gas for cooking				
House with natural gas				
House with internet				
House with cable TV				
Employed				
Unemployed				
Household occupation rate				
Household unemployment rate				
Enrolled in private health insurance				
Enrolled in public health insurance				
Enrolled in pension fund				
Good health				
Constant	−1.891***	0.172	−1.637***	0.189
FE past neighborhood	No		Yes	
FE current neighborhood	No		No	
N	18,715		17,651	

* Significantly at 10%
** Significantly at 5%
*** Significantly at 1%

Table 6.7 Life satisfaction models. Dependent variable equal to one if very satisfied (continued)

All sample

coef (iii)	se	coef (iv)	se	coef (v)	se	coef (vi)	se
0.000	0.004	0.000	0.004	0.002	0.005	0.003	0.005
−0.076	0.209	−0.088	0.210	−0.057	0.220	0.039	0.254
−0.000	0.000	−0.000	0.000	−0.000	0.000	−0.000**	0.000
−0.000	0.001	−0.000	0.001	−0.000	0.001	−0.001	0.001
0.161*	**0.052**					**0.134***	**0.060**
0.008	0.052	−0.026	0.053	−0.039	0.055	0.016	0.061
0.000***	0.000	0.000***	0.000	0.000***	0.000	0.000***	0.000
−0.047***	0.012	−0.047***	0.012	−0.058***	0.012	−0.058***	0.013
−0.007	0.006	−0.007	0.006	−0.012***	0.006	−0.010*	0.006
0.000	0.000	0.000	0.000	0.000**	0.000	0.000**	0.000
0.076**	0.042	0.077**	0.042	0.084***	0.042	0.058	0.046
−0.051	0.043	−0.051	0.043	−0.024	0.043	−0.041	0.046
−0.052	0.039	−0.050	0.039	−0.015	0.038	−0.053	0.042
−0.029	0.060	−0.031	0.061	−0.011	0.062	−0.042	0.067
−0.158***	0.064	−0.156***	0.064	−0.132***	0.064	−0.138**	0.072
0.063	0.061	0.063	0.061	0.043	0.062	0.069	0.070
−0.024	0.069	−0.022	0.069	0.006	0.070	0.019	0.077
−0.159**	0.082	−0.158**	0.082	−0.113	0.082	−0.090	0.087
0.032***	0.004	0.032***	0.004	0.021***	0.005	0.016***	0.005
0.270***	0.079	0.271***	0.079	0.202***	0.082	0.236***	0.087
−0.137	0.157	−0.147	0.157	−0.158	0.158	−0.219	0.176
0.014	0.119	0.021	0.118	0.000	0.121	0.010	0.133
0.185	0.146	0.187	0.145	0.171	0.147	0.161	0.164
0.090***	0.027	0.088***	0.027	0.083***	0.027	0.080***	0.030
				0.121	0.119	0.039	0.124
				0.325***	0.160	0.265*	0.166
				0.318**	0.172	0.246	0.178
				0.689***	0.176	0.657***	0.179
				0.206***	0.070	0.191***	0.083
				0.122	0.102	0.059	0.119
				0.048	0.075	0.018	0.088
				−0.000	0.086	−0.005	0.094
				0.084	0.087	0.087	0.093
				0.230***	0.043	0.196***	0.046
				0.097***	0.048	0.049	0.053
						−0.087**	0.049
						−0.178	0.143
						0.114**	0.060
						−0.255*	0.163
						0.080	0.059
						−0.138***	0.069
						0.095***	0.045
						0.286***	0.055
−2.779***	0.349	−2.628***	0.346	−2.609***	0.385	−2.784***	0.413
Yes		Yes		Yes		Yes	
Yes		Yes		Yes		Yes	
17,029		17,029		17,029		14,172	

(continued)

Table 6.7 Life satisfaction models. Dependent variable equal to one if very satisfied (continued)

| | Living in current neighborhood 10 or more years ago | | | |
| | coef | se | coef | se |
Variable	(vii)		(viii)	
Homicide rate	−0.004	0.006	−0.003	0.009
Capture rate/homicide rate	0.156	0.165	−0.236	0.235
Distance to crime	0.000***	0.000	0.000	0.000
Years living in this place	**−0.003*****	**0.001**	**−0.002***	**0.001**
Safe neighborhood	**0.103****	**0.057**	**0.164*****	**0.065**
Victim of offense	−0.035	0.065	−0.032	0.070
Household income	0.000***	0.000	0.000***	0.000
Number of persons in household	−0.046***	0.013	−0.041***	0.014
Age	0.007	0.008	−0.003	0.008
Age2	−0.000	0.000	0.000	0.000
Male	0.055	0.048	0.063	0.051
Household head with primary	−0.079**	0.047	−0.039	0.051
Household head with secondary	−0.068	0.049	−0.024	0.053
Hhold head with technique education	0.020	0.083	0.014	0.084
Household head single	−0.122*	0.075	−0.136**	0.081
Household head married	0.074	0.064	0.100	0.072
Household head separated	−0.046	0.077	−0.031	0.086
Household head lives with partner	−0.147*	0.091	−0.124	0.100
Educational attainment	0.052***	0.005	0.033***	0.005
House with fixed phone line				
House with electricity				
House with aqueduct				
House with sewerage				
Number of rooms in household				
Socioeconomic stratum 2				
Socioeconomic stratum 3				
Socioeconomic stratum 4				
Socioeconomic stratum 5 or 6				
Homeownership, house totally paid				
Homeownership, house partially paid				
Tenant				
House with gas for cooking				
House with natural gas				
House with internet				
House with cable TV				
Employed				
Unemployed				
Household occupation rate				
Household unemployment rate				
Enrolled in private health insurance				
Enrolled in public health insurance				
Enrolled in pension fund				
Good health				
Constant	−2.143***	0.249	−0.152	0.306
FE past neighborhood	No		Yes	
FE current neighborhood	No		No	
N	12,521		11,263	

* Significantly at 10%
** Significantly at 5%
*** Significantly at 1%

Table 6.7 Life satisfaction models. Dependent variable equal to one if very satisfied (continued)

Living in current neighborhood 10 or more years ago

coef	se	coef	se	coef	se	coef	se
(ix)		(x)		(xi)		(xii)	
−0.003	0.009	−0.002	0.009	−0.001	0.009	0.007	0.011
−0.219	0.236	−0.242	0.236	−0.181	0.237	−0.177	0.315
0.000	0.000	0.000	0.000	−0.000	0.000	−0.000	0.000
−0.002*	**0.001**	−0.002	0.001	−0.002	0.001	−0.002	0.002
0.165*	**0.064**					**0.134****	**0.076**
−0.033	0.071	−0.065	0.071	−0.076	0.074	0.034	0.085
0.000***	0.000	0.000***	0.000	0.000***	0.000	0.000***	0.000
−0.042***	0.014	−0.043***	0.014	−0.058***	0.014	−0.058***	0.015
−0.004	0.008	−0.004	0.008	−0.011	0.008	−0.007	0.009
0.000	0.000	0.000	0.000	0.000	0.000	0.000	0.000
0.067	0.051	0.067	0.051	0.067	0.052	0.042	0.060
−0.038	0.051	−0.040	0.051	−0.007	0.051	−0.025	0.053
−0.020	0.052	−0.020	0.052	0.028	0.054	−0.005	0.057
0.019	0.085	0.014	0.085	0.050	0.087	0.037	0.095
−0.140**	0.081	−0.138**	0.081	−0.107	0.081	−0.123	0.090
0.096	0.072	0.099	0.072	0.087	0.074	0.099	0.084
−0.032	0.086	−0.028	0.085	−0.001	0.087	0.053	0.095
−0.120	0.100	−0.116	0.100	−0.074	0.100	−0.101	0.109
0.032***	0.005	0.032***	0.005	0.021***	0.005	0.014***	0.006
0.215***	0.102	0.216***	0.102	0.142	0.106	0.177*	0.109
−0.152	0.191	−0.165	0.191	−0.178	0.194	−0.298*	0.202
0.043	0.132	0.055	0.132	0.029	0.136	0.054	0.151
0.253*	0.172	0.255*	0.172	0.252	0.179	0.238	0.189
0.072***	0.032	0.070***	0.032	0.065***	0.032	0.066**	0.035
				0.079	0.116	0.032	0.126
				0.215	0.153	0.198	0.161
				0.161	0.175	0.105	0.184
				0.635***	0.207	0.686***	0.214
				0.137**	0.083	0.136	0.098
				0.070	0.131	−0.012	0.158
				−0.004	0.092	−0.044	0.110
				0.029	0.110	0.007	0.122
				0.060	0.107	0.057	0.116
				0.278***	0.050	0.254***	0.053
				0.083*	0.055	0.016	0.061
						−0.047	0.064
						−0.055	0.175
						0.013	0.080
						−0.425**	0.218
						0.081	0.088
						−0.108	0.095
						0.133***	0.063
						0.301***	0.066
−0.306	0.322	−0.132	0.317	−0.461	0.375	−1.526***	0.516
Yes		Yes		Yes		Yes	
Yes		Yes		Yes		Yes	
11,263		11,263		11,263		9,192	

Table 6.8 Life satisfaction models. Dependent variable equal to one if very satisfied (continued)

| Variable | Living in current neighborhood 10 or more years ago, movers | | | |
| | coef | se | coef | se |
	(i)		(ii)	
Homicide rate	−0.010	0.008	**−0.028****	**0.015**
Capture rate/homicide rate	0.175	0.214	−0.214	0.357
Distance to crime	**0.000****	**0.000**	0.000	0.000
Years living in this place	−0.003	0.002	−0.001	0.003
Safe neighborhood	**0.134***	**0.083**	**0.192****	**0.095**
Victim of offense	−0.041	0.082	−0.039	0.094
Household income	0.000***	0.000	0.000***	0.000
Number of persons in household	−0.048***	0.016	−0.047***	0.018
Age	0.002	0.014	−0.011	0.017
Age2	0.000	0.000	0.000	0.000
Male	0.041	0.083	0.043	0.097
Household head with primary	−0.100	0.073	−0.063	0.081
Household head with secondary	0.094	0.089	0.129	0.095
Hhold head with technique education	0.109	0.131	−0.008	0.146
Household head single	−0.181**	0.110	−0.196*	0.128
Household head married	0.067	0.097	0.107	0.115
Household head separated	−0.210**	0.118	−0.228**	0.138
Household head lives with partner	−0.142	0.138	−0.107	0.168
Educational attainment	0.046***	0.007	0.025***	0.008
House with fixed phone line				
House with electricity				
House with aqueduct				
House with sewerage				
Number of rooms in household				
Socioeconomic stratum 2				
Socioeconomic stratum 3				
Socioeconomic stratum 4				
Socioeconomic stratum 5 or 6				
Homeownership, house totally paid				
Homeownership, house partially paid				
Tenant				
House with gas for cooking				
House with natural gas				
House with internet				
House with cable TV				
Employed				
Unemployed				
Household occupation rate				
Household unemployment rate				
Enrolled in private health insurance				
Enrolled in public health insurance				
Enrolled in pension fund				
Good health				
Constant	−1.936***	0.429	0.263	0.512
FE past neighborhood	No		Yes	
FE current neighborhood	No		No	
N	4,705		3,579	

* Significantly at 10%
** Significantly at 5%
*** Significantly at 1%

Table 6.8 Life satisfaction models. Dependent variable equal to one if very satisfied (continued)

Living in current neighborhood 10 or more years ago, movers

coef	se	coef	se	coef	se	coef	se
(iii)		(iv)		(v)		(vi)	
−0.028**	**0.015**	**−0.028****	**0.015**	**−0.026****	**0.014**	−0.015	0.019
−0.229	0.358	−0.233	0.359	−0.278	0.362	−0.108	0.425
0.000	0.000	0.000	0.000	0.000	0.000	0.000	0.000
−0.001	0.003	−0.001	0.003	−0.001	0.003	−0.005**	0.003
0.193***	**0.095**					**0.156***	**0.107**
−0.041	0.095	−0.079	0.092	−0.097	0.094	0.013	0.120
0.000***	0.000	0.000***	0.000	0.000**	0.000	0.000***	0.000
−0.048***	0.018	−0.050***	0.018	−0.067***	0.019	−0.073***	0.021
−0.011	0.017	−0.012	0.017	−0.022	0.017	−0.018	0.018
0.000	0.000	0.000	0.000	0.000	0.000	0.000	0.000
0.055	0.098	0.056	0.098	0.059	0.099	0.006	0.113
−0.067	0.082	−0.073	0.083	−0.051	0.084	−0.093	0.088
0.126	0.095	0.122	0.096	0.149*	0.098	0.137	0.104
−0.012	0.144	−0.031	0.144	−0.015	0.148	−0.086	0.171
−0.199*	0.128	−0.198*	0.128	−0.172	0.127	−0.082	0.139
0.096	0.116	0.095	0.116	0.071	0.119	0.116	0.132
−0.229**	0.139	−0.222*	0.138	−0.205*	0.139	−0.143	0.156
−0.108	0.169	−0.108	0.167	−0.092	0.167	−0.168	0.189
0.023***	0.008	0.023***	0.008	0.015**	0.009	0.005	0.010
0.331**	0.175	0.332**	0.175	0.266*	0.180	0.322*	0.198
−0.095	0.352	−0.115	0.351	−0.115	0.355	−0.006	0.395
−0.037	0.231	−0.021	0.233	−0.019	0.238	−0.058	0.257
−0.048	0.255	−0.027	0.253	−0.025	0.260	−0.154	0.276
0.053	0.046	0.052	0.046	0.046	0.047	0.035	0.055
				−0.097	0.145	−0.094	0.169
				0.080	0.216	0.095	0.253
				−0.024	0.252	0.085	0.263
				0.318	0.269	0.412	0.313
				0.097	0.139	0.015	0.157
				0.156	0.229	0.115	0.257
				−0.084	0.149	−0.186	0.172
				0.142	0.218	0.115	0.242
				−0.049	0.209	−0.056	0.233
				0.233***	0.080	0.253***	0.092
				0.099	0.081	0.084	0.089
						−0.005	0.114
						0.391	0.299
						−0.145	0.158
						−0.364	0.370
						0.020	0.161
						−0.223	0.161
						0.063	0.098
						0.364***	0.099
0.168	0.563	0.371	0.552	0.409	0.604	0.774	1.452
Yes		Yes		Yes		Yes	
Yes		Yes		Yes		Yes	
3,579		3,579		3,579		2,848	

(continued)

Table 6.8 Life satisfaction models. Dependent variable equal to one if very satisfied (continued)

Variable	Living in current neighborhood 10 or more years ago, always in current neighborhood			
	coef	se	coef	se
	(vii)		(viii)	
Homicide rate	−0.001	0.006	0.009	0.009
Capture rate/homicide rate	0.139	0.179	−0.104	0.322
Distance to crime	0.000***	0.000	−0.000	0.000
Years living in this place	−0.003***	0.001	−0.002	0.002
Safe neighborhood	**0.094**	**0.072**	**0.180*****	**0.083**
Victim of offense	−0.029	0.091	−0.029	0.097
Household income	0.000***	0.000	0.000***	0.000
Number of persons in household	−0.044***	0.018	−0.038**	0.020
Age	0.007	0.009	−0.002	0.010
Age2	0.000	0.000	0.000	0.000
Male	0.062	0.062	0.068	0.064
Household head with primary	−0.057	0.060	−0.006	0.069
Household head with secondary	−0.141***	0.052	−0.080	0.061
Hhold head with technique education	−0.017	0.095	0.000	0.102
Household head single	−0.071	0.103	−0.074	0.109
Household head married	0.095	0.084	0.142*	0.093
Household head separated	0.056	0.099	0.096	0.109
Household head lives with partner	−0.132	0.115	−0.107	0.128
Educational attainment	0.055***	0.006	0.040***	0.006
House with fixed phone line				
House with electricity				
House with aqueduct				
House with sewerage				
Number of rooms in household				
Socioeconomic stratum 2				
Socioeconomic stratum 3				
Socioeconomic stratum 4				
Socioeconomic stratum 5 or 6				
Homeownership, house totally paid				
Homeownership, house partially paid				
Tenant				
House with gas for cooking				
House with natural gas				
House with internet				
House with cable TV				
Employed				
Unemployed				
Household occupation rate				
Household unemployment rate				
Enrolled in private health insurance				
Enrolled in public health insurance				
Enrolled in pension fund				
Good health				
Constant	−2.187***	0.285	−0.870***	0.364
FE past neighborhood	No		Yes	
FE current neighborhood	No		No	
N	7,811		6,385	

*Significantly at 10%
**Significantly at 5%
***Significantly at 1%

Table 6.8 Life satisfaction models. Dependent variable equal to one if very satisfied (continued)

Living in current neighborhood 10 or more years ago, always in current neighborhood

coef	se	coef	se	coef	se	coef	se
(ix)		(x)		(xi)		(xii)	
0.009	0.009	0.009	0.009	0.011	0.010	**0.016***	**0.010**
−0.075	0.322	−0.116	0.323	−0.000	0.333	−0.100	0.407
−0.000	0.000	−0.000	0.000	−0.000	0.000	−0.000	0.000
−0.002	0.002	−0.002	0.002	−0.001	0.002	−0.002	0.002
0.183*	**0.082**					0.133	0.100
−0.028	0.098	−0.063	0.099	−0.070	0.102	0.029	0.114
0.000***	0.000	0.000***	0.000	0.000***	0.000	0.000***	0.000
−0.040***	0.020	−0.040***	0.020	−0.053***	0.021	−0.049***	0.021
−0.003	0.010	−0.003	0.010	−0.009	0.010	−0.007	0.011
0.000	0.000	0.000	0.000	0.000	0.000	0.000	0.000
0.065	0.064	0.064	0.064	0.059	0.064	0.066	0.076
−0.006	0.070	−0.005	0.069	0.039	0.070	0.061	0.076
−0.074	0.060	−0.071	0.060	−0.006	0.062	−0.040	0.071
0.009	0.103	0.010	0.103	0.067	0.108	0.067	0.123
−0.078	0.107	−0.076	0.106	−0.030	0.106	−0.077	0.123
0.143*	0.092	0.149*	0.092	0.155**	0.093	0.161*	0.112
0.092	0.108	0.095	0.107	0.133	0.110	0.195*	0.127
−0.101	0.127	−0.094	0.127	−0.025	0.126	−0.047	0.144
0.039***	0.006	0.038***	0.006	0.025***	0.007	0.019***	0.008
0.178	0.130	0.182	0.130	0.086	0.137	0.121	0.143
−0.193	0.240	−0.204	0.240	−0.218	0.247	−0.498**	0.255
0.101	0.168	0.115	0.167	0.077	0.173	0.105	0.204
0.472***	0.234	0.463***	0.233	0.456**	0.245	0.553***	0.252
0.087***	0.041	0.084***	0.041	0.081**	0.042	0.085**	0.046
				0.346*	0.219	0.275	0.216
				0.458**	0.236	0.427**	0.232
				0.419*	0.264	0.258	0.271
				0.977***	0.292	0.933***	0.290
				0.195**	0.112	0.238**	0.136
				0.047	0.181	−0.101	0.222
				0.061	0.124	0.070	0.147
				0.010	0.135	−0.013	0.160
				0.075	0.134	0.079	0.152
				0.322***	0.067	0.299***	0.071
				0.073	0.069	−0.050	0.076
						−0.087	0.079
						−0.275	0.259
						0.125	0.102
						−0.531*	0.329
						0.111	0.111
						−0.085	0.126
						0.169***	0.085
						0.276***	0.090
−1.129***	0.447	−0.908***	0.445	−2.034***	0.564	−2.777***	0.586
Yes		Yes		Yes		Yes	
Yes		Yes		Yes		Yes	
6,385		6,385		6,385		5,124	

feeling very satisfied, in contrast to the robust results found in Table 6.5 on life satisfaction.

When we compare the results obtained in Tables 6.6 and 6.8, we find that the effects of the homicide rate, the distance to crime, and feeling safe in the neighborhood are very similar; nonetheless, the arrest rates and having been a victim of an offense affected life satisfaction, but it does not affect the likelihood of feeling very satisfied.

4.3 The Role of the Type of Victimization

Tables 6.9 and 6.10 show the result of estimating Eq. 6.1, but now, splitting the variable victim of an offense into two variables, one that includes robbery (4.8% of households, most of the offenses in this subset), burglary (0.1% of households), and personal offenses (households with at least one member that has been threatened, blackmailed, murdered, kidnapped, or rapped; 0.8% of households), and the other includes the rest (households with at least one member that has been victim of car accidents, fights, gun shots, drugs, etc.; 2.5% of households).

The results of Tables 6.5 and 6.9 are very similar, meaning that both offenses included in Table 6.9 are important in the same models they were in Table 6.5, nonetheless, a comparison between Tables 6.6 and 6.10 reveals that although being a victim of an offense negatively affected life satisfaction in both populations, once we split the victimization variable, we find that the variable that includes robbery keeps affecting negatively life satisfaction in both populations, but the other variable only affects it on the population of *settlers* and not *previous movers*.

To have an idea of the magnitude of the effect of the homicide rate, the perception of security in the neighborhood and the two types of victimization, on life satisfaction, we reestimate, again, a few of the previous specifications by OLS and get standardized coefficients (not reported here). We find that a standard deviation increase in each of the homicide rate, the share of households feeling safe in their neighborhoods, the share of households reporting to have been a victim of burglary, and the share of households reporting to have been with a victim of other offenses implies a decrease of 5.3, −4.6 (that is, an increase), 2.1, and 0.3% of a standard deviation of life satisfaction, respectively.[29] That is, most of the effect found previously for the aggregate of all offenses can be explained by the ones that are mostly driven by burglary.

---

[29] This result was found, again, for the sample of previous movers with the specification in column (ii) in the tables, although other specification led to similar results.

5   Conclusions

Despite the empirical challenges faced to identify how crime affects life satisfaction, we exploit the large variation in the homicide rates between the different neighborhoods of Medellín, and a large data set with the census of its homicides over several years, to build homicide rates at the block level, and split the sample, in a way that allows us to get reasonable estimates of the effect of the homicide rate, individual's perception of security in their neighborhood of residence, and of the effect of their having been victimized, on life satisfaction.

We split our data in three subsets: (1) households who have always lived in their current houses, (2) households who have lived in their current houses for more than 10 years but moved there at some point in the past, and (3) households who have lived in their current houses less than 10 years ago. We find a negative effect of the homicide rate on life satisfaction for subsample (ii). The homicide rate affects their life satisfaction and their likelihood to feel very happy, that is, their likelihood to have very good quality of life conditions. That subsample of households is characterized for having the lowest quality of life conditions when compared to the other two subsamples. Note that not having found effects for the other two subsamples of households does not mean that no effect exists, but rather, that we could not identify one due to the challenge posed by households' self-selection into their current neighborhoods.

We also find a positive and robust effect of the perception of security in the households' neighborhood for the whole sample, and for each of the three subsamples described. Having been a victim of an offense is also robustly negatively related to life satisfaction, in particular, in the cases where the offense was robbery.

Our results show that a standard deviation increase in each of the homicide rate, the share of households feeling safe in their neighborhoods, and the share of households reporting to have been victimized implies a decrease of 5.3, −4.7 (that is, an increase), and 1.8% of a standard deviation of life satisfaction, respectively.

There are some caveats of our results worth mentioning. First, since our identification strategy was focused on subsample (ii) in order to sort out the endogeneity problem mentioned above, our results do not necessarily apply for the whole population. However, households in subsample (ii) are distributed across the entire city, and since security is a neighborhood's amenity, any policy aimed to attenuate the negative effects of crime on households' well-being would equally benefit households in that subsample or the other two.

Second, since we do not have data at different moments in time for the same individual, we cannot control for households fixed effects. Nonetheless, our data allow us to use fixed effects for current and previous household's neighborhood of residence.

Future research is needed to validate the robustness of our results using other identification strategies that avoid the problem of endogenous neighborhood selection. For example, Kling et al. (2005) use data from a randomized experiment in which some families were offered housing vouchers to enable them to move to

Table 6.9 Life satisfaction models. Dependent variable equal to one if satisfied. The role of the type of victimization

Variable	All sample			
	coef	se	coef	se
	(i)		(ii)	
Homicide rate	0.006*	0.004	0.007***	0.004
Capture rate/homicide rate	0.031	0.153	0.205	0.149
Distance to crime	0.000*	0.000	0.000	0.000
Years living in this place	−0.000	0.001	0.001*	0.001
Safe neighborhood	**0.316*****	**0.035**	**0.291*****	**0.034**
Victim of robbery, burglary, personal	**−0.161*****	**0.048**	**−0.194*****	**0.049**
Victim of other offenses	**−0.274*****	**0.071**	**−0.310*****	**0.079**
Household income	0.000***	0.000	0.000***	0.000
Number of persons in household	−0.067***	0.007	−0.069***	0.007
Age	−0.003	0.004	−0.005	0.004
Age2	0.000**	0.000	0.000	0.000
Male	0.092***	0.030	0.096***	0.032
Household head with primary	−0.105***	0.030	−0.065***	0.031
Household head with secondary	−0.083***	0.040	−0.036	0.040
Hhold head with technique education	0.012	0.073	0.050	0.075
Household head single	−0.243***	0.041	−0.232***	0.040
Household head married	0.050	0.041	0.058	0.043
Household head separated	−0.240***	0.043	−0.237***	0.045
Household head lives with partner	−0.198***	0.046	−0.140***	0.047
Educational attainment	0.070***	0.004	0.052***	0.004
House with fixed phone line				
House with electricity				
House with aqueduct				
House with sewerage				
Number of rooms in household				
Socioeconomic stratum 2				
Socioeconomic stratum 3				
Socioeconomic stratum 4				
Socioeconomic stratum 5 or 6				
Homeownership, house totally paid				
Homeownership, house partially paid				
Tenant				
House with gas for cooking				
House with natural gas				
House with internet				
House with cable TV				
Employed				
Unemployed				
Household occupation rate				
Household unemployment rate				
Enrolled in private health insurance				
Enrolled in public health insurance				
Enrolled in pension fund				
Good health				
Constant	0.116	0.145	0.364***	0.150
FE past neighborhood	No		Yes	
FE current neighborhood	No		No	
N	18,715		18,250	

* Significantly at 10%
** Significantly at 5%
*** Significantly at 1%

Table 6.9 Life satisfaction models. Dependent variable equal to one if satisfied. The role of the type of victimization (continued)

All sample							
coef	se	coef	se	coef	se	coef	se
(iii)		(iv)		(v)		(vi)	
0.002	0.006	0.003	0.006	0.001	0.005	0.004	0.007
0.120	0.227	0.106	0.227	0.098	0.210	−0.169	0.243
−0.000	0.000	−0.000	0.000	−0.000	0.000	−0.000	0.000
0.001**	0.001	0.002***	0.001	0.002***	0.001	0.002***	0.001
0.273*	**0.032**					**0.252***	**0.036**
−0.188*	**0.052**	**−0.250***	**0.053**	**−0.310***	**0.055**	**−0.262***	**0.057**
−0.266*	**0.081**	**−0.312***	**0.080**	**−0.293***	**0.079**	**−0.191***	**0.083**
0.000***	0.000	0.000***	0.000	0.000***	0.000	0.000***	0.000
−0.069***	0.007	−0.069***	0.007	−0.082***	0.007	−0.071***	0.008
−0.010***	0.005	−0.010***	0.005	−0.017***	0.005	−0.017***	0.005
0.000**	0.000	0.000**	0.000	0.000***	0.000	0.000***	0.000
0.118***	0.033	0.120***	0.033	0.131***	0.033	0.119***	0.036
−0.064**	0.033	−0.063**	0.033	−0.015	0.034	−0.042	0.037
−0.041	0.042	−0.037	0.042	0.035	0.046	−0.019	0.051
0.018	0.077	0.015	0.077	0.062	0.079	−0.027	0.092
−0.240***	0.042	−0.235***	0.041	−0.186***	0.043	−0.152***	0.047
0.031	0.044	0.030	0.044	−0.004	0.045	0.004	0.051
−0.252***	0.048	−0.252***	0.048	−0.233***	0.049	−0.186***	0.050
−0.137***	0.049	−0.137***	0.050	−0.109***	0.051	−0.067	0.055
0.044***	0.004	0.044***	0.004	0.027***	0.004	0.021***	0.005
0.396***	0.046	0.396***	0.046	0.293***	0.046	0.248***	0.050
−0.167	0.121	−0.179*	0.119	−0.183*	0.116	−0.202*	0.136
0.407***	0.074	0.418***	0.074	0.363***	0.075	0.324***	0.074
−0.047	0.107	−0.037	0.105	−0.045	0.104	−0.031	0.121
−0.044***	0.020	−0.047***	0.020	−0.052***	0.021	−0.042**	0.023
				0.037	0.068	−0.006	0.071
				0.163**	0.089	0.061	0.098
				0.569***	0.133	0.416***	0.146
				0.886***	0.156	0.685***	0.166
				0.296***	0.047	0.255***	0.051
				0.118*	0.074	0.063	0.080
				0.233***	0.057	0.203***	0.062
				−0.021	0.067	0.015	0.068
				0.200***	0.071	0.174***	0.074
				0.359***	0.034	0.311***	0.036
				0.328***	0.029	0.292***	0.031
						−0.181***	0.040
						−0.484***	0.086
						0.383***	0.067
						−0.420***	0.127
						0.250***	0.046
						−0.116***	0.046
						0.103***	0.040
						0.539***	0.035
−0.341	0.388	−0.128	0.396	−0.054	0.393	−0.423	0.448
Yes		Yes		Yes		Yes	
Yes		Yes		Yes		Yes	
17,936		17,936		17,936		15,228	

(continued)

Table 6.9 Life satisfaction models. Dependent variable equal to one if satisfied. The role of the type of victimization (continued)

| Variable | Living in current neighborhood 10 or more years ago | | | |
| | coef | se | coef | se |
	(vii)		(viii)	
Homicide rate	0.006	0.005	−0.006	0.005
Capture rate/homicide rate	−0.053	0.171	−0.059	0.283
Distance to crime	0.000*	0.000	−0.000	0.000
Years living in this place	0.000	0.001	0.001	0.001
Safe neighborhood	**0.289***	**0.042**	**0.257***	**0.041**
Victim of robbery, burglary, personal	**−0.125***	**0.060**	**−0.163***	**0.063**
Victim of other offenses	**−0.166**	**0.085**	**−0.189***	**0.091**
Household income	0.000***	0.000	0.000***	0.000
Number of persons in household	−0.063***	0.009	−0.066***	0.009
Age	0.002	0.005	−0.002	0.005
Age2	0.000	0.000	0.000	0.000
Male	0.082***	0.035	0.090***	0.037
Household head with primary	−0.094***	0.038	−0.036	0.040
Household head with secondary	−0.076	0.055	−0.016	0.056
Hhold head with technique education	0.024	0.096	0.084	0.105
Household head single	−0.260***	0.046	−0.257***	0.046
Household head married	0.061	0.050	0.058	0.051
Household head separated	−0.291***	0.050	−0.305***	0.053
Household head lives with partner	−0.169***	0.058	−0.115**	0.060
Educational attainment	0.068***	0.005	0.045***	0.005
House with fixed phone line				
House with electricity				
House with aqueduct				
House with sewerage				
Number of rooms in household				
Socioeconomic stratum 2				
Socioeconomic stratum 3				
Socioeconomic stratum 4				
Socioeconomic stratum 5 or 6				
Homeownership, house totally paid				
Homeownership, house partially paid				
Tenant				
House with gas for cooking				
House with natural gas				
House with internet				
House with cable TV				
Employed				
Unemployed				
Household occupation rate				
Household unemployment rate				
Enrolled in private health insurance				
Enrolled in public health insurance				
Enrolled in pension fund				
Good health				
Constant	−0.011	0.183	0.308	0.271
FE past neighborhood	No		Yes	
FE current neighborhood	No		No	
N	12,521		11,894	

* Significantly at 10%
** Significantly at 5%
*** Significantly at 1%

Table 6.9 Life satisfaction models. Dependent variable equal to one if satisfied. The role of the type of victimization (continued)

Living in current neighborhood 10 or more years ago							
coef	se	coef	se	coef	se	coef	se
(ix)		(x)		(xi)		(xii)	
−0.007	0.005	−0.007	0.006	−0.009*	0.006	−0.003	0.009
−0.072	0.284	−0.103	0.284	−0.067	0.270	−0.493**	0.297
0.000	0.000	0.000	0.000	−0.000	0.000	0.000	0.000
0.001	0.001	0.001	0.001	0.002***	0.001	0.002***	0.001
0.245*	**0.040**					**0.192***	**0.044**
−0.151*	**0.060**	**−0.212***	**0.061**	**−0.263***	**0.064**	**−0.188***	**0.071**
−0.137*	**0.091**	**−0.174***	**0.089**	**−0.162**	**0.087**	−0.103	0.098
0.000***	0.000	0.000***	0.000	0.000***	0.000	0.000**	0.000
−0.062***	0.009	−0.062***	0.009	−0.079***	0.009	−0.069***	0.009
−0.004	0.006	−0.004	0.006	−0.012***	0.006	−0.011**	0.006
0.000	0.000	0.000	0.000	0.000**	0.000	0.000**	0.000
0.106***	0.037	0.108***	0.037	0.116***	0.036	0.106***	0.040
−0.037	0.040	−0.036	0.040	0.022	0.041	−0.005	0.042
−0.024	0.056	−0.020	0.056	0.071	0.058	−0.012	0.063
0.069	0.105	0.061	0.104	0.138	0.109	0.043	0.123
−0.253***	0.047	−0.249***	0.047	−0.195***	0.050	−0.153***	0.055
0.030	0.051	0.029	0.051	−0.006	0.052	0.005	0.057
−0.298***	0.053	−0.298***	0.052	−0.280***	0.054	−0.236***	0.057
−0.125***	0.058	−0.124***	0.058	−0.102**	0.060	−0.072	0.064
0.043***	0.005	0.043***	0.005	0.024***	0.005	0.019***	0.006
0.441***	0.061	0.439***	0.060	0.335***	0.059	0.286***	0.066
−0.143	0.140	−0.154	0.138	−0.168	0.133	−0.193	0.165
0.422***	0.092	0.435***	0.091	0.368***	0.094	0.333***	0.094
−0.079	0.126	−0.070	0.124	−0.092	0.122	−0.081	0.144
−0.030	0.023	−0.034*	0.023	−0.043**	0.024	−0.023	0.026
				−0.008	0.087	−0.049	0.091
				0.108	0.106	0.013	0.111
				0.455***	0.166	0.292*	0.180
				0.901***	0.183	0.747***	0.196
				0.230***	0.050	0.173***	0.055
				0.030	0.098	−0.032	0.112
				0.197***	0.064	0.142***	0.068
				−0.088	0.085	−0.052	0.086
				0.275***	0.095	0.229***	0.095
				0.406***	0.042	0.332***	0.045
				0.343***	0.035	0.305***	0.038
						−0.181***	0.050
						−0.437***	0.103
						0.334***	0.082
						−0.501***	0.156
						0.259***	0.057
						−0.142***	0.060
						0.083**	0.049
						0.572***	0.041
−0.276	0.293	−0.833***	0.235	−1.178***	0.270	−0.161	0.390
Yes		Yes		Yes		Yes	
Yes		Yes		Yes		Yes	
11,894		11,894		11,894		9,875	

Table 6.10 Life satisfaction models. Dependent variable equal to one if satisfied. The role of the type of victimization

| Variable | Living in current neighborhood 10 or more years ago, movers | | | |
	coef	se	coef	se
	(i)		(ii)	
Homicide rate	−0.004	0.005	**−0.027*****	**0.011**
Capture rate/homicide rate	−0.063	0.235	**0.986*****	**0.364**
Distance to crime	**0.000*****	**0.000**	−0.000	0.000
Years living in this place	−0.002	0.002	−0.000	0.002
Safe neighborhood	**0.217*****	**0.069**	**0.195*****	**0.070**
Victim of robbery, burglary, personal	−0.118	0.086	**−0.177****	**0.096**
Victim of other offenses	−0.066	0.103	−0.010	0.117
Household income	0.000***	0.000	0.000***	0.000
Number of persons in household	−0.067***	0.014	−0.074***	0.014
Age	0.007	0.010	0.001	0.011
Age2	0.000	0.000	0.000	0.000
Male	0.048	0.058	0.090	0.065
Household head with primary	−0.107***	0.051	−0.042	0.061
Household head with secondary	−0.061	0.088	−0.033	0.107
Hhold head with technique education	−0.040	0.147	−0.030	0.179
Household head single	−0.149***	0.071	−0.192***	0.078
Household head married	0.123*	0.081	0.066	0.090
Household head separated	−0.309***	0.081	−0.367***	0.089
Household head lives with partner	−0.066	0.099	−0.050	0.108
Educational attainment	0.066***	0.008	0.042***	0.010
House with fixed phone line				
House with electricity				
House with aqueduct				
House with sewerage				
Number of rooms in household				
Socioeconomic stratum 2				
Socioeconomic stratum 3				
Socioeconomic stratum 4				
Socioeconomic stratum 5 or 6				
Homeownership, house totally paid				
Homeownership, house partially paid				
Tenant				
House with gas for cooking				
House with natural gas				
House with internet				
House with cable TV				
Employed				
Unemployed				
Household occupation rate				
Household unemployment rate				
Enrolled in private health insurance				
Enrolled in public health insurance				
Enrolled in pension fund				
Good health				
Constant	−0.158	0.340	−0.435	1.016
FE past neighborhood	No		Yes	
FE current neighborhood	No		No	
N	4,705		4,251	

* Significantly at 10%
** Significantly at 5%
*** Significantly at 1%

Table 6.10 Life satisfaction models. Dependent variable equal to one if satisfied. The role of the type of victimization (continued)

Living in current neighborhood 10 or more years ago, movers

coef (iii)	se	coef (iv)	se	coef (v)	se	coef (vi)	se
-0.028***	0.011	-0.027***	0.011	-0.029***	0.011	-0.025**	0.014
0.918***	0.358	0.886***	0.358	0.907***	0.362	0.517	0.431
-0.000	0.000	-0.000	0.000	-0.000	0.000	0.000	0.000
-0.000	0.002	0.000	0.002	0.000	0.002	-0.001	0.002
0.192***	0.071					0.145**	0.077
-0.159**	0.093	-0.198***	0.092	-0.231***	0.095	-0.209**	0.112
0.056	0.124	0.032	0.123	0.073	0.126	0.098	0.149
0.000***	0.000	0.000***	0.000	0.000***	0.000	0.000***	0.000
-0.072***	0.014	-0.072***	0.014	-0.091***	0.014	-0.085***	0.014
-0.001	0.011	-0.001	0.011	-0.013	0.011	-0.011	0.012
0.000	0.000	0.000	0.000	0.000	0.000	0.000	0.000
0.117**	0.066	0.114**	0.066	0.128***	0.065	0.172***	0.073
-0.042	0.060	-0.046	0.060	0.007	0.063	-0.041	0.068
-0.036	0.107	-0.041	0.107	0.029	0.112	-0.056	0.119
-0.025	0.180	-0.041	0.176	0.014	0.188	-0.059	0.242
-0.195***	0.079	-0.193***	0.078	-0.119*	0.080	-0.130*	0.089
0.029	0.090	0.032	0.090	-0.019	0.090	-0.089	0.102
-0.358***	0.089	-0.353***	0.089	-0.322***	0.092	-0.327***	0.095
-0.067	0.105	-0.066	0.106	-0.059	0.109	-0.122	0.121
0.039***	0.010	0.039***	0.010	0.023***	0.010	0.018*	0.012
0.449***	0.084	0.446***	0.083	0.303***	0.085	0.284***	0.098
-0.204	0.208	-0.213	0.206	-0.188	0.209	-0.338	0.289
0.399***	0.145	0.406***	0.146	0.355***	0.152	0.375***	0.163
-0.175	0.193	-0.156	0.192	-0.159	0.194	-0.108	0.225
-0.033	0.034	-0.034	0.035	-0.044	0.034	-0.033	0.039
				-0.001	0.092	-0.061	0.095
				-0.010	0.158	-0.122	0.167
				0.410**	0.244	0.233	0.262
				1.180***	0.295	1.195***	0.346
				0.276***	0.100	0.213***	0.104
				0.144	0.158	0.088	0.172
				0.200**	0.115	0.115	0.123
				-0.160	0.141	-0.182	0.157
				0.342***	0.155	0.395***	0.167
				0.370***	0.077	0.335***	0.092
				0.412***	0.055	0.373***	0.063
						-0.121*	0.078
						-0.221	0.191
						0.389***	0.117
						-0.662***	0.291
						0.182***	0.081
						-0.250***	0.096
						0.036	0.091
						0.626***	0.063
-0.814	1.022	-0.716	0.985	-0.775	0.991	-0.868	0.816
Yes		Yes		Yes		Yes	
Yes		Yes		Yes		Yes	
4,251		4,251		4,251		3,567	

(continued)

Table 6.10 Life satisfaction models. Dependent variable equal to one if satisfied. The role of the type of victimization (continued)

| Variable | Living in current neighborhood 10 or more years ago, always in current neighborhood | | | |
	coef	se	coef	se
	(vii)		(viii)	
Homicide rate	0.012*	0.007	−0.000	0.008
Capture rate/homicide rate	−0.036	0.165	−0.309	0.353
Distance to crime	0.000	0.000	−0.000	0.000
Years living in this place	−0.002	0.001	0.000	0.001
Safe neighborhood	**0.343***	**0.053**	**0.318***	**0.058**
Victim of robbery, burglary, personal	**−0.113***	**0.074**	**−0.151****	**0.080**
Victim of other offenses	**−0.243***	**0.118**	**−0.326***	**0.136**
Household income	0.000***	0.000	0.000***	0.000
Number of persons in household	−0.063***	0.010	−0.062***	0.011
Age	0.001	0.007	−0.001	0.007
Age2	0.000	0.000	0.000	0.000
Male	0.104***	0.052	0.088**	0.052
Household head with primary	−0.097**	0.053	−0.026	0.057
Household head with secondary	−0.094*	0.064	−0.001	0.069
Hhold head with technique education	0.040	0.118	0.143	0.129
Household head single	−0.332***	0.065	−0.328***	0.071
Household head married	0.013	0.072	0.026	0.074
Household head separated	−0.283***	0.065	−0.285***	0.069
Household head lives with partner	−0.246***	0.077	−0.167***	0.080
Educational attainment	0.067***	0.006	0.049***	0.006
House with fixed phone line				
House with electricity				
House with aqueduct				
House with sewerage				
Number of rooms in household				
Socioeconomic stratum 2				
Socioeconomic stratum 3				
Socioeconomic stratum 4				
Socioeconomic stratum 5 or 6				
Homeownership, house totally paid				
Homeownership, house partially paid				
Tenant				
House with gas for cooking				
House with natural gas				
House with internet				
House with cable TV				
Employed				
Unemployed				
Household occupation rate				
Household unemployment rate				
Enrolled in private health insurance				
Enrolled in public health insurance				
Enrolled in pension fund				
Good health				
Constant	0.084	0.212	0.650***	0.221
FE past neighborhood	No		Yes	
FE current neighborhood	No		No	
N	7,811		7,181	

* Significantly at 10%
** Significantly at 5%
*** Significantly at 1%

Table 6.10 Life satisfaction models. Dependent variable equal to one if satisfied. The role of the type of victimization (continued)

Living in current neighborhood 10 or more years ago, always in current neighborhood

coef	se	coef	se	coef	se	coef	se
(ix)		(x)		(xi)		(xii)	
−0.002	0.008	−0.001	0.008	−0.005	0.009	−0.003	0.010
−0.304	0.347	−0.342	0.348	−0.335	0.361	−0.816***	0.408
0.000	0.000	−0.000	0.000	−0.000	0.000	−0.000	0.000
0.000	0.001	0.001	0.001	0.002*	0.001	0.002*	0.001
0.299*	**0.057**					**0.246***	**0.070**
−0.146	**0.078**	**−0.228***	**0.077**	**−0.304***	**0.082**	**−0.181**	**0.093**
−0.281*	**0.138**	**−0.333***	**0.136**	**−0.344***	**0.128**	**−0.241**	**0.142**
0.000***	0.000	0.000***	0.000	0.000***	0.000	0.000	0.000
−0.058***	0.011	−0.057***	0.011	−0.073***	0.011	−0.061***	0.013
−0.002	0.007	−0.002	0.007	−0.008	0.007	−0.008	0.008
0.000	0.000	0.000	0.000	0.000	0.000	0.000	0.000
0.096**	0.051	0.099**	0.050	0.104***	0.050	0.076	0.055
−0.029	0.058	−0.024	0.057	0.043	0.057	0.033	0.059
−0.017	0.067	−0.006	0.067	0.093	0.068	0.007	0.073
0.115	0.130	0.111	0.129	0.206*	0.133	0.107	0.145
−0.318***	0.072	−0.311***	0.072	−0.268***	0.076	−0.179***	0.083
0.006	0.075	0.003	0.075	−0.036	0.076	0.030	0.085
−0.275***	0.069	−0.281***	0.069	−0.274***	0.072	−0.175***	0.082
−0.172***	0.080	−0.172***	0.080	−0.151**	0.082	−0.064	0.088
0.047***	0.006	0.047***	0.006	0.027***	0.006	0.023***	0.007
0.454***	0.076	0.455***	0.076	0.360***	0.076	0.301***	0.085
−0.065	0.211	−0.077	0.208	−0.108	0.196	−0.117	0.220
0.443***	0.110	0.465***	0.109	0.398***	0.111	0.342***	0.113
−0.065	0.168	−0.064	0.165	−0.107	0.156	−0.105	0.180
−0.036	0.031	−0.040	0.031	−0.051*	0.032	−0.018	0.037
				−0.014	0.136	−0.052	0.143
				0.184	0.147	0.105	0.154
				0.533***	0.210	0.415**	0.235
				0.747***	0.232	0.557***	0.262
				0.199***	0.060	0.141***	0.068
				−0.053	0.128	−0.149	0.145
				0.202***	0.074	0.175***	0.082
				−0.065	0.103	0.005	0.109
				0.280***	0.110	0.190**	0.114
				0.449***	0.052	0.354***	0.060
				0.321***	0.051	0.279***	0.057
						−0.240***	0.063
						−0.553***	0.129
						0.309***	0.111
						−0.503***	0.198
						0.339***	0.074
						−0.077	0.074
						0.078	0.063
						0.557***	0.058
−1.074	0.858	0.594***	0.222	0.865***	0.259	0.536**	0.321
Yes		Yes		Yes		Yes	
Yes		Yes		Yes		Yes	
7,181		7,181		7,181		5,897	

neighborhoods with better socio-economic conditions, to evaluate the existence, magnitude, and direction of neighborhood effects for some socioeconomic and health outcomes.[30] Since neighborhoods having better socioeconomic conditions usually have lower crime rates, an experiment like the one they study could be used to inquire for individual's life satisfaction and assess the effect of crime on it once endogenous location is controlled for, in order to provide additional support to our findings. Alternatively, a potential new experimental design could randomize households living in high homicide rate neighborhoods into low homicide rate neighborhoods, and then proceed to assess the relationship between crime and life satisfaction.

Other interesting questions to investigate in future research include the study of the effects on life satisfaction of other types of crimes such as robbery, drug trafficking, etc. This chapter provides evidence of a negative effect of the homicide rate on life satisfaction; however, we do not know how the incidence of other crimes affects life satisfaction of individuals; in particular, considering that different types of crimes often affect different populations. For example, Gaviria and Velez (2001) find that in Colombia, homicides and domestic violence are disproportionately borne by the poor, and property crime and kidnappings by the rich. Di Tella et al. (2010) find that in Argentina, the poor are more vulnerable to being victimized in general and are more affected by home robberies, but as affected as the rich by street robberies.

Finally, this research provides some key policy implications. First, our results are consistent with the existence of a substitution effect between the homicide rates and income; to keep their life satisfaction constant when households choose to live in neighborhoods with lower homicide rates, they end up with lower disposable income and vice versa. That is, individuals are in fact paying with their income an economic cost in order to avoid crime and, in particular, to avoid high homicide rates. This result is in line with Gaviria et al. (2010a) who find evidence for Bogotá of the capitalization of lower homicide rates in higher property values. This chapter provides further evidence of how imperfectly security is provided across neighborhoods in the main Colombian cities and the way households privately and endogenously auction it. The negative capitalization of crime, and particularly of homicides, reflects an institutional limitation of the authorities to provide an equitable access to public goods. Map 6.3 shows that in fact the homicide rate is concentrated among some specific areas, which turn out to be the poorest ones. Even though many households are willing to pay to avoid crime (homicides), just a few are actually able to pay for it, what leads on the one hand to the emergence of urban private markets for security (a supposedly pure public good), while on the other hand prevents the poorest from getting security. Second, we find a measure of the impact of the cost of crime to societies that go beyond the traditional economic measures like its impact on earnings, wealth, its fiscal impact or its impact on economic growth, to an intangible one, like it is life satisfaction. Since life satisfaction is a much broader concept, it

---

[30] The research design is based on comparisons of three groups to which households were randomly assigned in the moving to opportunity social experiment, operated in five cities of the USA: Baltimore, Boston, Chicago, Los Angeles, and New York.

might also be capturing psychological, mental, social, and other relevant dimensions on which higher homicide rates affect welfare.

Acknowledgments We thank the Judicial Police Sectional of the National Police Department, (SIJIN), and the Administrative Department of Municipal Planning of Medellín, for providing the data; and Jorge Eliécer Giraldo for assistance. We also thank comments received by two anonymous referees. The opinions expressed here are those of the authors and not of the *Banco de la República de Colombia* nor of its Board.

Appendix 1

We use a bivariate kernel density estimator to construct the variables used in our estimations (homicide rate, distance to crime, and arrest rates), and the maps. We use two variables: the distance, in meters, from the centroid of each block to the place where the homicide was committed, and numbers of months elapsed between the date of each homicide and the date the survey was carried out. Given random r-vectors $X_1, X_2, \ldots, X_n$, the multivariate kernel density estimator is defined as

$$\hat{p}_H(x) = \frac{1}{n|H|} \sum_{i=1}^{n} K\left(H^{-1}(x - X_i)\right), \quad x \in \mathfrak{R}^r,$$

where H is a $(r \times r)$ nonsingular matrix that generalizes the window width and K is a multivariate function with mean 0 and integrates to 1. We tried with Bartlett Epanechnikov kernel since it is the one with the minimal asymptotic integral squared error, and Gaussian kernel. We use *rule-of-thumb method* and likelihood cross-validation to the window width.

Appendix 2

Variable	Description
Homicide rate	Homicide rate per 10,000 inhabitants, by block of each individual interviewed by ECV 2008 (constructed with Kernel procedure)
Capture rate/homicide rate	Homicide rate per 10,000 inhabitants divided by capture rate per 10,000 inhabitants of the block where the individual live (constructed with Kernel procedure)
Distance to crime	Average distance between the centroid of each block where individual interviewed by ECV 2008 live and the place where homicides occurred (Estimated using the Kernel)
Years living in this place	ECV 2008 asked how many year the people have been living in the place where they are actually living

(continued)

(continued)

Variable	Description
Safe neighborhood	We constructed a dummy variables that is 1 if individuals answered to have "very safe" and "safe" feeling perceptions of the neighborhood or district where you live
Victim of robbery, burglary, personal	We constructed a dummy variable that is 1 if individuals interviewed or other member of their household were victims of robbery, burglary, personal.
Victim of other offenses	We constructed a dummy variable that is 1 if individuals interviewed or other member of their household were victims of other offenses
Household income	The sum of the income of the members of the household.
Number of persons in household	Number of persons living currently in the same home
Age	Age of the interviewed individual
Age 2	Age of the interviewed individual squared
Male	Dummy variable if the interviewed individual is male
Household head with primary	Dummy variable equal to 1 if educational level of the household head is at least primary studies
Household head with secondary	Dummy variable equal to 1 if educational level of the household head is at least secondary studies
Hold head with technique education	Dummy variable equal to 1 if educational level of the household head is at least technique studies
Household head single	Dummy variable equal to 1 if the household head is single
Household head married	Dummy variable equal to 1 if the household head is married
Household head separated	Dummy variable equal to 1 if the household head is separated
Household head lives with partner	Dummy variable equal to 1 if the household head lives with partner
Educational attainment	Educational attainment
House with fixed phone line	Dummy variable equal to 1 if the house has fixed phone line
House with electricity	Dummy variable equal to 1 if the house has electricity
House with aqueduct	Dummy variable equal to 1 if the house has aqueduct
House with sewerage	Dummy variable equal to 1 if the house has sewerage
Number of rooms in household	Number of rooms in household
Socioeconomic stratum 2	Dummy variable equal to 1 if socioeconomic stratum where individual live is equal to 2
Socioeconomic stratum 3	Dummy variable equal to 1 if socioeconomic stratum where individual live is equal to 3
Socioeconomic stratum 4	Dummy variable equal to 1 if socioeconomic stratum where individual live is equal to 4
Socioeconomic stratum 5 or 6	Dummy variable equal to 1 if socioeconomic stratum where individual live is equal to 5 or 6
Homeownership, house totally paid	Dummy variable equal to 1 if the house is own and totally paid
Homeownership, house partially paid	Dummy variable equal to 1 if the house is own and partially paid
Tenant	Tenant
House with gas for cooking	Dummy variable equal to 1 if the house has gas for cooking
House with natural gas	Dummy variable equal to 1 if the house has gas natural gas
House with internet	Dummy variable equal to 1 if the house has internet

(continued)

(continued)

Variable	Description
House with cable TV	Dummy variable equal to 1 if the house has cable TV
Employed	Dummy variable if individual is employed
Unemployed	Dummy variable if individual is unemployed
Household occupation rate	Number of people with employment divided by the number of persons in household
Household unemployment rate	Number of people unemployment divided by the number of persons in household
Enrolled in private health insurance	Dummy variable equal to 1 if interviewed is enrolled in private health insurance
Enrolled in public health insurance	Dummy variable equal to 1 if interviewed is enrolled in public health insurance
Enrolled in pension fund	Dummy variable equal to 1 if interviewed is enrolled in pension fund
Good health	Dummy variable equal to 1 if the interviewed answer to has "very good" health or "good" health
Constant	Constant
FE past neighborhood	Fixed effect of past neighborhood
FE current neighborhood	Fixed effect of current neighborhood

References

Alesina, A., Di Tella, R. & MacCulloch, R. (2004). Inequality and happiness: are Europeans and Americans different? *Journal of Public Economics, 88*(9–10), 2009–2042.

Blanchflower, D. G., & Oswald, A. J. (2004). Well-being over time in Britain and the USA. *Journal of Public Economics, 88*(7–8), 1359–1386.

Bullinton, B. (1992). A smuggler's paradise: cocaine trafficking through the Bahamas. In A. W. McCoy & A. A. Block (Eds.), *War on drugs: Studies in the failure of U.S. narcotics policy* (pp. 209–236). Boulder: Westview Press.

Buvinic, M., Morrison, A., & Orlando, M. B. (2005). Violencia, crimen y desarrollo Social en América Latina y el Caribe. *Papeles de Población, 043*, 167–214.

Clark, A. E., & Oswald, A. J. (1994). Unhappiness and unemployment. *The Economic Journal, 104*(424), 648–659.

Cohen, M. A. (2008). The effect of crime on life satisfaction. *The Journal of Legal Studies, 37*(S2), S325–S353.

Cohen, M., & Rubio, M. (2007). *Violence and crime in Latin America*. Solution Paper, Copenhagen Consensus and Inter-American Development Bank, San José.

Cutrona, C. E., Russella, D. W., Hesslinga, R. M., Brown, P. A., & Murryc, V. (2000). Direct and moderating effects of community context on the psychological well-being of African American women. *Journal of Personality and Social Psychology, 79*, 1088–1101.

Deaton, A. (2008). Income, health, and well-being around the world: evidence from the gallup world poll. *Journal of Economic Perspectives, 22*(2), 53–72.

Di Tella, R., MacCulloch, R. J., & Oswald, A. J. (2001). Preferences over inflation and unemployment: Evidence from surveys of happiness. *The American Economic Review, 91*(1), 335–341.

Di Tella, R., MacCulloch, R. J., & Oswald, A. J. (2003). The macroeconomics of happiness. *The Review of Economics and Statistics, 85*(4), 809–827.

Di Tella, R., MacCulloch, R., & Ñopo, H. (2008). *Happiness and beliefs in criminal environments*. RES Working Paper (IADB), 4605.

Di Tella, R., Galiani, S., & Schargrodsky, E. (2010). Crime distribution and victim behavior during a crime wave. In R. Di Tella, S. Edwards, & E. Schargrodsky (Eds.), *The economics of crime: Lessons for and from Latin America* (pp. 175–204). Chicago: National Bureau of Economic Research and The University of Chicago Press.

Diener, E., Suh, E. M., Lucas, R. E., & Smith, H. L. (1999). Subjective well-being: Three decades of progress. *Psychological Bulletin, 125*(2), 276–302.

Easterlin, R. A. (1974). Does economic growth improve the human lot? In P. A. David & M. W. Reder (Eds.), *Nations and households in economic growth: Essays in honour of Moses Abramowitz* (pp. 89–125). New York: Academic.

Easterlin, R. (2001). Income and happiness: Towards a unified theory. *The Economic Journal, 111*(473), 465–484.

Ferrer-i-Carbonell, A., & Frijters, P. (2004). How important is methodology for the estimates of the determinants of happiness? *The Economic Journal, 114*(497), 641–659.

Franzini, L., Caughy, M., Murray, S., & O'Campo, P. (2008). Perceptions of disorder: Contributions of neighborhood characteristics to subjective perceptions of disorder. *Journal of Environmental Psychology, 28*, 83–93.

Frey, B. S., & Stutzer, A. (1999). Measuring preferences by subjective well-being. *Journal of Institutional and Theoretical Economics, 155*(4), 755–788.

Gamarra, E. A. (2003). La diáspora colombiana en el sur de la Florida. In *Memorias del Seminario sobre Migración Internacional Colombiana y la Conformación de Comunidades Transnacionales*. Bogotá: Ministerio de Relaciones Exteriores.

Gaviria, A., & Vélez, C. E. (2001). *Who bears the burden of crime in Colombia?* Fedesarrollo: Informes de Investigación.

Gaviria, A., Medina, C., Morales, L., & Núñez, J. (2010a). The cost of avoiding crime: The case of Bogotá. In R. Di Tella, S. Edwards, & E. Schargrodsky (Eds.), *The economics of crime: Lessons for and from Latin America* (pp. 175–204). Chicago: National Bureau of Economic Research and The University of Chicago Press.

Gaviria, A., Medina, C., & Tamayo, J. A. (2010b). *Assessing the link between adolescent fertility and urban crime*. Borradores de Economía, 594.

Geis, K. J., & Ross, C. E. (1998). A new look at urban alienation: The effect of neighborhood disorder on perceived. *Social Psychology Quarterly, 61*(3), 232–246.

Giraldo, J. (2008). Urban armed conflict and homicidal violence: The Medellín case Urvio. *Revista Latinoamericana de Seguridad Ciudadana, 5*, 99–113.

Giraldo, J. E., Medina, C., & Tamayo, J. A. (2010). A characterization of crime in Medellín. Borradores de Economía, Banco de la República (forthcoming).

Graham, C., & Pettinato, S. (2002). *Happiness and hardship: Opportunity and insecurity in new market economies*. Washington, DC: Brookings Institution Press.

Gugliotta, G., & Leen, J. (1989). *Kings of cocaine inside the Medellín cartel an astonishing true story of murder, money and international corruption*. New York: Simon and Schuster.

Heckman, J. J., & Masterov, D. V. (2007). The productivity argument for investing in young children. *Review of Agricultural Economics, 29*(3), 446–493.

Helburn, N. (1982). Geography and quality of life. *Annals of the Association of American Geographers, 72*(4), 445–456.

Information System for Security and Coexistence – SISC. (2009). Boletín Semestral de Violencia Homicida en Medellín, Primer Semestre de 2009. Alcaldía de Medellín.

Kling, J. R., Liebman, J. B., & Katz, L. F. (2005). Experimental analysis of neighborhood effects. *Econometrica, 75*(1), 83–119.

Krug, E. G., Dahlberg, L. L., Mercy, J. A., Zwi, A. B., & Lozano, R. (2002). *World report on violence and health*. Geneva: World Health Organization.

Latkin, C. A., & Curry, A. D. (2003). Stressful neighborhoods and depression: A prospective study of the impact of neighborhood disorder. *Journal of Health and Social Behavior, 44*(1), 34–44.

Latkin, C. A., German, D., Hua, W., & Curry, A. D. (2009). Individual-level influences on perceptions of neighborhood disorder: A multilevel analysis. *Journal of Community Psychology, 37*(1), 122–133.

Layard, R. (2005). *Happiness: Lessons from a new science.* New York: The Penguin Books.

Lochner, L., & Moretti, E. (2004). The effect of education on crime: Evidence from prison inmates, arrests, and self-reports. *The American Economic Review, 94*(1), 155–189.

McBride, M. J. (2001). Relative income effects on subjective well-being in the cross-section. *Journal of Economic Behavior and Organization, 45*(3), 251–278.

Medina, C., Morales, L., & Núñez, J. (2010). Quality of life in urban neighborhoods of Bogotá and Medellín, Colombia. In E. Lora, A. Powell, B. Praag, & P. Sanguinetti (Eds.), *The quality of life in Latin American cities: Markets and perceptions* (pp. 117–160). Washington, DC: Inter-American Development Bank and the World Bank.

Michalos, A. C., & Zumbo, B. D. (2000). Criminal victimization and the quality of life. *Social Indicators Research, 50,* 245–295.

Palau, J. C., & Llorente, M. V. (2009). Reintegración y seguridad ciudadana en Medellín: Un balance del programa de paz y reconciliación (2004–2008). Informes FIP, 8.

Parkes, A., Kearns, A., & Atkinson, R. (2002). What makes people dissatisfied with their neighborhoods? *Urban Studies, 39*(13), 2413–2438.

Powdthavee, N. (2005). Unhappiness and crime: Evidence for South Africa. *Economica, 72*(3), 531–547.

Riley, K. J. (1996). *Snow job? The war against international cocaine trafficking.* New Brunswick: Transaction Publishers.

Ross, C. E., & Jang, S. J. (2000). Neighborhood disorder, fear, and mistrust: The buffering role of social ties with neighbors. *American Journal of Community Psychology, 28*(4), 401–420.

Ross, C. E., Reynolds, J. R., & GeisSource, K. J. (2000). The contingent meaning of neighborhood stability for residents' psychological well-being. *American Sociological Review, 65*(4), 581–597.

Sampson, R. J., & Raudenbush, S. W. (2004). Seeing disorder: Neighborhood stigma and the social construction of "Broken Windows". *Social Psychology Quarterly, 67*(4), 319–342.

Scarborough, B. K., Like-Haislip, T. Z., Novak, K. J., Lucas, W. L., & Alarid, L. F. (2010). Assessing the relationship between individual characteristics, neighborhood context, and fear of crime. *Journal of Criminal Justice, 38,* 819–826.

Sirgy, M. J., & Cornwell, T. (2002). How neighborhood features affect quality of life. *Social Indicators Research, 59*(1), 79–114.

Soares, R., & Naritomi, J. (2010). Understanding high crime rates in Latin America: The role of social and policy factors. In R. Di Tella, S. Edwards, & E. Schargrodsky (Eds.), *The economics of crime: Lessons for and from Latin America* (pp. 175–204). Chicago: National Bureau of Economic Research and the University of Chicago Press.

Thoumi, F. (1995). *The political economy of illegal drugs in Colombia.* Boulder: Lynne Rienner Press.

Villamarin, L. A. (1996). *The FARC cartel.* Editions The Pharaoh, Bogotá, Colombia.

Winkelmann, L., & Winkelmann, R. (1998). Why are the unemployed so unhappy? *Economica, 65*(257), 1–15.

Chapter 7
State of Affliction: Fear of Crime and Quality of Life in South Africa

Benjamin J. Roberts

1 Introduction

> Everywhere I went, the issue of crime was raised, alongside issues like unemployment and the cost of living… When the people talk to me I can see the fear in their eyes and hear the desperation in their voices (*President Jacob Zuma, The Star, 29th December 2008*)

Few issues in South Africa today provoke as emotive a response as that of crime. Since the release of official crime statistics in late 2006, the country has witnessed a vigorous and intensifying public debate about the credibility of the emerging trends and the efficacy of the policy and programmatic responses. Crime persistently features as a pressing national priority area among citizens in public opinion surveys. In addition, media images of violent criminal acts and mounting public disaffection abound. Yet, this chapter is not primarily concerned with the actual levels of victimisation in South Africa but rather with the fear of crime, which remains an increasingly salient though largely under-researched related social phenomenon in the country.

Interest in people's anxieties about personal safety seems to have derived, at least in part, from recognition of the complex and detrimental effects that fear of criminal violence imparts on quality of life at the individual, community and societal levels. These include a reliance on racial stereotypes in discussion on crime, constraints on people's mobility and ability to socialise, a hastening retreat from public space and the proliferation of gated communities, high walls and fences and an array of private security measures (Louw 1997; Lemanski 2004). Such anxieties may also diminish the sense of trust and cohesion within communities, as well as provide mounting

B.J. Roberts (✉)
Democracy, Governance and Service Delivery Research Programme,
Human Sciences Research Council (HSRC), Private Bag X07, Dalbridge,
Durban 4014, South Africa
e-mail: broberts@hsrc.ac.za

D. Webb and E. Wills-Herrera (eds.), *Subjective Well-Being and Security*,   149
Social Indicators Research Series 46, DOI 10.1007/978-94-007-2278-1_7,
© Springer Science+Business Media B.V. 2012

appeals for punitive measures such as the death penalty and lend credibility to vigilante violence (Jackson 2006; Møller 2005). As Valji et al. (2004, p. 3) reflect, these forms of behaviour pose a threat in terms of fuelling cycles of violence, challenging the entrenchment of a culture of human rights and ultimately acting as an impediment to further progress in reconciliation in the country.

Concern about personal safety can clearly exert an influence at the policy level too. For example, in a situation where a sizable proportion of the public views migrants and political refugees from other countries as a threat in respect of criminal activity, then public fears could impose pressure for the adoption of rather protectionist immigration policy. Public demands for the government and the South African Police Service to better manage the crime situation, coupled the seeming refusal of many people to accept the official message that crime rates are not rising, may be seen as indicative of the relative influence of public's views about safety and security (Jackson 2006, p. 253).

For many of the reasons articulated above, the fear of crime has become a prominent social and political problem in international circles. This is especially true of Britain, the USA and Europe, where it has frequently been heralded as a public concern that is at least as pressing as crime itself (Gilchrist et al. 1998). Since the 1960s, the fear of crime in its own right has been the focus of increasing attention of researchers and policymakers. Countless studies have been conducted with the aim of understanding, monitoring and evaluating fear of crime, with many concluding that 'such fear continues to impinge upon the well-being of a proportion of the population' (Gilchrist et al. 1998, p. 283). This body of work has additionally pointed to an unequal distribution of both crime and the fear of crime, with some people demonstrating increased risk of victimisation while others are more acutely and regularly fearful (Farrall and Gadd 2004, p. 499). This finding and recognition of the harm that fear can cause to individuals and communities has led some governments to respond by establishing the reduction of the fear of crime as a social objective distinct from reducing actual crime and warranting specific government interventions (see, for example, Home Office 2004). The South African government appears to be following suit, with one of the twelve high-level priority outcomes that were adopted by the new Zuma administration following the 2009 general elections focusing on the objective that 'all people in South Africa are and feel safe'.

This chapter begins by briefly reviewing previous research on fear of crime and its effect of quality of life, followed by a methodological section that critically reflects on the limitations associated with measuring fear of crime and describes the data and principal measures available for the analysis. It then focuses on estimates of worry about crime using a newly developed categorical scale. This is followed by sections attempting to discern significant demographic, social and spatial differentials in these perceptions and establish the extent to which crime-related variables (including fear) explain global indicators such as satisfaction with life. By so doing, this investigation hopes to make a modest contribution to the evidence base about the nature of fear of crime in non-Western countries.

2 Prior Research on Fear of Crime and Quality of Life

Despite the proliferation of scholarship on criminal victimisation, personal safety and fear of crime over the last few decades, a review of more than 6,000 publication abstracts conducted a decade ago by Michalos and Zumbo (2000, p. 246) revealed that scant attention had been devoted to studying the interconnections between measures of individual criminal victimisation and quality of life. Five years later, Møller (2005) supplemented this literature search by examining approximately 600 journals published by Kluwer between 1997 and 2004 and identified a mere three articles in addition to the Michalos and Zumbo (2000) paper that probe the crime–quality-of-life relationship. If one were to narrow the search terms to focus more explicitly on the relationship between fear of crime and quality of life, the accumulated empirical evidence on this admittedly complex phenomenon remains highly circumscribed, somewhat contradictory and based predominantly on local area studies.

In the last decade, there has been a modest expansion in published research on crime and quality of life. In their influential investigation in Prince George, British Columbia, Michalos and Zumbo (2000) demonstrated that fear and experience of criminal victimisation, together with other crime-related measures, accounted for less than ten percent of variation in happiness, life satisfaction and satisfaction with quality of life scores. In a study conducted in the Los Angeles Metropolitan Area, Adams and Serpe (2000) show that fear of crime is negatively correlated with social integration, control or mastery over one's environment, and life satisfaction. Multivariate analysis, however, shows that fear of crime does not have a significant direct effect on life satisfaction but instead appears to indirectly influence life satisfaction by reducing one's senses of control over their life. Kitchen and Williams (2010) analyse data from telephonic surveys and in-depth interviews that were conducted among residents of Saskatoon, Canada, in 2001, 2004 and 2007 and show that the odds of being more fearful rises significantly as level of satisfaction with life falls in rounds of interviewing.

There has also been recent attention to the effects of fear of crime in the British research literature. Jackson et al. (2007) analyse the 2003/2004 British Crime Survey and find statistically significant associations ($p < .001$) between level of worry over specific types of criminal victimisation and perceived impact of crime on individual quality of life. In addition, the study provides evidence that the frequency of worry about crime is inversely related to quality of life, with a greater detrimental impact being reported among those who stated they worried often about robbery, burglary, and car crime increase during the year prior to being interviewed. Other studies have revealed the damaging effect of fear of crime on psychological well-being and physical functioning (Stafford et al. 2007; Jackson and Stafford 2009). Jackson and Gray (2010) differentiate between dysfunctional and functional fear of crime, the former referring to worry that erodes quality of life and the latter relating to situations where the fearful adopt precautionary measures that offset the potential negative effect on quality of life. Their investigation in parts of London shows that about three-quarters of the fearful were in the dysfunctional category and a quarter in the functional.

Building on this work, Jackson and Kuha (2010) examine cross-national European Social Survey (ESS) data and find a positive correlation between frequency of worry and perceived seriousness of its impact of quality of life, and conclude that 20–30% of citizens in the surveyed countries experience some form of 'dysfunctional or damaging fear of crime' that imparts moderate to serious effects on quality of life. Moore (2006) also uses ESS data to show that fear of crime has a significant negative association with happiness.

Of particular relevance to the current study are the studies that have begun to investigate the crime–quality-of-life nexus in developing country contexts. In South Africa, Møller (2005) finds that fear of crime and worry about personal safety in Nelson Mandela Metropolitan Municipality exerts a more negative impact on satisfaction with life as a whole relative to the experience of criminal victimisation. In fact, in a number of instances, victims of crime reported equivalent or higher levels of life satisfaction and domain satisfaction than non-victims. This notable study has since been complemented with other research based on national survey data. Using the nationally representative 1993 SALDRU study, Kingdon and Knight (2006) find that safety from criminal victimisation had a small but statistically significant negative effect on life satisfaction. Based on an assessment of the 1997 October Household Survey (OHS), conducted by Statistics South Africa, Powdthavee (2005) further analyses the relationship between victimisation and perceived quality of life. Unlike Møller (2005), he finds that life satisfaction is significantly lower among victims of crime than non-victims when controlling for household expenditure and other related characteristics. Also in line with expectations, he shows that non-victims are less satisfied with life when they reside in areas with a higher incidence of crime.

Based on data from the 2005 South African Social Attitudes Survey (SASAS), Roberts (2010) provides mixed evidence on the relationship between conventional single-item fear of crime measures and quality of life. While a significant, negative relationship was apparent between feeling personally safe on most days and life satisfaction, those who were more fearful of walking alone in their neighbourhood after dark were not significantly less satisfied with life than those who were unafraid. Examples of other evidence from developing countries include findings from Ghana that found that satisfaction with community quality of life was a predictor of fear of crime (Adu-Mireku 2002) and the Malawian study by Davies and Hinks (2010), which shows a strong negative relationship between feeling unsafe and life satisfaction on aggregate and irrespective of wealth status.

3   Method

3.1   On Measuring Fear of Crime

The swift growth, complexity and sophistry of research on fear of crime in recent years have been accompanied by an inevitable increase in methodological reflection on the adequacy of the instruments traditionally used to examine this phenomenon.

Out of this endeavour, a literature has developed that proposes various refinements to early measures employed in the field of study. Following a useful review by Farrall et al. (1997), the principal methodological objections raised in relation to quantitative examinations of fear of crime relate to the generally static nature of surveys and their capacity to capture complex social processes, *conceptual* ambiguity of what is meant by 'fear of crime' and *operational* concerns about the design and phrasing of survey questions. Cumulatively, these problems have sowed doubts about the extent to which estimates of the incidence of fear of crime serve as valid representations of a social event or alternatively whether they are being distorted by shortcomings in the measurement instruments and techniques (Farrall et al. 1997, p. 672).

One of the earliest and most common questions used by researchers to gauge fear of crime enquires about how safe an individual felt in their local area, and surveys have typically included variants on the following form: 'How safe do you feel walking alone in this area after dark?'. Ferraro and LaGrange (1987) have classified this line of questioning as measuring 'formless' fears that relate to a vague threat to personal security and distinguish it from measures aimed at capturing 'concrete' fears that refer to a particular crime (e.g. types of property crime or individual/personal crime). This distinction has also been dubbed as being between 'global' and 'crime-specific' measures. Some of the criticisms that have tended to be levelled at the global questions include:

- Failing to make direct reference to crime at all
- Using a rather imprecise geographical reference – the 'neighbourhood' or 'local area'
- Asking about an activity which many people may rarely do ('walking alone after dark'), either out of preference or do due to physical limitation (especially for the elderly)
- Referring neither to a specific time period nor the frequency of fearful experiences (e.g. number of times in the past year that the person felt unsafe) (Farrall and Gadd 2004, pp. 494–95; Hale 1996; Ferraro and LaGrange 1987).

One common response to such criticisms of the global measure of fear of crime has been to make mere phrase changes to include words that more explicitly refer to fear (e.g. asking about how *afraid* or *fearful* rather than how *unsafe*). Another has been for surveys to ask respondents a broader range of questions, such as asking directly about concern over becoming a victim of different types of crime rather than crime in general (i.e. concrete or crime-specific fears) or referring to general feelings of unsafety when at home alone at night (Pantazis 2000). There does, however, remain scepticism about whether such refinements have in fact done much to overcome the methodological limitations of the global measures (Farrall et al. 1997).

There has been some recent experimental research aimed at improving the conceptualisation of fear of crime in addition to the validity of the measurement tools. A full review is not possible here, but arguably the most salient new body of work is that by Stephen Farrall, Jonathan Jackson and colleagues in the UK that was supported by Economic and Social Research Council (ESRC). This research has demonstrated the conceptual complexities inherent in responses to general fear of crime questions. The quantitative studies by Jackson (2004, 2006), Farrall et al. (2009), Gray et al. (2008a, b) and Jackson and Gray (2010) suggest that fear of crime is an expressive in addition to an experiential phenomenon. The expressive component is akin to 'a more diffuse/ambient anxiety'. It is a general awareness of the likelihood or risk of victimisation that is informed by evaluations of many interrelated insecurities about social and physical change in domains such as social cohesion and interpersonal trust, community values, norms and moral standards, as well as declining neighbourhood conditions and disorder. Alternatively, experiential fear is seen as 'an everyday worry', a set of tangible emotions deriving from a feeling that one's personal safety is being directly threatened.

What does this conceptual distinction mean for measuring the fear of crime? Farrall and Gadd (2004), Jackson (2004) and Gray et al. (2008a, b) all argue that the conventional survey-based questions on the *intensity* of fear of crime ('*how* worried or afraid are you?') are tapping into more general anxiety or expressive fear. As such, it is argued that the prevalence of fear may be overestimated since these measures fail to take into account the *frequency* of fear ('*how often* are you worried or afraid?') or the *impact* of such worries on everyday life. Empirical results suggest that intensity and frequency measures do not closely correspond, with many people scoring highly on intensity of fear measures but reporting low scores on the frequency items, i.e. they are generally quite worried about being victimised but this worry is not regularly manifest (Farrall and Gadd 2004; Gray et al. 2008a, b; Farrall et al. 2009). With their narrower focus on episodic experiences of fear, it has been suggested that the frequency of worry questions appear to be more effective at capturing experiential fear (Jackson 2004).

A further complication in understanding fear of crime is the difference between functional and dysfunctional fear (Jackson and Gray 2010). The implication being that not all fear may be damaging, and that in certain instances, it may provoke precautionary behaviour and measures that buffer against the potentially negative consequences of worries about crime on quality of life.

These conceptual developments in understanding worries about crime have led to the proposal that in combining responses to frequency and impact of fear measures, more precise estimates of the everyday experience of the fear of crime can be derived that focus on the emotional experience that adversely affects well-being. As Jackson and Kuha (2010, p. 5) assert, 'if we – as a community of scholars – are interested in fear of crime as a serious social problem, it is important to measure both the frequency of worry (to capture the pattern of lived experience) and negative impact (to capture the corrosive effect of such experience)'. Rounds 3 and 4 of the European Social Survey (2006 and 2008) incorporated a set of four new items alongside old walking-alone measure that encompass the frequency and impact of burglary and violent crime. The specific form of these questions is as follows:

1. 'How often, if at all, do you worry about your home being burgled?', with the response categories 'All or most of the time', 'Some of the time', 'Just occasionally' and 'Never'.

2. (If the answer is other than 'Never') 'Does this worry about your home being burgled have a serious effect on the quality of your life, some effect or no real effect on the quality of your life?'.

3–4. Two questions with similar phrasing, though 'your home being burgled' is substituted with 'becoming a victim of violent crime'.

It is this more experientially based definition and measurement approach to fear of crime that is adopted in this chapter and applied to the South African context.

3.2   Data

The present study draws on data from the 2009 round of the South African Social Attitudes Survey (SASAS), a repeated cross-sectional survey that has been conducted annually by the Human Sciences Research Council (HSRC) since 2003. The survey round consists of nationally representative probability samples of 3,305 South African adults aged 16 years and over living in private households. Each SASAS round of interviewing consists of a sub-sample of 500 Population Census enumeration areas (EAs), stratified by province, geographical subtype and majority population group. Designed as a time series, SASAS aims to providing a unique, long-term account of the speed and direction of change in underlying public values and the social fabric of modern South Africa. Apart from a standard set of demographic and background variables, the questionnaires contain a core module, which is repeated each round, with the aim of monitoring change and continuity in a variety of socioeconomic and sociopolitical variables over time. In addition to the core module, each round of interviewing accommodates rotating modules on specific themes, the aim being to provide detailed attitudinal evidence to inform policy and academic debate. The study design and research tools were approved by the HSRC's Research Ethics Committee (REC). Participants are asked for written informed consent, while written permission for young South Africans less than 18 years is also secured from their parents/guardians.

While recognising the salience of crime-related issues as a national priority in the South African context and the consequent need to include appropriate measures as part of the core SASAS module, the survey does not purport to be a national victimisation survey that can accommodate a broad range of questions on the experience and perceptions of crime. In an attempt to include a suitably broad set of social attitudes, the space available for a fairly exhaustive attitudinal investigation of fear of crime is unfortunately quite constrained. Therefore, since Round 3 (2005), the survey has included several global measures, as follows:

• How safe or unsafe do you feel personally on most days?
• How safe or unsafe do you feel walking alone in this area after dark?
• How safe or unsafe do you feel walking alone in this area during the day?

The rationale for including the first of the three measures was due to its inclusion in earlier annual HSRC attitudinal surveys. Between 1991 and 1997, the phrasing of the question was 'How safe do you feel in South Africa today?', but the current form was introduced in 1998. The other two measures have been included in previous national Victims of Crime Surveys.

Due to concerns about the adequacy of the SASAS fear of crime measures, these standard items have recently begun to be supplemented by the experimental fear of crime measures derived from the European Social Survey (as discussed above). The fifth round of SASAS in 2007 introduced the two ESS frequency items concerning worry about burglary and violent crime, together with the experience of victimisation question. In both sixth and seventh SASAS rounds (2008 and 2009), the remaining two ESS impact on quality of life questions were also added, opening up possibilities for replicating the Jackson and Kuha (2010) fear of crime classification approach based upon these variables.

In terms of quality of life, all rounds of the survey have included the common satisfaction with life-as-a-whole measure using a five-point Likert scale. In the tradition of Andrews and Withey (1976), this global measure of life satisfaction employs a single-item, unitary approach. However, increasing attention has been devoted to measuring life satisfaction as an aggregate of various individual life domains, with specific domain scores being averaged to yield a measure of global subjective well-being (Cummins 1996b). This is partly due to the recognition that the global question is unable to provide meaningful information on the life components that contribute to an individual's overall sense of well-being. With this in mind, the 2009 SASAS round included the Personal Wellbeing Index (*PWI*) (Cummins et al. 2003), an example of a multi-item, quality of life instrument. This represented the first occasion the PWI was tested in a national probability sample in the country.

The PWI was developed as part of a barometer to measure satisfaction with life among Australians that evolved from the Comprehensive Quality of Life Scale (ComQol) (Cummins et al. 1994). Drawing on empirical and theoretical literature, the PWI consists of eight life domains which are conceived as the first-level deconstruction of satisfaction with life as a whole, namely, standard of living, health, achieving in life, relationships, safety, community connectedness, future security and spirituality/religion (Cummins et al. 2003). Respondents are asked to rate their satisfaction on an 11-point (0–10) end-defined response scale (Jones and Thurstone 1955), ranging from 0 (extremely dissatisfied) to 10 (extremely satisfied), after which respondent-level data from the eight domains is averaged and transformed into a 0–100 scale. The first four of the aforementioned domains were shown to be common to many multidimensional quality of life measures. So too was emotional well-being, of which the spirituality domain is an example. The safety and community domains were new additions, the former being proposed to incorporate concepts such as security, personal control, independence and autonomy, and residential stability, while community connectedness is intended to tap into concepts such as social class, community involvement and integration (Cummins 1996a, b). Although the safety domain has tended not to make a unique contribution to the explained variance in global life satisfaction in the Australian context, it has been retained due to the unique contribution it has been shown to make in other countries, such as Argentina and Slovakia (International Wellbeing Group 2006). Testing of the PWI to date has demonstrated it to be a reliable indicator of well-being, with cross-cultural validity (Lau et al. 2005; Tiliouine et al. 2006).

The PWI is based on the theoretical model of subjective well-being homeostasis (Cummins 1998; Cummins and Nistico 2002; Cummins et al. 2002). This derives from the observation from comparative data for Western countries that responses to the general satisfaction-with-life question are remarkably stable, with a tendency to range within a narrow band at the positive end of the satisfaction continuum. Accordingly, homeostasis theory postulates that SWB is 'actively controlled and maintained by a set of psychological devices…that function under the control of personality' (Cummins et al. 2003, p. 162), such that positive or negative life events produce transitory fluctuations in satisfaction with life prior to the devices returning it to the individual's homeostatic 'set point'. While processes of adaptation typically facilitate the recovery back to set-point level following the experience of negative events or emotions, Cummins (2010) argues that in situations where these experiences are chronic and strong, as is the case with extreme poverty or anxiety, then homeostasis may be continually defeated and the capacity to recover frustrated. Though satisfaction with 'life as a whole' is considered an approximation of the homeostatic set point, the domains are considered less abstract, more distant from the homeostatic influence, and thus more sensitive to life conditions (Cummins et al. 2003).

In this chapter, the PWI, together with a satisfaction with life question that similarly uses an 11-point (0–10) end-defined response scale transformed into a 0–100 scale, will serve as the quality of life measures used for analysis.

4 Fear of Crime at the National Level

The pattern of responses to the four ESS survey questions on the frequency of worry and its impact on quality of life from the 2009 SASAS round is presented in Table 7.1. Approximately a third of adult South Africans indicated that they never worried about their home being burgled or becoming a victim of violent crime, while nearly half expressed worry either 'just occasionally' or 'some of the time'. For both types of crime, around a quarter of adults indicated that their worry was a constant presence in their lives. A similar distribution of responses is evident in relation to the items addressing the impact of worry on one's quality of life. For those that expressed some level of worry about the two crime types, only around a tenth (12%) felt it had 'no real effect', with a significant proportion (33% in the case of burglary and 31% for violent crime) acknowledging at least 'some effect'. This means that an estimated quarter of the adult population in South Africa (23% for burglary; 25% for violent crime) believes that the worries harboured about becoming victims of specific forms of crime are having a serious adverse impact on the quality of life.

Table 7.1 Frequencies and proportions of responses to four questions on worry about crime in South Africa, 2009

SASAS 2009	Worry about burglary		Worry about violent crime	
	Frequency	Weighted %	Frequency	Weighted %
	Frequency of worry		*Frequency of worry*	
Never	998	32.3	995	32.6
Just occasionally	596	17.6	556	15.7
Some of the time	928	28.7	977	30.2
All or most of the time	762	21.4	754	21.5
Total	3,284	100.0	3,282	100.0
(Missing)	21		23	
	Effect of worry on quality of life		*Effect of worry on quality of life*	
(Never worry)	998	32.7	995	32.7
No real effect	373	11.8	367	11.6
Some effect	1,097	32.8	1,076	30.5
Serious effect	786	22.7	824	25.2
Total	3,254	100.0	3,262	100.0
(Missing)	51		43	

Source: South African Social Attitudes Survey, Round 7 (2009)

Table 7.2 Estimated proportions of different effects on quality of life given frequency of worry about crime in South Africa, 2008–2009 (row %)

SASAS 2009	Effect of worry on quality of life				
	(Never worry)	No real effect	Some effect	Serious effect	Total
Worry about burglary					
Never	100				100
Just occasionally		40.0	51.0	9.0	100
Some of the time		12.8	69.8	17.4	100
All or most of the time		5.9	19.5	74.6	100
Total	32.7	11.8	32.8	22.7	100
Worry about violent crime					
Never	100				100
Just occasionally		44.8	46.6	8.6	100
Some of the time		12.3	65.9	21.9	100
All or most of the time		4.4	15.8	79.9	100
Total	32.7	11.6	30.5	25.2	100

Data: South African Social Attitudes Survey, Round 7 (2009)

Cross tabulations of the frequency and impact questions, as presented in Table 7.2, confirm what one would intuitively expect of the measures, namely that the more often one feels fearful of victimisation, the higher the perceived detrimental effect on quality of life. Bivariate analysis confirms the strong positive association between the frequency of worry and perceived impact on quality of life variables, with a Pearson Product-Moment Correlation Coefficient of 0.80 in relation to home burglary and 0.81 for violent crime. Both are statistically significant at the 0.01 level of confidence.

Following the model-assisted scoring method based on latent class modelling devised by Jackson and Kuha (2010), responses to the four items were combined into a single categorical fear of crime variable consisting of the six classes.[1] On aggregate, the 2009 data show that 34% of respondents were unworried, while 13% worried occasionally only about home burglary or only about violent crime (6% and 7%, respectively). A quarter of the adult population (23%) displayed moderate levels of worry, 4% had a fairly high level, while 27% were classified as having very high levels of worry.[2]

From a comparative perspective, these results suggest that South Africans are significantly more fearful than a majority of their counterparts in Europe. Comparing the 2009 SASAS results against those from 23 other developing and industrialised countries in Europe included in the 2006 round of the European Social Survey, South Africa is ranked as having the highest level of fear. On average for the ESS countries, 59% of respondents were unworried, with 28% falling in classes 4–6 combined and only 5% in class 6 (Jackson and Kuha 2010). By contrast, in South Africa, the share of respondents falling in the most worried category is, at 27%, more than five times higher than the ESS average, while the share in classes 4–6 is approximately double the ESS average. Therefore, from a cross-country perspective, fear of crime persists as a phenomenon that affects a sizable proportion of the South African population and, as such, warrants serious policy attention.

4.1   Contrasting Old and New Fear of Crime Measures

How does the new multi-item fear of crime measure relate to the old measures? Table 7.3 presents the joint distribution of the new measure and two of the standard measures, specifically the 'personally safe on most days' and the 'walking alone after dark' items. The new measure shows that 47% of the population was classified into the three least worried categories, with 53% in the three most worried categories. By comparison, 50% were safe or very safe on the personal safety item, with 32% feeling unsafe or very unsafe (the balance were neutral). Moreover, 69% felt unsafe on the walking-alone question relative to 31% feeling safe. This suggests

---

[1] In this chapter, use has been made of the classification derived by Jackson and Kuha (2010) using the pooled European Social Survey data from Round 3, which was shown to 'work in consistent and comparable ways in different countries' with country-level analysis suggesting that the 'measurement models show reasonable configural equivalence across the 23 countries' (p.11). Future methodological testing will need to be undertaken to fit a 6-class model using SASAS data exclusively and checking this against the general ESS classification for consistency.

[2] Estimates using weighted 2008 SASAS data show a similar pattern, though with some differences at the tail ends of the distribution. In that survey round, 43% of the adult population was unworried, 11% was worried only about one of the two types of crime, 21% was mildly worried, 5% was fairly worried, and 21% was highly worried.

Table 7.3 Levels of fear of crime in South Africa using new categorisation compared to old single-item measures, 2009 (col %)

	Class based on four new fear of crime questions						
	1	2	3	4	5	6	
	(Unworried)	(Burglary only)	(Violent crime only)	(Mild worry)	(Fairly high worry)	(Most worried)	Total
Old question: 'How safe do you feel personally on most days?'							
Very safe	21.1	11.2	8.8	4.0	3.2	3.6	10.4
Safe	56.4	38.6	48.4	33.0	27.8	24.7	39.8
Neither nor	12.3	26.3	21.5	26.0	19.8	13.9	17.5
Unsafe	8.9	22.1	18.6	31.5	41.4	37.3	24.4
Very unsafe	1.3	1.9	2.7	5.5	7.8	20.5	7.9
Total	100	100	100	100	100	100	100
(Row %)	(34.1)	(5.7)	(6.6)	(22.7)	(3.6)	(27.3)	(100)
Old question: 'How safe or unsafe do you feel walking alone in this area after dark?'							
Very safe	19.6	1.6	4.5	2.7	3.7	3.4	8.7
Fairly safe	42.2	22.1	23.3	16.4	5.5	4.8	22.4
Bit unsafe	22.9	31.1	34.1	33.8	27.2	19.8	25.9
Very unsafe	15.4	45.3	38.1	47.1	63.6	72.1	43.0
Total	100	100	100	100	100	100	100
(Row %)	(34.1)	(5.7)	(6.6)	(22.7)	(3.6)	(27.3)	(100)

Data: South African Social Attitudes Survey, Round 7 (2009)

that the new measure is capturing a greater level of fear than the personal safety item but lower fear relative to the walking-alone indicator.

Bivariate analysis indicates that there is a moderate association between the different items, with a correlation coefficient of $r=0.47$ between responses to the new measure and the old personal safety question and a coefficient of $r=0.50$ in relation to the walking-alone measure. The table shows that there is a reasonable degree of correspondence at the margins but that the measures may be identifying different groups of people as fearful. For instance, of those designated unworried (class 1) according to the new measure, 10% felt personally unsafe on most days while a considerable 38% said they felt afraid of walking alone in their area at night. The fact that a contingent of those professing they do not worry about becoming a victim of specific crimes and that fear of crime has no impact on their quality of life should feel unsafe walking alone after dark is not surprising given that Ferraro and LaGrange (1987, p. 76) assert that the walking-alone question judges the likely risk of victimisation rather an emotional reaction to crime. Simply put, a person who states they feel unsafe walking alone in their area at night may in reality be unafraid of crime because they merely avoid walking alone in their neighbourhood at night. They do, however, recognise that they would be unsafe if they were to engage in such an activity. At the other end of the scale, of those identified as most worried (class 6), only a small share (8%) felt safe walking alone after dark, but nearly a third (29%) declared they felt personally safe on most days. This could possibly be attributable to the imprecision of the old measure, which makes no reference to crime at all.

5 Sociodemographic Correlates of Fear

Having discussed fear of crime at the national level, this section examines important disparities in perceptions of safety amongst various groups in the population. Central to most attempts at explaining such observed sub-group differences in fear of crime has been the concept of vulnerability. The basic premise is that fear of victimisation is likely to be more salient for those who feel incapable of adequately protecting themselves. This may be due to physical limitations such as an inability to run fast or the lack of physical prowess to fend off attackers, or social factors such as having the financial means to protect one's property, or living alone. It has been suggested that three dimensions of vulnerability interact to promote fear of crime, namely, (a) exposure to risk (of victimisation), (b) the anticipation of serious consequences, and (c) the loss of control, which translates as the lack of effective defence, protective measures or prospect of escape (Killias 1990; Hale 1996). Gender, age, race and socioeconomic factors are key variables in the research literature that have been identified as fulfilling the aforementioned conditions and extensively used to explain fear of crime, and are explored below.

5.1 Reviewing the Evidence Base

Numerous studies have demonstrated that women tend to report higher levels of fear relative to men, to the extent that gender has been seen as the foremost social divider on fear of crime (Gilchrist et al. 1998). This observation has been considered surprising, as men are considerably more likely to be at risk of criminal victimisation (Hale 1996). This gender differential in fear of crime has been attributed to factors such as vulnerability, environmental cues, victimisation, an inability of men to accurately assess the risks confronting them as well as their relative reluctance to admit their fears (Sutton and Farrall 2005, p. 212). Age has also featured extensively in fear of crime research, with an emphasis on the elderly and the impact such worries may have on their quality of life. It has been conventionally assumed that as people grow older, the more vulnerable and hence more fearful they become, which has prompted concerns about behaviour modification and self-imposed confinement in their own homes (Hale 1996; Fattah and Sacco 1989; Chadee and Ditton 2003). In practice, evidence of the professed relationship between age and fear of crime remains inconsistent and contested. Some studies have supported the existence of a positive relationship between the two (Clemente and Kleiman 1977; Braungart et al. 1980; Warr 1984; Baldassare 1986), but there is mounting evidence that one's age is of negligible or limited significance to explaining overall fear of crime (Ferraro and LaGrange 1988, 1992; Chadee and Ditton 2003; Sutton and Farrall 2005).

Research primarily from the USA and UK has suggested that race, social class and socioeconomic status are salient covariates of fear of crime, with the excluded, poor and less educated relatively more fearful of victimisation (see, for example, Clemente and Kleiman 1977; Ortega and Myles 1987; Liska et al. 1988; Box et al.

1988; Hale 1996). Explanations for this finding have focused on environmental and contextual factors, including the likelihood that these groups reside in areas where incivilities and crime are high and have an associated lack of resources to protect themselves and their property. Given South Africa's apartheid history and persisting poverty and inequality, one would expect a similar class gradient in fear of crime. Møller's (2005, p. 292) study in Nelson Mandela Metropolitan Municipality provides some confirmation of this, by showing that victimisation and fear of crime were associated with socioeconomic status. White, wealthier households were significantly more likely to experience household crime, less fearful of crime and misfortune and more satisfied with life. Conversely, fear of crime and dissatisfaction with personal safety emerged as more prominent among black African respondents and those with lower living standards.

5.2   Explaining Fear of Crime

Regression analysis was undertaken using the 2009 SASAS data to explore the relationships between the new fear of crime measure and basic characteristics of the survey respondents and the households in which they reside. Since the new fear of crime measure is inherently ordinal rather than cardinal, use is made of ordered probit equations, which explore the probability that an individual will place him or herself in a particular response category. A stepwise approach was used for the modelling, introducing firstly socioeconomic variables, followed by victimisation and crime attitudes variables, and lastly the Personal Wellbeing Index and social trust variables.

The ordered probit results are presented in Table 7.4. Model I includes just individual and household-level socioeconomic attributes and confirms that women express greater levels of worry over crime than men, Indian adults are more fearful than black adults, while coloured adults are less fearful. Importantly, age and educational attainment do not emerge as significant predictors of fear of crime, *ceteris paribus*. Those who were never married reported higher levels of fear than those who were unmarried but living with a partner, while discouraged work-seekers (unemployed not looking for work) were less fearful than those in full-time unemployment. Household size appears to be inversely related to fear, and although level of living standard did not emerge as a significant predictor, place of residence did. Those residing in informal urban settlements and formal urban areas were significantly more fearful than those in rural, traditional authority areas.

When adding in the crime-related variables (Model II), sex remains a significant determinant of fear, though the nature of racial differences changes somewhat. Coloured respondents are no longer significantly different from black respondents in terms of levels of fear, though Indian respondents continue to exhibit higher levels of worry about crime than black respondents. The same relationships hold in relation to marital and employment status, household size and geographic location, though living standard level now becomes a significant predictor of fear, with those

Table 7.4 Ordered probit on fear of crime in South Africa, 2009

	Fear of crime (6-point scale)					
	Model I		Model II		Model III	
	Coef.	Signif.	Coef.	Signif.	Coef.	Signif.
(A) Respondent's characteristics						
Age (years)	−0.001	*n.s.*	0.005	*n.s.*	0.001	*n.s.*
Age sq.	0.010	*n.s.*	0.004	*n.s.*	0.006	*n.s.*
Female	0.165	***	0.116	**	0.135	**
Race: coloured	−0.218	**	−0.136	*n.s.*	−0.086	*n.s.*
Race: Indian	0.384	**	0.304	*	0.386	**
Race: white	0.031	*n.s.*	0.156	*n.s.*	0.223	**
Married	0.020	*n.s.*	−0.055	*n.s.*	0.006	*n.s.*
Living together with partner	−0.170	*	−0.252	**	−0.243	**
Widower/widow	0.050	*n.s.*	−0.024	*n.s.*	0.021	*n.s.*
Divorced/separated	0.010	*n.s.*	−0.032	*n.s.*	0.006	*n.s.*
Education: primary	0.058	*n.s.*	0.090	*n.s.*	0.123	*n.s.*
Education: grades 8–11 or equivalent	−0.085	*n.s.*	−0.094	*n.s.*	−0.017	*n.s.*
Education: matric or equivalent	−0.008	*n.s.*	−0.039	*n.s.*	0.030	*n.s.*
Education: tertiary	−0.041	*n.s.*	0.062	*n.s.*	0.168	*n.s.*
Employed part time	0.063	*n.s.*	0.015	*n.s.*	0.012	*n.s.*
Unemployed looking for work	0.064	*n.s.*	0.057	*n.s.*	0.007	*n.s.*
Unemployed not looking for work	−0.333	***	−0.244	**	−0.288	***
Pensioner	−0.203	*n.s.*	−0.185	*n.s.*	−0.199	*n.s.*
Student/learner	−0.033	*n.s.*	0.039	*n.s.*	0.047	*n.s.*
(B) Household characteristics						
Household size	−0.022	**	−0.022	**	−0.028	***
Medium living standards	−0.012	*n.s.*	−0.184	**	−0.123	*n.s.*
High living standards	−0.037	*n.s.*	−0.218	*	−0.124	*n.s.*
Formal urban area	0.275	***	0.206	**	0.183	**
Informal urban settlement	0.523	***	0.424	***	0.389	***
Rural farm-worker households	−0.148	*n.s.*	−0.010	*n.s.*	−0.003	*n.s.*
(C) Crime-related variables						
Victim of (household or individual crime)			0.556	***	0.596	***
Neighbourhood crime increased			0.378	***	0.358	***
Confidence in the police			−0.030	*n.s.*	−0.022	*n.s.*
Satisfaction with government crime reduction efforts in neighbd			−0.063	**	−0.051	*
(D) Satisfaction						
Personal Wellbeing Index (*PWI*)					−0.010	***
(E) Social integration						
Social trust					−0.007	*n.s.*

Reference variables are black (race), never married (marital status), no schooling (education level), employed full-time (employment status), low living standards and rural traditional authority areas (geographic location)
*, **, ***, *n.s.* Significant difference at the 0.05, 0.01 and 0.001 levels, not significant

with medium and high living standards generally less fearful than those with low living standards. Being a victim of (household or individual) crime and believing that neighbourhood crime has increased are both positively related to levels of fear, while satisfaction with local crime reduction efforts by the government is negatively related to fear.

The final model shows that once the Personal Wellbeing Index and social trust variables are introduced, the personal characteristics associated with fear remain largely the same. The main difference is that white adults emerge as more fearful than black adults, with Indian respondents demonstrating a similar pattern. At the household level, household size and geographic location remain unchanged although living standard level again becomes insignificant. Perceptions of increasing neighbourhood crime, experience of victimisation and satisfaction witch government's crime reduction efforts remain significant. Higher levels of personal well-being is related to moderately lower levels of fear, while social trust does not enter significantly into the fear of crime equation.[3]

What can be inferred from these regression results? The statistically significant gender difference in the new fear of crime measure, with adult women more worried than adult men, conforms to international evidence. Yet, if one observes the actual percentages of men and women classified into each of the six new fear of crime categories (results not shown), it is apparent that the differences are not particularly large – a few percentage points at each end of the distribution. This is important in that it draws attention to the feeling of vulnerability experienced by men, rather than portraying them solely as the aggressor and perpetrator (Goodey 1997). Adult South African men in fact seem to be *almost as afraid* as adult women, implying that we need to be careful in portraying anxieties about crime as an issue pertaining predominantly to women (Gilchrist et al. 1998). The South African data also corroborate the emerging international finding of a weak association between fear of crime and age.

The results on the relationship between fear of crime and race, class and socioeconomic status are somewhat surprising and pose important challenges to prevailing stereotypes. Race has been prominent in the South African debate on crime and fear of crime. Racial segregation effectively insulated white South Africans from the political violence and high crime rates experienced by township dwellers during apartheid. After the 1994 transition, the location of crime has shifted, with white people more likely to be experiencing higher victimisation than before, which has fostered the view that they are the primary targets of criminal activity (Leggett 2005; Møller 2005). Politically, there have been signs of frustration with the persisting public fears over safety and the perception of the country as an especially violent place. For instance, the 1997 and 2002 ANC National Conferences explicitly mentioned fear among segments of the population, especially the contrast between the

---

[3]The regression model was replicated with the satisfaction-with-life in general variable replacing the Personal Wellbeing Index. The results were virtually identical, both in terms of the coefficients and levels of significance.

hope and aspirations of the majority of South Africans and the ambivalence and fear of minority communities (ANC 2002a, b; Mbeki 2007). Also, former President Mbeki made strong pronouncements about 'white fears', crime as a justification for racism and fear mongering (Mbeki 2004a, b, 2007). The SASAS modelling shows that Indian respondents consistently express significantly higher level of fear for personal safety relative to other respondents, while there was no significant difference between black and white respondents with regard to levels of concern over personal safety in two of the three models. These results refute the popular notion of fear of crime in South Africa as predominantly 'white fear' and suggest the need to move beyond a 'racialised discourse' of crime as this 'not only misrepresents whites as the predominant victims, but conversely portrays blacks as the primary perpetrators', which propagates suspicion and 'stranger danger' and disrupts social cohesion (Valji et al. 2004, p. 3).

The SASAS results further indicate that the other socioeconomic status variables included in the analysis, namely living standards level[4] and educational attainment, generally do not have a significant effect on fear of crime. This absence of a strong association adds credence to the contention that South Africans across the socioeconomic divide are fearful.

The analysis points to the importance of environmental context, with rural residents less concerned about their personal safety than their urban counterparts. This is not unexpected since people in rural communities tend to be more geographically dispersed than urban residents, and previous international research has found there to be a positive relationship between community size and fear of crime (Clemente and Kleiman 1977; Hale 1996). What is interesting is the deeply entrenched fear among residents of the country's informal settlements. This finding challenges the conventional portrayal of fearful suburbanites and the manifold target hardening measures they have installed in response. The sobering reality is that people living in informal settlements cannot afford to adorn their properties with razor-wire or electric fencing, burglar bars, state-of-the-art alarm systems, or hire private security to supplement police services. These areas often lack street lighting or ready access for police and other emergency services, which may further be conducive to heightened concerns of safety. The relative cost of crime to residents of informal settlements is also likely to be substantively higher than for middle- and upper-class residents in the suburbs. This is because they are less likely to be able to replace lost assets, and the impact of physical injury is likely to be more debilitating due to a greater reliance on their ability to perform manual, unskilled labour as a

---

[4]The Living Standards Measure (LSM) has been used as a proxy for material well-being due to high non-response in the reporting of household income (23% refused or were uncertain), which raised concerns about the variable's reliability. The LSM is a form of household-level asset index that was developed by the South African Advertising Research Foundation (SAARF) and combines together responses to 29 variables to classify the population into 10 LSM groups, where 10 is the highest and 1 is the lowest. Essentially, the LSM is a wealth measure based on standard of living rather than income. In the analysis presented here, low living standards correspond to LSMs 1–3, medium living standards refer to LSMs 4–6 and high living standards to LSMs 7–10.

primary livelihood strategy (May 2000). There is also a certain irony in the observation that residents of informal settlements are the most fearful, as previous research has found that concern over crime can readily become a manifestation of generalised fear of squatters and that rising crime levels reinforce negative views of squatters (Ballard 2004). The crime-related variables in the models reaffirm the role of context, as perceptions of neighbourhood crime and crime reduction efforts in addition to the direct experience of criminal victimisation all contribute significantly to the prediction of fear.

6 Fear of Crime and Quality of Life: Bivariate and Multivariate Relationships

Having explored individual variables associated with the new fear of crime measure and undertaken a preliminary examination of its determinants using multivariate analysis, the task which is addressed in this section is to employ bivariate and multivariate methods to measure the relationships between sociodemographic and crime-related variables on the one hand and the general indicators of life satisfaction and personal well-being included in the survey on the other. Preliminary results are presented in Table 7.5, which reports on basic bivariate analysis. A total of 24 independent variables were included in the analysis, consisting of eight demographic variables (including four race dummy variables), seven household attributes and nine crime-related variables.

The table shows that for most of the independent variables, there were significant relationships with life satisfaction and personal well-being. With regard to individual characteristics, men were moderately more likely to be satisfied with life or possess a higher sense of personal well-being than women. Educational attainment, being coloured, Indian or white and being married were also positively related to life satisfaction and personal well-being, while age and being black were negatively associated with these quality of life variables. In terms of household-level socioeconomic characteristics, living standard level, household income and being a resident in a formal urban area, all exhibited relatively robust positive correlations with the dependent variables, while living in a rural traditional authority area or informal settlement, and household size were negatively related.

In terms of the crime-related variables, the strongest relationship is between respondents' satisfaction with how safe they feel and the dependent variables. The Pearson Product-Moment Correlation for this relationship is highest for the Personal Wellbeing Index (0.60), meaning that the more the respondent feels satisfied with personal safety, the more she or he feels a greater sense of personal well-being. It is important to mention that the 'satisfaction with how safe you feel' variable is one of the satisfaction domains that forms part of the PWI calculation. Apart from this item, the more respondents were worried, based on the new fear of crime measure and the two principal conventional fear measures used in the survey series, the lower their satisfaction with personal well-being and life satisfaction.

Table 7.5 Correlations among crime-related and demographic variables and life satisfaction and personal well-being

	Life satisfaction[a]: (0–100 scale)	Personal Wellbeing Index (PWI)[b]
(A) Demographic variables		
Sex (male)	*n.s.*	0.04
Age (years)	−0.08	−0.08
Race: black	−0.24	−0.29
Race: coloured	0.09	0.12
Race: Indian	0.07	0.10
Race: white	0.21	0.24
Marital status	0.06	0.12
Education level	0.27	0.31
(B) Household attributes		
Household size	−0.12	−0.10
Household income	0.33	0.36
Living standard	0.39	0.38
Formal urban area	0.23	0.19
Informal urban settlement	−0.10	−0.13
Rural communal areas	−0.19	−0.13
Rural farm-worker households	*n.s.*	*n.s.*
(C) Crime-related variables		
New fear of crime measure	−0.10	−0.18
Old measure: afraid personally on most days	−0.14	−0.23
Old measure: fear of walking alone in neigbourhd. at night	−0.12	−0.25
Victim of (household or individual) crime	*n.s.*	0.05
Neighbourhood crime increased	−0.06	−0.20
Confidence in the police	0.10	0.07
Satisfaction with government crime reduction efforts in neighbd.	0.04	0.14
Satisfaction with how safe you feel	0.34	0.60
Support for the death penalty	*n.s.*	*n.s.*

All entries significant at 0.05 or better; *n.s.* = not significant
[a]Values of the satisfaction with life-as-a-whole question that are less than 50 are classified as 'dissatisfied', while those greater than 50 are categorised as 'satisfied'. The neutral middle category (life satisfaction = 50) is omitted
[b]Values of the PWI that are less than 50 are classified as 'dissatisfied', while those greater than 50 are categorised as 'satisfied'. The neutral middle category (PWI = 50) is omitted

The correlations between these three fear variables and respondents' personal well-being and life satisfaction were all moderately negative, ranging between −0.12 and −0.25, with slightly higher reported coefficients again evident when the PWI is the dependent variable.

A surprising finding, though manifests also in Møller's (2005) study, is the fact that experience of criminal victimisation was positively related to the two quality of life measures, with those reporting that they or a member of their household had been a victim of burglary or assault in the last five years slightly more satisfied with life.

Police confidence and satisfaction with the state's local crime reduction efforts both displayed small but significant positive associations with the quality of life variables, and perceived rise in neighbourhood crime produced a small negative relationship with personal well-being and life satisfaction. Support for the death penalty was not associated with life satisfaction or personal well-being.

Turning to multivariate level, following the broad approach adopted by Michalos and Zumbo (2000), a set of step-wise multivariate regression analyses were conducted to examine with more precision the relationship between crime-related variables and the global life satisfaction measure (Table 7.6). Three regressions were conducted. In the first instance, satisfaction with life was regressed on a set of demographic and socioeconomic variables, together with crime-related variables (Model I). Secondly, the global measure was regressed on the same demographic and socioeconomic variables, and a set of domain satisfaction variables, but omitting the crime-related block of items (Model II). The final regression was conducted with the demographic and socioeconomic variables, the domain satisfaction variables and the crime-related variables (Model III). This modelling method enables one to ascertain the additional explanatory power that the crime-related variables provide in terms of explaining levels of life satisfaction among the survey respondents (Michalos and Zumbo 2000, p. 279). In presenting the regression results, only those variables that had a statistically significant ($p<0.05$) effect on the global indicators were retained.

Model I shows that many of the demographic and household socioeconomic variables were statistically significant predictors. Women were more satisfied with life than men, while coloured, Indian and white respondents were more satisfied than black respondents. Those who were married or widowed were found to report higher satisfaction levels compared to those who have never been married, while those with a primary or higher education provided more positive evaluations than those with no schooling. In contrast with full-time employees, being an unemployed work-seeker reduces life satisfaction. Household size is also negatively related with life satisfaction, though a positive relationship is observed in terms of living standard level. People living on rural commercial farms were also found to express higher levels of satisfaction than those in rural traditional authority areas. Of the five crime-related variables, all except satisfaction with government's local crime reduction efforts were significantly related to life satisfaction. The new fear of crime measure and perceptions of increasing neighbourhood crime have negative regression coefficients, meaning that being more fearful and believing that local crime is escalating depress one's satisfaction with life. As with the bivariate analysis, a positive relationship is observed between experience of victimisation and life satisfaction, while higher confidence in police performance is also linked to higher satisfaction. Finally, interpersonal or social trust is shown to be positively related to life satisfaction. Combined, these variables account for 26% of the total variance in life satisfaction scores.

Model II in the second column of the table demonstrates that when the crime variables are dropped and replaced with a set of satisfaction domains, almost all the sociodemographic variables become insignificant. Only sex and geographic location

Table 7.6 Regression of satisfaction with life as a whole on demographic, crime-related and domain satisfaction variables

	Satisfaction with life as a whole (0–100 scale)		
Model:	I	II	III
Explanatory variables in equation	*Beta*	*Beta*	*Beta*
(A) Respondent's characteristics			
Age (years)	a	a	a
Age sq.	−0.144	a	a
Female	2.806	2.044	1.673
Race: coloured	4.356	a	a
Race: Indian	6.066	a	a
Race: white	6.570	a	a
Married	2.616	a	a
Widower/widow	4.468	a	a
Education: primary	4.429	a	a
Education: grades 8–11 or equivalent	10.509	a	a
Education: metric or equivalent	11.195	a	a
Education: tertiary	17.663	a	2.344
Unemployed looking for work	−6.926	a	a
(B) Household characteristics			
Household size	−0.637	a	a
Medium living standards	7.660	a	a
High living standards	14.135	a	a
Formal urban area	a	2.003	2.079
Rural farm-worker households	3.620	4.012	3.798
(C) Crime-related variables			
Fear of crime (6-item scale)	−1.278	a	−0.409
Victim of (household or individual crime)	4.306	a	a
Neighbourhood crime increased	−1.503	a	a
Confidence in the police	0.933	a	0.813
Satisfaction with government crime reduction efforts in neighbd.	a	a	−1.248
(D) Satisfaction domains			
Standard of living	a	4.296	4.191
One's health	a	1.047	1.068
One's achievement in life	a	1.739	1.733
One's personal relationships	a	0.775	0.811
How safe you feel	a	0.765	0.729
Feeling part of one's community	a	0.348	0.437
One's future security	a	0.470	0.411
One's spirituality or religion	a	a	a
(E) Social integration			
Social trust	1.942	0.700	0.740
Constant	38.944	−1.518	0.142
Number of observations	2983	3081	2968
Adj R-squared	0.2639	0.6170	0.6245

Reference variables are black (race), employed full-time (employment status), no schooling (education level), never married (marital status) and rural traditional authority area (location)
The symbol 'a' means that the variable is not in the equation

continue to exhibit any explanatory power. Seven of the eight satisfaction domains are significantly related to life satisfaction, the exception being satisfaction with one's spirituality or religion. Satisfaction with one's standard of living ($\beta=0.43$) and achievement in life ($\beta=0.17$) were the most powerful predictors from among the domain set. By including the satisfaction domains, the model is able to explain 62% of the variance in life satisfaction scores.

The full set of sociodemographic, crime-related and domain satisfaction regressors are included in model III. Sex, tertiary education and geographic location are the only sociodemographic variables achieving statistical significance. Of the crime variables, the fear of crime measure has a small, negative effect on life satisfaction ($\beta=-0.04$), as does satisfaction with government's local crime reduction efforts ($\beta=-0.13$). Police confidence again has a positive influence on life satisfaction. The crime-related variables only increase the explained variance by less than a percent over and above model II, suggesting that collectively, these measures do not have an appreciable impact on life satisfaction in the South African context.

7 Conclusion

This exploratory study set out to investigate the extent and nature of fear of crime in South Africa after nearly two decades of democracy, as well as to build on recent empirical studies by exploring the impact of crime-related issues on quality of life in a developing country context. The study also contained an element of experimentation by being one of the first applications in a non-Western setting of new multiple-item survey measures of worry about crime that were developed and validated using the European Social Survey. These measures, together with the single, six-category scale that is derived from them, aim to overcome conceptual and measurement limitations associated with conventional measures by probing both the frequency and impact of worry.

At the national level, the 2009 round of the South African Social Attitudes Survey found that between 50% and 60% of adults in the country were characterised by some level of dysfunctional or damaging fear of crime. This was based on the broadly equivalent shares expressing worries 'some of the time' or 'all or most of the time' about becoming a victim of violent crime or house robbery and that claimed such worry had 'some' or a 'serious' impact on their quality of life. Following the methodological approach proposed by Jackson and Kuha (2010), the four ESS measures were reduced to a single item that indicated that 34% of respondents were unworried, 13% worried occasionally only about home burglary or only about violent crime, 23% possessed a moderate level and 4% a fairly high level of worry, while 27% had very high levels of worry. From a comparative perspective, findings from the 2006 European Social Survey round suggest that South Africans are significantly more fearful than a majority of citizens from other parts of the world.

In terms of understanding the personal attributes associated with fear of crime, the survey results pose critical challenges to some of the prevailing stereotypes of who the fearful in the country are and provide further support for other national and sub-national surveys that have arrived at similar conclusions. Firstly, while women are shown to be more fearful of crime higher than men, the difference is modest with a considerable proportion of male adults openly expressing worries about crime. This finding is noteworthy in that it draws attention to the vulnerabilities experienced by men rather than portraying them solely as aggressors and perpetrators. Secondly, multivariate modelling suggested that in many instances, there is no significant difference in fear of crime between black and white respondents, with Indian respondents constantly displaying the highest levels of fear. Given this finding, the popular reference to fear of crime in the country as predominantly 'white fear' is lamentable in that it is misleading and neglects the needs of a majority who are less able to adequately voice their concerns. Thirdly, other socioeconomic status variables included in the analysis, namely living standard level, educational attainment and employment status, exhibited only weak associations with worry about crime. There is nonetheless support for the relationship between fear and place of residence. While it was unsurprising to find that people residing in rural areas tend to experience less fear of victimisation than their urban counterparts, a significant finding is that it is in the country's informal settlements that fear seems most pervasive. This is likely to be related to a lack of basic policing, services and infrastructure in such areas, as well as inability to afford target hardening measures, all of which increase the risk of victimisation (Richards et al. 2007).

Actual experience of victimisation and perceptions of rising neighbourhood crime were both shown to be significant, positive predictors of fear of crime. A weaker but statistically significant relationship was also present between quality of life measures and fear of crime. Those with higher satisfaction with life and Personal Wellbeing Index scores tended to be less fearful in general.

When life satisfaction is treated as a dependent variable, the findings provide further support for the conclusion from earlier studies that fear of crime has only a small negative effect on quality of life. In fact, multivariate analysis shows that in South Africa, fear of crime together with other crime-related variables, such as victimisation and perceptions of changing levels of neighbourhood crime, collectively account for substantially less than five percent of total variance in life satisfaction. Interestingly, the analysis also provides confirmatory evidence for the finding by Møller (2005) that those having experienced criminal victimisation are actually more rather than less satisfied with life compared to non-victims.

From a methodological and analytical standpoint, the present research has been limited by several factors. Given the availability of comparable cross-country data, it would be useful to conduct further comparative analysis to better understand how the nature of fear of crime and quality of life in the country differs from other contexts. This would include further validation of the new fear of crime measure by re-performing the latent class analysis to determine whether the scaling derived for Europe is apposite in the South African case. In addition, the fear of crime regression results point to the salience of ecological traits, so in accordance with suggestions by Adams and Serpe (2000) and Adu-Mireku (2002), future work should attempt to incorporate neighbourhood or community characteristics alongside individual and household traits. While it is argued that the new fear of crime classification is based on 'a more fully-specified conceptual definition' (Jackson and Kuha 2010, p. 15), further research is required to tease out more fully the patterns of difference in the old and new fear of crime measures, even though the broad identification of the fearful and unworried appears broadly complimentary between the two.

In conclusion, the study has confirmed that deep-seated fears about personal safety continue to be shared by a sizable contingent of South Africans across the socioeconomic and demographic spectrum. Yet, South Africans have shown resilience and resolve by not allowing such insecurities and both direct and indirect experiences of crime to impact to any significant degree on their life satisfaction. However, from the results presented in the chapter, it is readily apparent that the fear equation remains of considerable importance for policy discussion. Identifying, testing out and evaluating strategies for reducing the fear of crime should need to be increasingly recognised as a priority in the country alongside that of reducing crime itself. While this task is likely to be rendered difficult by the social, economic and political insecurity that tends to underscore fear of crime, it is only by doing so that we can expect to dislodge the shadow of anxiety that looms over the 'rainbow nation'.

References

Adams, R. E., & Serpe, R. T. (2000). Social integration, fear of crime, and life satisfaction. *Sociological Perspectives, 43*(4), 605–629.

Adu-Mireku, S. (2002). Fear of crime among residents of three communities in Accra, Ghana. *International Journal of Comparative Sociology, 43*(2), 153–168.

African National Congress (ANC). (2002a). *Umrabulo*: Special 51st National Conference Edition, No. 16, August. http://www.anc.org.za/show.php?id=2932. Accessed May 3, 2011.

African National Congress (ANC). (2002b). *Umrabulo*: Special edition: National Policy Conference, No. 17, October. http://www.anc.org.za/show.php?id=2931. Accessed May 3, 2011.

Andrews, F. M., & Withey, S. B. (1976). *Social indicators of well-being: American's perceptions of life quality*. New York: Plenum Press.

Baldassare, M. (1986). The elderly and fear of crime. *Sociology and Social Research, 70*(3), 218–221.

Ballard, R. (2004). Middle class neighbourhoods or 'African kraals'? The impact of informal settlements and vagrants on post-apartheid white identity. *Urban Forum, 15*(1), 48–73.

Box, S., Hale, C., & Andrews, G. (1988). Explaining fear of crime. *British Journal of Criminology, 28*(3), 340–356.

Braungart, M. M., Braungart, R. G., & Hoyer, W. J. (1980). Age, sex and social factors in fear of crime. *Sociological Focus, 13*(1), 55–66.

Chadee, D., & Ditton, J. (2003). Are older people most afraid of crime? Revisiting Ferraro and Le Grange in Trinidad. *British Journal of Criminology, 43*(2), 417–433.

Clemente, F., & Kleiman, M. B. (1977). Fear of crime in the United States: A multivariate analysis. *Social Forces, 56*(2), 519–531.

Cummins, R. A. (1996a). Assessing quality of life. In R. I. Brown (Ed.), *Quality of life for people with disabilities: Models, research and practice* (pp. 116–150). London: Chapman & Hall.

Cummins, R. A. (1996b). The domains of life satisfaction: An attempt to order chaos. *Social Indicators Research, 38*(3), 303–332.

Cummins, R. A. (1998). The second approximation to an international standard of life satisfaction. *Social Indicators Research, 43*(3), 307–334.

Cummins, R. A. (2010). Subjective wellbeing, homeostatically protected mood and depression: A synthesis. *Journal of Happiness Studies, 11*(1), 1–17.

Cummins, R. A., & Nistico, H. (2002). Maintaining life satisfaction: The role of positive cognitive bias. *Journal of Happiness Studies, 3*(1), 37–69.

Cummins, R. A., McCabe, M. R., Romeo, Y., & Gullone, E. (1994). The comprehensive quality of life scale: Instrument development and psychometric evaluation on tertiary staff and students. *Educational and Psychological Measurement, 54*(2), 372–382.

Cummins, R. A., Gullone, E., & Lau, A. L. D. (2002). A model for subjective wellbeing homeostasis: The role of personality. In E. Gullone & R. A. Cummins (Eds.), *The universality of subjective well-being indicators* (Social indicators research book series, pp. 7–46). Dordrecht: Kluwer.

Cummins, R. A., Eckersley, R., Pallant, J., van Vugt, J., & Misajon, R. (2003). Developing a national index of subjective wellbeing: The Australian unity wellbeing index. *Social Indicators Research, 64*(2), 159–190.

Davies, S., & Hinks, T. (2010). Crime and happiness amongst heads of households in Malawi. *Journal of Happiness Studies, 11*(4), 457–476.

Farrall, S., & Gadd, D. (2004). Evaluating crime fears: A research note on a pilot study to improve the measurement of the 'fear of crime' as a performance indicator. *Evaluation, 10*(4), 493–502.

Farrall, S., Bannister, J., Ditton, J., & Gilchrist, E. (1997). Questioning the measurement of the 'fear of crime': Findings from a major methodological study. *British Journal of Criminology, 37*(4), 658–679.

Farrall, S., Jackson, J., & Gray, E. (2009). *Social order and the fear of crime in contemporary times.* Oxford: Oxford University Press, Clarendon Studies in Criminology.

Fattah, E. A., & Sacco, V. F. (1989). *Crime and victimisation of the elderly.* New York: Springer.

Ferraro, K. F., & LaGrange, R. L. (1987). The measurement of fear of crime. *Sociological Inquiry, 57*(1), 70–101.

Ferraro, K. F., & LaGrange, R. L. (1988). Are older people more afraid of crime? *Journal of Aging Studies, 2*(3), 277–287.

Ferraro, K. F., & LaGrange, R. L. (1992). Are older people more afraid of crime? Reconsidering age differences in fear of victimisation. *Journal of Gerontology, 47*(5), S233–S244.

Gilchrist, E., Bannister, J., Ditton, J., & Farrall, S. (1998). Women and the 'fear of crime': Challenging the accepted stereotype. *British Journal of Criminology, 38*(2), 283–298.

Goodey, J. (1997). Boys don't cry: Masculinities, fear of crime and fearlessness. *British Journal of Criminology, 37*(3), 401–418.

Gray, E., Jackson, J., & Farrall, S. (2008a). Reassessing the fear of crime. *European Journal of Criminology, 5*(3), 363–80.

Gray, E., Jackson, J., & Farrall, S. (2008b). Researching everyday emotions: Towards a multi-disciplinary investigation of the fear of crime. In H. Kury & T. Hartnagel (Eds.), *Fear of crime, punitivity: New developments in theory and research* (pp. 3–24). Bochum: Universitatsverlag Brockmeyer.

Hale, C. (1996). Fear of crime: A review of the literature. *International Review of Victimology, 4*(2), 79–150.

Home Office. (2004). Confident communities in a secure Britain: The home office strategic plan 2004–08. London: Her Majesty's Government. http://www.archive2.official-documents.co.uk/document/cm62/6287/6287.pdf. Accessed May 3, 2011.

International Wellbeing Group. (2006). *Personal wellbeing index manual.* Melbourne: Deakin University. http://www.deakin.edu.au/research/acqol/instruments/wellbeing-index/. Accessed May 3, 2011.

Jackson, J. (2004). Experience and expression: Social and cultural significance in the fear of crime. *British Journal of Criminology, 44*(6), 946–66.

Jackson, J. (2006). Introducing fear of crime to risk research. *Risk Analysis, 26*(1), 253–264.

Jackson, J., & Gray, E. (2010). Functional fear and public insecurities about crime. *British Journal of Criminology, 50*(1), 1–21.

Jackson, J., & Kuha, J. (2010). Worry about crime among European citizens: A latent class analysis of cross-national data. London: Methodology Institute, London School of Economics. http://ssrn.com/abstract=1603465. Accessed May 3, 2011.

Jackson, J., & Stafford, M. (2009). Public health and fear of crime: A prospective cohort study. *British Journal of Criminology, 49*(6), 832–847.

Jackson, J., Farrall, S., & Gray, E. (2007). Experience and expression in the fear of crime. Experience & expression in the fear of crime (Working Paper No. 7). Swindon: ESRC

Jones, L. V., & Thurstone, L. L. (1955). The psychophysics of semantics: An experimental investigation. *The Journal of Applied Psychology, 39*(1), 31–36.

Killias, M. (1990). Vulnerability: Towards a better understanding of a key variable in the genesis of the fear of crime. *Violence and Victims, 5*(2), 97–108.

Kingdon, G. G., & Knight, J. (2006). Subjective well-being poverty vs. income poverty and capabilities poverty? *Journal of Development Studies, 42*(7), 1199–1224.

Kitchen, P., & Williams, A. (2010). Quality of life and perceptions of crime in Saskatoon, Canada. *Social Indicators Research, 95*(1), 33–61.

Lau, A. L. D., Cummins, R. A., & McPherson, W. (2005). An investigation into the cross-cultural equivalence of the personal wellbeing index. *Social Indicators Research, 72*(3), 403–430.

Leggett, T. (2005). The state of crime and policing. In J. Daniel, R. Southall, & J. Lutchman (Eds.), *State of the nation: South Africa 2004–2005* (pp. 144–176). Cape Town: HSRC Press.

Lemanski, C. (2004). A new apartheid? The spatial implications of fear of crime in Cape Town, South Africa. *Environment and Urbanization, 16*(2), 101–111.

Liska, A. E., Sanchirico, A., & Reed, M. D. (1988). Fear of crime and constrained behaviour: Specifying and estimating a reciprocal effects model. *Social Forces, 66*(3), 827–837.

Louw, A. (1997). Surviving the transition: Trends and perceptions of crime in South Africa. *Social Indicators Research, 41*(1–3), 137–168.

May, J. (Ed.). (2000). *Poverty and inequality in South Africa: Meeting the challenge.* Cape Town/London: David Phillip/Zed Press.

Mbeki, T. (2004a). Letter from the President: Voters will not be swayed by fear or fiction. *ANC Today, 4*(9), 5–11. http://www.anc.org.za/docs/anctoday/2004/at09.htm. Accessed May 3, 2011.

Mbeki, T. (2004b). Letter from the President: When is good news bad news? *ANC Today, 4*(39), 1–7. http://www.anc.org.za/docs/anctoday/2004/at39.htm. Accessed May 3, 2011.

Mbeki, T. (2007, March). Letter from the President: Freedom from racism – a fundamental human right. *ANC Today, 7*(10), 16–22. http://www.anc.org.za/docs/anctoday/2007/at10.htm. Accessed May 3, 2011.

Michalos, A. C., & Zumbo, B. D. (2000). Criminal victimization and the quality of life. *Social Indicators Research, 50*(3), 245–295.

Møller, V. (2005). Resilient or resigned? Criminal victimization and quality of life in South Africa. *Social Indicators Research, 72*(3), 263–317.

Moore, S. C. (2006). The value of reducing fear: An analysis using the European Social Survey. *Applied Economics, 38*(1), 115–117.

Ortega, S. T., & Myles, J. L. (1987). Race and gender effect on the fear of crime: An interactive model with age. *Criminology, 25*(1), 133–152.

Pantazis, C. (2000). 'Fear of crime', vulnerability and poverty: Evidence from the British Crime Survey. *British Journal of Criminology, 40*(3), 414–436.

Powdthavee, N. (2005). Unhappiness and crime: Evidence from South Africa. *Economica, 72*(287), 531–547.

Richards, R., O'Leary, B., & Mutsonziwa, K. (2007). Measuring quality of life in informal settlements in South Africa. *Social Indicators Research, 81*(2), 375–388.

Roberts, B. (2010). Fear factor: Perceptions of safety in South Africa. In B. J. Roberts, J. M. Kivilu, & Y. D. Davids (Eds.), *South African social attitudes, the 2nd report: Reflections on the age of hope* (pp. 250–275). Cape Town: HSRC Press.

Stafford, M., Chandola, T., & Marmot, M. (2007). Association between fear of crime and mental health and physical functioning. *American Journal of Public Health, 97*(11), 2076–2081.

Sutton, R. M., & Farrall, S. (2005). Gender, socially desirable responding and the fear of crime: Are women really more anxious about crime? *British Journal of Criminology, 45*(2), 212–224.

Tiliouine, H., Cummins, R. A., & Davern, M. (2006). Measuring wellbeing in developing countries: The case of Algeria. *Social Indicators Research, 75*(1), 1–30.

Valji, N., Harris, B., & Simpson, G. (2004). Crime, security and fear of the other. *SA Reconciliation Barometer, 2*(1), 3–4.

Warr, M. (1984). Fear of victimisation: Why are women and the elderly more afraid? *Social Science Quarterly, 65*(3), 681–702.

Chapter 8
The Relationship Between Perceptions of Insecurity, Social Capital, and Subjective Well-Being: Empirical Evidences from Areas of Rural Conflict in Colombia

Eduardo Wills-Herrera, Luz E. Orozco, Clemente Forero-Pineda, Oscar Pardo, Venetta Andonova

> *"Security must be measured in the lives of the people, not by the weaponry of State"*
>
> *Mahbub-ul Haq*

1 Introduction

Development studies have suffered from a materialistic bias (Easterlin 2001, 1995). For instance, the predominant emphasis on economic growth has neglected other important issues such as peace and security which have been previously studied as public goods, not as commodities, and thus have not been measured as contributing to development. In contrast to seeing societal development as economic growth, other conceptual streams, such as the human development movement (Sen 1999; Haq 1999a, b), refer to development "of, by and for the people." This approach understands societal development as the promotion and advance of human and social well-being. Subjective well-being – SWB – explores the self-evaluations carried out by people of how satisfied they are with their lives, including both positive and negative evaluations. It is a subjective appraisal which includes a cognitive and an affective dimension (Wills 2009). For instance, individuals measure their SWB in a number of different ways (Kim-Prieto 2005), rating their satisfaction with different life domains in a bottom-up procedure (Cummins 1996; Brief et al. 1993). Individuals

---

Wills-Herrera, E., Orozco, L. E., Forero, C., Pardo, O., & Andonova, V. (2011, February). The relationship between perceptions of insecurity, social capital and subjective well-being: Empirical evidences from areas of rural conflict in Colombia. *Journal of Socio-Economics, 40*(1), 88–96. Printed with permission of the publisher ©Elsevier Inc.

E. Wills-Herrera (✉) • L.E. Orozco • C. Forero-Pineda • O. Pardo • V. Andonova
School of Management, Universidad de los Andes, Calle 21 # 1-10, Bogotá, Colombia
e-mail: ewills@uniandes.edu.co

evaluate their well-being in different setting and contexts, including their subjective evaluation of security (Wills-Herrera et al. 2009). In this chapter, we argue that the perception of satisfaction with security is one of the important life domains which influence evaluations of subjective well-being. We also state that social connections, social capital, play an important role in influencing perceptions of insecurity. Belongingness to social networks is one of the main facets of social capital. Social capital entails the capital that can be accumulated in social relationships and can be conceptualized as a resource for action (Coleman 1988). Social capital flows through social connections and individuals' potential to make connections.

Prior to the emergence of the human development concept (Sen 2006; Jolly and Ray 2007), development largely meant progress. Well-being was related to a person's income levels and other non-material values such as belonging to social networks and social connections were not taken into account. Under the human development approach (Gasper 2005), the definition of well-being includes particular facets or dimensions of life, including feelings of security. Feelings of security can be seen as part of a human security concept which has been proposed as an individual-centered process diverging from the security notion derived from the military forces available to protect a specific nation or country (Gasper et al. 2008; Gasper 2010). For instance, the commission on human security (Ogata and Sen 2003) defines it as "protecting the vital core of all humans' lives in ways that enhance human freedoms and human fulfillment." So, human security is not limited to the negative dimension of the absence of violent conflict but includes safeguarding opportunities for people to build their strengths and aspirations. We distinguish insecurity as the opposite variable of security. It is a people-centered and multidimensional concept. We explore this concept in rural settings of conflictive Colombia where political and social conflicts have pervaded the economic activity over the last 50 years. We hypothesize that subjective insecurity is a different variable from objective facts of violent conflict and state that subjective perception of insecurity is negatively correlated with an individual's well-being. We propose that social capital as personal connections and a sense of belonging to social networks moderates the relationship between subjective insecurity and subjective well-being. Thus:

H1: Perceptions of security are a different construct than objective indicators of insecurity, and both constructs are poorly correlated.
H2: SWB is negatively influenced by levels of perceived insecurity (personal, community, and political).
H3: Social capital, as membership of voluntary associations, and trust and reciprocity, is positively associated with subjective well-being, and it moderates the relationship between perceptions of insecurity and SWB.
H4: SWB is significantly different for women as compared to men, to highly educated individuals as compared to less educated individuals, to married couples as compared to other marital status, and is positively associated with income.

This research is important because it tests with empirical evidence from a conflictive environment how subjective insecurity as a component of human security influences SWB and how such relationship is moderated by social capital. It is also important because it states that people construct safeguards against violence and conflict through participation in community networks and activities (social capital) which generates feelings of protection for the individual. Results of this relationship have both theoretical and practical implications for public policy.

2   Theoretical Framework

2.1   Subjective Well-Being

Subjective well-being (SWB), the self-evaluation that people carry out of their lives, has been proposed (Agner 2010; Diener 1984, 2000; Cummins 2004) as an alternative measure to track the development of societies instead of economic growth and other related objective indicators such as population health, crime, and objective security. SWB as a subjective appraisal from people themselves includes cognitive judgments and affective reactions. People rate their satisfaction with life as a whole or in relation with specific life domains such as family life, goal pursuit, social relationships, security, and many others (Diener and Seligman 2004). SWB is a multidimensional construct, and it is influenced by individual, social, cultural, and environmental variables (Wills-Herrera et al. 2009). SWB has been measured in the literature as a top-down global measure, satisfaction with life as a whole – SWLS – (Diener et al. 1985) a five-item scale as well as a bottom-up measure (Cummins et al. 2003) by which different facets of life satisfaction are considered to add significantly to the overall level of SWB. Cummins et al. (2003) have proposed the Personal Well-being Index – PWI – which consists of seven facets which have been consistently tested in 19 waves in Australia in order to perform intertemporal and interpersonal comparisons. The seven facets that have shown a significant contribution to the PWI are: (1) satisfaction with health, (2) personal relationships, (3) safety, (4) standard of living, (5) achieving goals, (6) community connectedness, and (7) future security. Other authors have replicated and validated the PWI in different contexts such as urban Bogotá, Colombia, showing a significant contribution of other facets such as satisfaction with religiosity/spirituality (Wills 2009). In this chapter, we are interested in exploring the influence of community connectedness and perceptions of insecurity on SWB under extreme conditions of objective insecurity. We propose in accordance to Cummins et al. (2003) that despite the occurrence of a conflictive scenario, individuals held a fairly constant level of SWB that is influenced by contextual and social variables. Perceptions of insecurity influence SWB because insecurity manifests a lack of control or autonomy of the person in relation to managing his environment. Perceptions of insecurity are manifested to the person as fears of losing control of their lives, loss of property, loss of social relationships, or even their life. Presence of present dangers and lack of control affects SWB. However, an adaptation process may also occur under severe environmental conditions. Many people live under violent circumstances yet are able to maintain a stable level of SWB or they develop strategies to reduce its impact. This stable level may be influenced by variables such as community connectedness and social capital. We researched the influence of subjective insecurity on SWB in areas of rural conflict in Colombia that have maintained a prolonged social and political conflict over the last 50 years. Therefore, we hypothesize that subjective perceptions of insecurity are a better predictor of SWB than objective measures of crime and insecurity.

2.2 Objective/Subjective Security

The discourse about security has evolved from an external, objective view to one which considers personal and social insecurities. The definition of objective security prevailed with an emphasis on national security from a military point of view. This vision expressed security/insecurity through objective indicators of crime and events that threatened societies or communities. On the other hand, the concept of human security has been proposed as an umbrella concept to emphasize the relationship between individual and social insecurities in the tradition of the human development discourse (Sen 1999). Mahbub-ul Haq introduced this concept in the Human Development Reports (UNDP 2000) in order to humanize the treatment of security, distinguishing the security of nations or regions from the security of individuals. It is an integrative rather than a defensive concept. He proposed not to focus on the physical aspect of personal security but to redefine it to include the capacity and abilities of individuals and communities to control their environments and secure basic conditions for a good life. Human security refers to confident social actors who possess enough capabilities and freedoms and whose agency enables them to successfully operate in the public domain. The idea is to liberate the individual from fears about harm and consequent ill-being. In that order of ideas, human security is a concept that is essentially subjective. It expresses the abilities of an individual to withstand threats arising from social conflict, political repression, and crime. It is measured by asking people directly how they feel in terms of handling and controlling their basic conditions for life, expressing their political views, and having the freedom to meet and associate to pursue their own interests.

In the Colombian context, objective indicators of violence have been proposed for security/insecurity at both the municipal and national levels, including indexes of homicides by 100,000 inhabitants, number of events related to kidnappings, clashes of legal military groups with illegal armed groups (guerrilla and paramilitary), and number of displaced individuals from municipality. We consider that perceptions of insecurity will closely predict SWB rather than objective measures of security, because "objective" indicators may be underrepresented, people may become accustomed, whereas perceptions include not only the perception of an external threat but also the ability and capacity the individual has in order to confront such a threat as well as the coping strategies that individuals and communities use to reduce external threats or the removal of vulnerabilities.

We make a distinction between objective measures of violence, as reflected in official reports, and the subjective perceptions of personal, political, economic, and communitarian insecurity, as reported by the heads of rural production units. Evidence suggests that answers to questions about perceptions of insecurity may reflect a psychological mindset rather than real objective threats to security (Diprose 2007).

2.3 Perceptions of Insecurity and Coping Strategies

Wood (2006) proposes that in countries such as Ethiopia, Perú, and Colombia, poor people may secure some kind of informal protection in return for dependence on patrons for security. He identifies several mechanisms by which poor people may improve security: (1) altering time-preference behavior; (2) enhancing capacities to prepare for hazards, one of these capacities may be capacity to associate; (3) formalizing rights, particularly in rural areas; (4) "de-clientilizing"; (5) enlarging choice via pooling of resources; (6) improving predictability of institutional performance; and (7) strengthening the membership of well-functioning collective organizations such as meso-organizations.

As part of a larger research (Forero et al. 2009), we proposed and tested that perceived insecurity may foster organizational hybrids (conceived as collective associations involving several parties, long-contracting, and associated decisions) as a strategic response to insecurity. We also tested that voluntary association to well-functioning organizations, as social capital, may influence perceptions of insecurity. That is to say, that individuals and communities develop different coping strategies to face insecurity. Strategies such as enhancing capacities to face external threats through association, enlarging choice by pooling of resources of different producers and strengthening membership in collective associations, are all buffer mechanisms that may reduce perceptions of insecurity.

2.4 Social Capital

Social capital has been variously defined; its value relies on the positive consequences of sociability and the importance of nonmonetary forms of capital as a source of influence and as a resource for action. Bourdieu (1986) originally defined it as "the aggregate of actual or potential resources which are linked to a possession of a durable network of more or less institutionalized relationships of mutual acquiescence or recognition" (Bourdieu 1986). It stresses the importance of social connections for the individual in order to access valuable resources. Its main idea is that involvement and participation in groups can have positive consequences for both the individual and the community to which they have voluntarily associated. It places those positive consequences in a nonmonetary form of capital. Social capital includes interpersonal trust, the sense of belonging to a social network, and reciprocity behaviors. We used as the measure of social capital the subject's voluntary association to social, cultural, or environmental organizations at the local level. People with a larger network of social contacts may provide ample material and affective support to individual members, adding to their subjective well-being. Social networks may also provide diverse knowledge and information for work opportunities and possibilities for association to develop productive projects. People and communities with higher levels of social capital have higher levels of health and therefore of SWB.

Social capital has been related to SWB in different forms. Previous empirical research from international samples (Helliwell 2005) has shown that measures of social capital, including specific and general trust, have substantial effects on well-being way beyond those flowing from economic benefits. Trust is seen as a facilitator, a lubricant of voluntary associations and networks. SWB appears to be related to various sorts of trust and also to the networks that may support such trust. Additionally, the voluntary association to cultural, social, and economic organizations provides the person with a safety network, information about possible threats to his/her security, and support in the case of crisis. Therefore, we state that the higher the social capital of the individual, the higher his perception of security.

3   Method

Seven hundred and forty two surveys were applied to owners or managers of rural productive properties in 2006. These properties are located in 25 different municipalities (see Annex 1) that belong to five different geographical regions of the country (see Annex 2). The five regions were chosen according to different levels of objective insecurity items as well as the type of production (large "haciendas" – large estate farming; and "minifundios" – small holdings). We choose municipalities with high, medium, and low objective insecurity indexes. Objective insecurity indexes included the following items per 100,000 inhabitants for 5 years: (1) number of homicides, (2) number of kidnappings, (3) number of armed clashes, and (4) total number of displaced people out of the region. The participation of leaders of local organizations in the survey was important to obtain truthful answers, especially in municipalities with high level of violence where the informal pressure of violent groups to the general population may affect the answers.

We performed both multiple and multilevel regressions. Multilevel regression included data of three levels: (1) individual, (2) municipal, and (3) regional.

3.1   Individual Level Data

We used perceptions of insecurity at the individual level as our independent variable and SWB at the individual level as our dependent variable. SWB was measured with

Table 8.1 Principal components analysis for subjective insecurity

Constructs	Questions	Loads
Personal insecurity (PERINS)	In this municipality, people fear for their life	.761
Crombach's alpha: 0.713	You fear robberies or physical aggression at home	.646
	In this municipality, my life has been threatened by illegal armed groups	.613
	People in this municipality have to bribe to produce	.597
	In this municipality, I feel safe to leave at night and my children can play in the neighborhood	.590
Political insecurity (POLINS)	People are free to practice their politics or religion	.745
Crombach's alpha: 0.595	People can associate to develop productive projects	.635
	I have felt persecuted by my politics or religious beliefs	.595
	People can participate in every kind of meeting	.583
Economical insecurity (ECOINS)	I can obtain a suitable income in this municipality to have an acceptable standard of living	.813
Crombach's alpha: 0.573	In this municipality, there is a good climate to start businesses	.778
Communitarian insecurity (COMINS)	I belong to social or religious groups which lead me to feel safe	.777
Crombach's alpha: 0.481	It is necessary to be armed in this municipality	.531
	Do your family and neighbors make you feel safe	.487

four items of the Personal Well-being Index – PWI – (Cummins et al. 2003) in a five-point Likert scale. The four items were named as follows: (1) satisfaction with life as a whole, (2) satisfaction with being part of a community, (3) satisfaction with personal achievements, and (4) satisfaction with political or religious beliefs. Satisfaction with personal security and future security, which are items that belong to the PWI scale, were not included because our independent variable was perception of insecurity and it could generate co-linearity problems between the independent and dependent variable. We performed an exploratory factor analysis using analysis of principal components and obtained one factor with eigenvalue higher than 1 and Crombach's alpha of 0.72.

For perceptions of insecurity, the factorial analysis with principal components, performed with 14 items, produced four different components which we named: (1) perceptions about personal safety (PERINS), (2) perceptions about political freedom of voice and expressions (POLINS), (3) perceptions of economic security (ECOINS), and (4) perceptions of security provided by the community (COMINS). Table 8.1 shows how items loaded in each factor of insecurity. Although Crombach's alphas are low, especially for the last component, we decided to use the four components because of two reasons: (1) this is the first empirical approach in which the scale is used in different contexts and (2) the affirmations conceptually match. For both, SWB and perceptions of insecurity, missing values were replaced with the municipal average for each item.

The measurement of social capital at the individual level included two items: (1) strength of the relationships of ego as part of the community network (RELAT) (see Annex 3) and (2) perception of trust and reciprocity among group members

(TRU/REC). This latter item (Crombach's alpha 0.641) included perceptions about (1) the willingness of people in the municipality to help when it is necessary and (2) feelings of trust within the community.

We also included the following independent variables as control variables: the perception about how much non-governmental organizations, such as associations or cooperatives, promote collective actions (MESOCOLLEC); demographical variables of rural owners/managers such as (1) gender (GEN), (2) age (AGE), (3) educational level (EDUTIME), (4) marital status (MARSTAT), (5) individual income level (INCOM), (6) number of children per household (CHILD), (7) period of time the individual has lived in the municipality (RESIDTIME), (8) property size (SIZE), and (9) distance to the nearest town (DIST).

We used multiple regressions as follows:

$$SWB = \beta_0 + \beta_1 * PERINS + \beta_2 * POLINS + \beta_3 * ECOINS + \beta_4 * COMINS$$
$$+ \beta_5 * RELAT + \beta_6 * TRUREC + \beta_7 * MESOCOLLEC + \beta_8 * AGE + \beta_9 * EDUTIME$$
$$+ \beta_{10} * INCOM + \beta_{11} * CHILD + \beta_{12} * RESIDTIME + \beta_{13} * GEN + \beta_{14} * MARSTAT$$
$$+ \beta_{15} * SIZE + \beta_{16} * DIST \tag{8.1}$$

3.2 Multilevel Contextual Data

We included demographical variables in second and third levels as contextual variables that may explain differences in SWB. Second-level variables include data for each of the 25 chosen municipalities, and third-level variables aggregate data of municipalities to create a region. See Annex 1.

Variables in the municipal level include (1) objective insecurity indexes, (2) life quality index, (3) education level of individuals aged 12 years and over (EDUAVE), (4) total municipal income, (5) per capita municipal income, and (6) proportion of people of working age. Variables included in both levels were: (1) average age (AGEAVE), (2) proportion of men, (3) proportion of literate children of 7 years old and over (LITERPROP), (4) proportion of people belonging to ethnic groups, (5) people currently employed, (6) unemployed people, and (7) people who cannot work.

Objective insecurity indexes include: (1) homicides (HOMAVE), (2) kidnappings (KIDNAVE), (3) armed clashes (CLASHAVE), and (4) displaced people (DISPAVE).

Equations 8.2–8.4 show our multilevel model including three levels: individual (i), municipal (j), and regional (k). Only significant results are included.

$$SWB_{ijk} = \beta_{0jk} + \beta_{100} * POLINS + \beta_{200} * ECOINS + \beta_{300} * COMINS$$
$$+ \beta_{400} * POLINS * RELAT + \beta_{500} * COMINS * TRUREC + \beta_{600} * MESOCOLLEC + e_{ijk} \tag{8.2}$$

$$\beta_{0jk} = \beta_{00k} + \beta_{010} * EDUAVE + \mu_{0jk} \tag{8.3}$$

$$\beta_{00k} = \beta_{000} + \beta_{001} * AGEAVE + \beta_{002} * LITERPROP + \mu_{00k} \tag{8.4}$$

4 Results

Significant results were found for the relationship between perceptions of insecurity, social capital, and SWB. Subjective perceptions of insecurity did not correlate well with objective hard data of violent events. Another important result found is the positive effect of social capital on SWB and its moderating effect on the relationship between insecurity perceptions and SWB. The contribution of the two variables of social capital to the model is around 6%.

Our sample of 742 observations allowed us to develop a multiple regression model with a low size effect and high power, near to 80%. In consequence, it is a robust model about the relationships between SWB, subjective insecurity, and social capital that can be further explored in future research. Another important result is that perceptions of political, economic, and communitarian insecurities affect SWB, which is consistent with our definition of SWB. In this study, perceptions of political insecurity have the highest contribution to SWB due to the particular conflictive environment.

Correlations among objective and subjective insecurities. Results of the correlations between subjective perceptions of insecurity and objective hard data of violent events at the municipal level were mixed. In general, there are no significant correlations between hard data of violent events and subjective perceptions of insecurity. Nevertheless, perceptions of insecurity did correlate with two variables: the number of armed clashes and the number of homicides in the last year. Additionally, personal insecurity did correlate with the number of homicides in the last year. We also found that the number of homicides and armed clashes, respectively, explained 34.2% and the 30.5% of the variance of communitarian insecurity. Finally, the number of homicides in the last year explained 25.1% of the variance of subjective personal insecurity.

These results show that perception about insecurity is not necessarily related to violent facts and that some recent violent events have more influence in some insecurity perceptions than past violent events (Table 8.2).

4.1 Results at the Individual Level

Table 8.3 shows the mean, standard deviation, and correlations for the involved variables. As expected, SWB and subjective perceptions of insecurity were negatively correlated. These relationships were found to be significant. Non-significant correlations among SWB and variables related with economical status of individuals such as income (INCOM), education time (EDUTIME), property size (SIZE), and distance to the nearest town (DISTANCE) were found.

There is a significant correlation among number of children per family, CHILD, and INCOM with social capital variables. CHILD positively correlates

Table 8.2 Correlations among objective and subjective insecurities – 25 municipalities

Independent variables	SWB	2	3	4	5	6	7
1. POLINS	.648**	–	–	–	–	–	–
2. ECOINS	0.386	0.3	–	–	–	–	–
3. COMINS	.627**	.471*	0.048	–	–	–	–
4. HOMAVE	0.102	0.153	−0.321	0.262	–	–	–
5. KIDNAVE	−0.088	−0.06	−0.298	−0.063	.761**	–	–
6. CLASHAVE	0.289	0.163	−0.064	.598**	.623**	.407*	–
7. DISPAVE	−0.062	−0.028	−0.053	−0.095	.539**	.703**	.406*
	SWB	2	3	4	9	10	11
8. HOM2005	.531**	0.302	0.031	.608**	–	–	–
9. KIDN2005	−0.109	−0.121	−0.279	0.034	0.346	–	–
10. CLASH2005	0.393	0.217	0.085	.578**	.787**	0.3	–
11. DIS2005	0.316	0.249	0.202	0.227	0.446	0.025	.666**

*Pearson correlation. It is significant at 0.05
**Pearson correlation. It is significant at 0.01

with the effort to strengthen relationships (RELAT) and trust and reciprocity (TRU-REC) because most of the communitarian activities (sports, cultural, civic, scholar) focus on the development of infants. INCOM negatively correlates with the same variables, suggesting that higher levels of social capital are found in low-income individuals.

Results of multiple regressions are shown in Table 8.4. Perception of political, economic, and communitarian insecurity explains 24.1% of the SWB variance. Capital social variables and cooperation promoted by organizations contribute 5.6% and 1.3% of the variance, respectively. Political insecurity is the most important variable; it explains 15.3% of SWB. Each of the two social capital variables contributed 2.8% of the SWB variance.

Two demographical variables, marital status and gender, consistently correlate with SWB. This result is consistent with other international findings. It is important to highlight the positive and significant effect of female gender on SWB. The main result with marital status indicates that married people who have formalized their status have a more positive perception of well-being (+0.083) than other kinds of union. Other demographical variables did not show any significant correlation with SWB (Table 8.5).

A positive moderating effect of social capital on the relationship between subjective insecurity and SWB was found. When perceptions of insecurity are low, SWB is higher and it increases even more if social capital is present. This important result shows that the strength of relationships developed as being a part of the community moderates the influence of personal, political, and economic insecurity and that perception of trust and reciprocity among community members moderates the economic and communitarian insecurity influence to explain SWB (Table 8.6).

Table 8.3 Mean, standard deviation, and correlations among variables at the individual level and SWB

	Mean	s.d.	1	2	3	4	5	6	7	8	9	10	11	12	13	14
1. SWB	4.309	0.661														
2. PERINS	2.304	0.881	−.188**													
3. POLINS	1.825	0.666	−.403**	.433**												
4. ECOINS	2.429	0.937	−.274**	.240**	.208**											
5. COMINS	2.022	0.746	−.369**	.400**	.358**	.125**										
6. AGE	45.504	13.077	.015	.086*	.013	−.089*	.031									
7. RESIDTIME	2.904	0.357	−.026	.013	.017	.098**	−.041	.051								
8. CHILD	3.490	2.556	.037	.082*	.041	−.055	−.009	.599**	.082*							
9. EDUTIME	2.625	0.956	.048	−.035	−.045	−.102**	.010	−.305**	−.117**	−.347**						
10. INCOM	2.201	1.180	.042	−.023	−.034	−.278**	.143**	.136**	−.083*	−.041	.350**					
11. DIST	13.212	37.676	−.006	.056	.072*	−.011	.012	−.017	.026	.016	.004	.033				
12. SIZE	75.761	261.767	−.014	.054	.011	−.050	.019	−.014	−.056	−.010	.164**	.167**	.046			
13. RELAT	0.115	0.133	.217**	.101**	−.054	.018	−.154**	−.046	.101**	.093*	.012	−.103**	−.007	.046		
14. TRU-REC	3.885	0.812	.365**	−.242**	−.274**	−.151**	−.341**	.043	.008	.121**	−.077*	−.167**	−.040	−.034	.105**	
15. MESOCOLLEC	0.407	0.611	.196**	.033	−.078*	.030	−.092*	−.135**	.051	−.048	.030	−.121**	.019	.024	.249**	.119**

*Correlation is significant at 0.05 (bilateral)
**Correlation is significant at 0.01 (bilateral)

Table 8.4 Multiple regression model: SWB as explained by types of insecurity, types of social capital, and collective actions by meso-organizations

Variable	Beta		Sig.	R2	Change in F for the model	Significance of F change
POLINS	B$_2$	−0.237	0.000	0.158	139,553	0.000
ECOINS	B$_3$	−0.179	0.000	0.195	34,579	0.000
COMINS	B$_4$	−0.168	0.000	0.248	53,025	0.000
RELAT	B$_5$	0.134	0.000	0.276	29,171	0.000
TRU-REC	B$_6$	0.188	0.000	0.308	35,291	0.000
MESOCOLLEC	B$_7$	0.112	0.000	0.319	12,505	0.000

Model 2: Basic model plus demographical data (marital status, gender)

Variable	Beta		Sig.	R2	Change in F	Significance of F change
MARSTAT – formal marriage	β_{14}	0.083	0.007	0.316	7.330	0.007
GEN – female	β_{13}	0.088	0.004	0.317	8.168	0.004

Table 8.5 Multiple regression model with SWB as dependent variable including non-significant variables

Variable		Beta std	P value
PERINS	B1	0.076	0.040
POLINS	B3	−0.253	0.000
ECOINS	B3	−0.159	0.000
COMINS	B4	−0.199	0.000
RELAT	B5	0.127	0.000
TRU-REC	B6	0.210	0.000
MESOCOLLEC	B7	0.115	0.000
AGE	B8	0.004	0.918
EDUTIME	B9	0.011	0.754
INCOME	B10	0.084	0.022
CHILD	B11	0.015	0.699
RESIDTIME	B12	−0.030	0.332
DIST	B15	0.013	0.662
SIZE	B16	−0.041	0.194

4.2 Results for the Municipal and Regional Levels

The results for the three-level models are included in Table 8.7 and in Eqs. 8.2–8.4. We found a high correlation between personal insecurity and political insecurity with SWB at the second and third level.

The meaning of the results at the second (Eq. 8.3) and third (Eq. 8.4) models is as follows: Aggregated SWB for individuals in one municipality differs from the SWB level in other municipalities. Aggregated SWB level for individuals in one region is different from the SWB for other regions. We tried to identify some variables at each level that explain those differences. At the second level, represented in

Table 8.6 Moderating effect of social capital and subjective insecurity on SWB

Model	Standard B	Significance level	$R2$	Significance level in $R2$ change
PERINS (a)	−.278	.000	.031	***
RELAT(e)	.030	.758	.084	***
(a)×(e)	.238	.026	.089	**
POLINS (b)	−.455	.000	.156	***
RELAT (e)	.005	.957	.193	***
(b)×(e)	.208	.047	.196	**
ECOINS (c)	−.358	.000	.073	***
RELAT (e)	−.004	.967	.121	***
(c)×(e)	.254	.013	.127	**
COMINS (d)	−.320	.000	.131	***
RELAT (e)	.223	.028	.156	***
(d)×(e)	−.064	.525	.155	
PERINS (a)	−.186	.245	.031	***
TRU-REC (f)	.264	.008	.122	***
(a)×(f)	.087	.599	.121	
POLINS (b)	−.469	.000	.153	***
TRU-REC (f)	.162	.068	.213	***
(b)×(f)	.153	.258	.213	
ECOINS (c)	−.657	.000	.071	***
TRU-REC (f)	.051	.555	.160	***
(c)×(f)	.480	.002	.170	**
COMINS (d)	−.658	.000	.130	***
TRU-REC (f)	.014	.882	.183	***
(d)×(f)	.383	.008	.190	*

*Correlation is significant at 0.1 (bilateral)
**Correlation is significant at 0.05 (bilateral)
***Correlation is significant at 0.01 (bilateral)

Eq. 8.3 by β_{0jk}, we found a significant effect of school time spent on SWB. The higher the municipal average of educational levels, the higher the SWB at the same level. At the highest level, represented in Eq. 8.4 by β_{00k}, our results included a positive effect of AGE average on the aggregated level of SWB and a negative effect of the Proportion of Literate People at the regional level on aggregated SWB.

It is important to note that the multilevel regression model asserts the findings in the multiple regression model to the extent that there was no influence of objective indexes of violence as source of variation of SWB. Although the power level of this model is further limited because the sample size in each municipality is reduced (25 observations as minimum per municipality), we call the attention on the fact that both the environment for the individual (the municipality) and a distant environment (the region) affect SWB via different variables and in different depths. The variance at the municipal level represents 14.28% of the initial variance and is explained in 80% by the average level of education of people in the municipality. The variance at the regional level, which is 4.76% of the initial variance, is explained by the average age in the region.

Table 8.7 Multilevel regression model at levels *i*, *j*, and *k* for SWB

Variable	Stimated β
Intercept	0.018
POLINS-*i*	(0.286)***
POLINS*RELAT-*i*	0.372***
ECOINS-*i*	(0.123)***
COMINS-*i*	(0.422)***
COMINS*(TRU-REC)-*i*	0.365***
MESOCOLLEC-*i*	0.086***
EDUAVE-*j*	0.206***
AGEAVE-*k*	1.194***
LITERPROP-*k*	(0.303)*
Explained variance	
i level (individual)	33.3%
j level (municipal)	80%
k level (regional)	86.7%

According to Snijders and Bolkster (1999)
*Correlation is significant at 0.1 (bilateral)
**Correlation is significant at 0.05 (bilateral)
***Correlation is significant at 0.01 (bilateral)

5 Discussion

This research focused on the relationship between subjective insecurity and subjective well-being and the moderating effect of social capital on that relationship. Both models (multiple and multilevel) confirm the hypothesis that perception of insecurity influences negatively SWB. Individuals with lower perception of insecurity have higher levels of SWB. This important result stresses the idea that insecurities are held in people's minds and subjective perceptions, not only objective events, influence the individual well-being of people.

Social capital at the individual, municipal, and regional level has significant effects on both perceptions of insecurity and SWB in the sense that the higher the level of social capital, the lower the influence of insecurities on SWB. This result corroborates previous research in the sense that people use networks or associations as a buffer effect against insecurity through the spreading of information in close networks about events that affect people's fears and insecurities. SWB is influenced in a positive way by the existence of social networks and the trust and reciprocity levels that exist in the community. These variables reduce the negative effect of insecurity over SWB.

This is an important result because it corroborates previous theoretical findings of the positive influence of social connections on well-being and suggests that to associate and act collectively is a strategic response to insecurities and violent events at the contextual level. It has also important practical implications for public policy, empowerment of communities, and strengthening of voluntary associations at the local level.

Three main facets of perceptions of insecurity were found: political, economical, and communitarian. These three items combined explain more than 30% of the variance of SWB. Political insecurity includes not only feelings of fear to exert civil rights but also fear to lose one's own life. Communitarian insecurity contributes to explain

5.1% of SWB. In rural zones, people feel more well-being when they participate freely in a community and also when they participate in the construction of strong ties within their community. We also note that communitarian subjective insecurity correlated positively with political insecurity. Perceptions of economic insecurity explained 3.8% of SWB. It is a small contribution, a result which is coherent with results found in previous research in the sense that individual incomes do not explain SWB after a certain level of income (Easterlin 1995). People need to develop social capacities and maintain social relationships above income generation to feel well.

Our results confirm another set of previous research in the sense that satisfaction with security is a dimension of the Personal Well-being Index (PWI) (Cummins et al. 2003). If SWB is measured from a bottom-up approach, with facets, and not as a global measure of satisfaction (Diener et al. 1985), security becomes an important dimension of the SWB construct. Previous research has suggested that SWB may have an individual stable level due to homeostasis or a treadmill effect (Cummins et al. 2003; Brickman et al. 1978). This treadmill effect suggests that people adapt to hard conditions of life, showing resilience to overcome conflictive events and situations and accommodate to new conditions of life in conflictive environments. Our results show that as rural producers have to survive because migrating or displacing is not an option for everybody, people develop strategic responses via social capital and association to conflictive environments. This strategic response may explain why SWB is maintained at a constant level despite negative insecurity conditions.

Correlations between subjective perceptions of insecurity and objective hard data of violent events were mixed. Objective hard data of insecurity and violence did not correlate significantly with subjective well-being, suggesting that cognitive representations and feelings of insecurity influence people's evaluations of satisfaction with their lives. We propose that an adaptation effect to insecurity takes place in the minds of people living in regions with conflict. People adapt their minds to objective data that signal potential insecurities and develop survival strategies. Future research is needed in order to define how particular survival strategies influence perceptions of insecurity and consequent actions.

Political insecurity explained a larger part of the variance found in SWB as compared to economic or communitarian insecurity. This result signals the importance of viewing the Colombian conflict as a political conflict where individuals fear to express their political views or belonging to a political movement. Future research is needed to explain why some objective indicators of insecurity explain some of the subjective insecurities and others not.

Regarding the influence of demographic variables on subjective well-being, two interesting effects were found: Less educated people showed significantly higher levels of SWB, and people not formally married showed lower levels of subjective well-being. To find that SWB is influenced by contextual dimensions, not just by dispositional factors, is an important result that adds to our current knowledge. These results give interesting insights of how demographical variables at multiple levels influence levels of SWB. Older people experience higher levels of SWB which may also signal the process of becoming accustomed to adverse contextual environments. Older people may learn how to adapt to extreme conditions and develop coping strategies to deal with insecurities such as creating associations for producing and distributing agricultural goods.

As a synthesis, the findings of this research let us conclude that individual SWB is influenced by perceptions of insecurity and that these perceptions are influenced by their social connections and life experiences. For instance, in environments with high political conflicts, it is expected that individuals have difficulties to exert their civil and political rights so that political insecurity may prevail over other kinds of insecurities.

Finally, these results highlight the importance of integrating two conceptual streams that have been developed independently: The stream found in human development and human security thinking led by Amartya Sen and Mahbub-ul Haq and the recent research in subjective well-being and happiness found in the social-psychological literature (Diener 2000; Veenhoven 2000; Cummins et al. 2003), economics (Easterlin 2001; Oswald 2003), and in journals such as the Journal of Happiness Studies. By the integration of concepts such as human security as part of the multidimensional construct of subjective well-being, theoretical and practical implications of these streams of research may be furthered.

The relationship between social capital and SWB may also be extrapolated to other contexts. Although some empirical studies have found no differences between rural and urban levels of SWB, in this study, we found that social capital (trust, reciprocity, and social network) in the Colombian context has a higher impact on rural people than on urban people. Urban people are less dependent of their closest community to survive.

The fact that violence facts have a limited influence over perception of insecurity shows that the existence of insecurity perceptions is not limited to violent environments; other causes should be analyzed to explain those perceptions. However, the important point is that at the extent of insecurity, perceptions are higher in the people's life; their feelings of SWB as an integral construct will tend to be lower.

The relationship between social capital and SWB may also be extrapolated to other contexts. Although some empirical studies have found no differences between rural and urban observations in reference to SWB, the rural conditions could represent a limit for the generalization of this result because the social capital (trust, reciprocity, and social network), at least in the Colombian context, has a higher impact on rural people than it is on urban people. Urban people are less dependent of the closest community to survive.

Finally, results in this research have practical implications for public policies such as strengthening communitarian networks as buffer mechanisms against violent events, strengthening trust in associations through more education and training, and strengthening networks for production as a strategy to survive conflictive environments in rural areas.

Our research has limitations that must be considered: Representativeness of the sample was partial. We could not have a complete inventory of households in the rural areas because survey information at this level is not complete. This creates external validity restrictions. With regard to SWB as a dependent variable, we could not use all the items of the PWI because of budget and time limitations in a survey that included more than 50 questions. Therefore, we worked with a proxy for SWB.

Multilevel analysis was made in its most simple way, with random effect only in intercepts. To deepen our theoretical and practical understanding, it is necessary to know in detail the random effect not only for the studied variables at the second and third levels but also in relation to other control variables that were not considered in this research.

Annex 1. Municipalities Per Region and Chosen Municipalities

Region	Municipalities in region for third-level variables	Chosen municipalities
Montes de María	Córdoba, Carmen de Bolívar, Guamo, María la baja, San Jacinto, San Juan Nepomuceno, Zambrano, Colosó, Chalán, Morroa, Ovejas, Palmito, Los Palmitos, San Onofre, Tolú Viejo	Carmen de Bolívar, Guamo, San Juan Nepomuceno, Los Palmitos, Tolú Viejo
Magdalena Medio	Regidor, Tiquisio, Rio Viejo, Arenal, Morales, Santa Rosa del Sur, Simití, San Pablo, Cantagallo, La Gloria, Gamarra, Aguachica, San Martín, San Alberto, Puerto Wilches, Sabana de Torres, Rionegro, Yondó, Barrancabermeja, San Vicente de Chucurí, Betulia, El Carmen de Chucurí, Puerto Berrio, Puerto Nare, Bajo Simacota, Puerto Parra, Landazuri, Cimitarra, Bolívar, El Peñón	San Pablo, San Alberto, Puerto Wilches, Sabana de Torres, Cimitarra
Nariño	Pasto, Alban, Aldana, Ancuya, Arboleda, Barbacoas, Belen, Buesaco, Colon, Consaca, Contadero, Cordoba, Cuaspud, Cumbal, Cumbitara, Chachag?I, El Charco, El Peñol, El Rosario, El Tablon De Gomez, El Tambo, Funes, Guachucal, Guaitarilla, Gualmatan, Iles, Imues, Ipiales, La Cruz, La Florida, La Llanada, La Tola, La Union, Leiva, Linares, Los Andes, Magi, Mallama, Mosquera, Nariño, Olaya Herrera, Ospina, Francisco Pizarro, Policarpa, Potosi, Providencia, Puerres, Pupiales, Ricaurte, Roberto Payan, Samaniego, Sandona, San Bernardo, San Lorenzo, San Pablo, San Pedro De Cartago, Santa Barbara, Santacruz, Sapuyes, Taminango, Tangua, Tumaco, Tuquerres, Yacuanquer	La Unión, Los Andes, Policarpa, Ricaurte, San Pablo
Huila	Neiva, Acevedo, Agrado, Aipe, Algeciras, Altamira, Baraya, Campoalegre, Colombia, Elias, Garzon, Gigante, Guadalupe, Hobo, Iquira, Isnos, La argentina, La plata, Nataga, Oporapa, Paicol, Palermo, Palestina, Pital, Pitalito, Rivera, Saladoblanco, San Agustin, Santa Maria, Suaza, Tarqui, Tesalia, Tello, Teruel, Timana, Villavieja, Yaguara	Algeciras, Iquira, Oporapa, San Agustín, Santa María
Meta	Villavicencio, Acacias, Barranca De Upia, Cabuyaro, Castilla La Nueva, Cubarral, Cumaral, El Calvario, El Castillo, El Dorado, Fuente De Oro, Granada, Guamal, Mapiripan, Mesetas, La Macarena, Uribe, Lejanias, Puerto Concordia, Puerto Gaitan, Puerto Lopez, Puerto Lleras, Puerto Rico, Restrepo, San Carlos De Guaroa, San Juan De Arama, San Juanito, San Martin, Vistahermosa	Acacias, El Castillo, Lejanías, San Carlos de Guaroa, San Martín

Annex 2

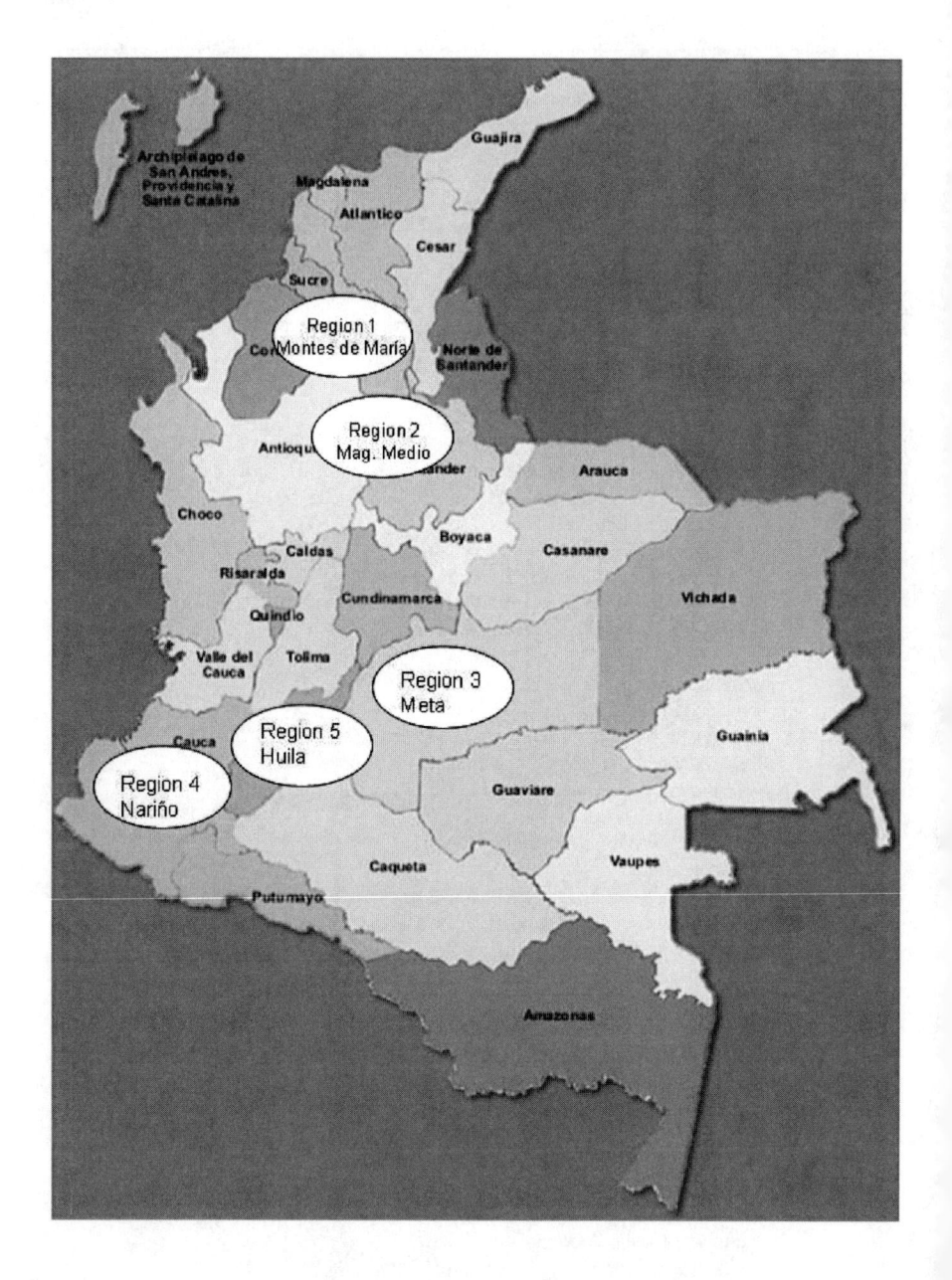

Annex 3. Belongingness to Associations in Order to Measure Social Capital?

1. Groups for community action
2. Neighbor associations
3. Parents associations
4. Sport teams
5. Chorus and groups of music, theatre, and literature
6. Labor unions
7. Communitarian mothers associations
8. Women associations
9. Alumni associations
10. Association in pro of any cause
11. Users associations
12. Consumers associations
13. Citizenships oversight
14. Social clubs
15. Religious communities
16. None
17. Other. Which?

References

Andrew, O. (2003). How much do external factors affect wellbeing? A way to use 'happiness economics' to decide. *The Psychologist, 16*, 140–141.

Bourdieu, P. (1986). The forms of capital. In J. Richardson (Ed.), *Handbook of theory and research for the sociology of education* (pp. 241–258). New York: Greenwood.

Brickman, P., Coates, D., & Bulman, J. R. (1978). Lottery winners and accident victims: Is happiness relative? *Journal of Personality and Social Psychology, 36*, 917–927.

Brief, A. P., Butcher, A. H., George, J. M., & Link, K. E. (1993). Integrating bottom-up and top-down theories of subjective well-being: The case of health. *Journal of Personality and Social Psychology, 64*, 646.

Coleman, J. S. (1988). Social capital in the creation of human capital. *The American Journal of Sociology, 94*, 95.

Cummins, R. A. (1996). The domains of life satisfaction: An attempt to order chaos. *Social Indicators Research, 38*(3), 303.

Cummins, R. A., Eckersley, R., Pallant, J., Van Vugt, J., & Misajon, R. (2003). Developing a national index of subjective wellbeing: The Australian unity wellbeing index. *Social Indicators Research, 64*(2), 159.

Diener, E. (1984). Subjective well-being. *Psychological Bulletin, 95*(3), 542–575.

Diener, E. (2000). Subjective well-being: The science of happiness and a proposal for a national index. *American Psychologist, 55*(1), 34–43.

Diener, E., & Seligman, M. E. P. (2004). Beyond money: Toward an economy of well-being. *Psychological Science in the Public Interest, 5*(1), 1–31.

Diener, E. D., Emmons, R. A., Larsen, R. J., & Griffin, S. (1985). The satisfaction with life scale. *Journal of Personality Assessment, 49*, 71–75.

Diprose, R. (2007, December). Safety and security: A proposal for internationally comparable indicators of violence [Special issue]. *Oxford Development Studies on Values and Multidimensional Poverty, 35*(4), 431–458.

Easterlin, R. A. (1995). Will raising the incomes of all increase the happiness of all? *Journal of Economic Behavior & Organization, 27*(1), 35.

Easterlin, R. A. (2001). Income and happiness: Towards a unified theory. *The Economic Journal, 111*(473), 465.

Forero, C., Wills-Herrera, E., Andonova, V., Orozco, L., Pardo, O. (2009). *Violence, personal and political insecurity and hybrid organizational forms: A study in conflict-ridden zones in Colombia.* Paper submitted to the International Society for New Institutional Economics, ISNIE, Toronto.

Gasper, D. (2005). Securing humanity: Situating human security as concept and discourse. *Journal of Human Development, 6*(2), 221–245.

Gasper, D. (2010). Understanding the diversity of conceptions of well being and quality of life. *Journal of Socio-Economics, 39*(3), 351–360.

Gasper, D,, & Thanh-Dam, T. (2008). *Development ethics through the lenses of caring, gender, and human security, Institute of Social Studies* (Working Paper, No. 459). The Hague.

Gasper, D., Van der Maesen, L., Truong, T. D., & Walker, A. (2008). *Human security and social quality: Contrasts and complementarities, Institute of Social Studies* (Working Papers, No. 462). The Hague

Haq, M-Ul. (1999a). *Reflections on human development* (2nd ed.). New York/Delhi: Oxford University Press.

Haq, M-Ul. (1999b). *Reflections on human development* (2nd ed.). Oxford: Oxford University Press.

Helliwell, J. F. (2005). *Wellbeing, social capital and public policy. What's new? National Bureau of Economic Research* (Working Paper No 11807).

Islam, G., Wills, E., & Hamilton, M. (2009). Objective and subjective indicators of happiness in Brazil. The mediating effect of social class. *Journal of Social Psychology, 149*(2), 267–271.

Jolly, R., & Ray, D. B. (2007). Human security - national perspectives and global agendas: Insights from national human development reports[dagger]. *Journal of International Development, 19*(4), 457.

Kim-Prieto, Ch, Diener, E., Tamir, M., Scollon, C. H., & Diener, M. (2005). Integrating the diverse definitions of happiness: A time-sequential framework of subjective wellbeing. *Journal of Happiness Studies, 6*(3), 261–300.

Ogata, S, & Sen, A. (2003). *Final report of the Commission on Human Security*, http://www.humansecurity-chs.org/finalreport/index.html

Sen, A. (1999). *Development as freedom*. New York: Oxford University Press.

Sen, A. (2006). *Identity and violence: The illusion of destiny*. New York: W. W. Norton.

Snijders, T. A. B., & Bosker, R. J. (1999). *Multilevel analysis: An introduction to basic and advanced multilevel modeling*. London/Thousand Oaks: Sage Publications.

Veenhoven, R. (2000). The four qualities of life: Ordering concepts and measures of the good life. *Journal of Happiness Studies, 1*, 1–39.

Wills, E. (2009). Spirituality and subjective well-being: Evidences for a new domain in the personal well-being index. *Journal of Happiness Studies, 10*(1), 49.

Wills-Herrera, E., Islam, G., & Hamilton, M. (2009). Subjective wellbeing in cities: A multidimensional concept of individual, social and cultural, variables. *Applied Research in Quality of Life, 4*(2), 201–221.

Wood, G. (2006). *Using security to indicate wellbeing, wellbeing in developing countries, University of Bath* (Working Paper 22). England.

Chapter 9
The Linkages Between Insecurity, Health, and Well-Being in Latin America: An Initial Exploration Based on Happiness Surveys[*]

Carol Graham and Juan Camilo Chaparro

1 Introduction

Crime and insecurity are increasingly common features of life in Latin America and the Caribbean, particularly in urban areas. Victimization rates in the region are among the highest in the world, with the exception of Sub-Saharan Africa (Fig. 9.1). The proportion of the population in the region that feels safe walking at night in their neighborhood is the lowest in the world, as is the proportion that trusts the police (Fig. 9.2). These phenomena affect the quality of life of all of the region's citizens, although some cohorts (and particularly the wealthy) have more means to protect themselves than do others. Concurrently, no country in the region has managed to achieve a security climate in its urban areas that approximates that of the developed economies (IADB 2008, Chapter 8).

Despite the generally high perceptions of insecurity in the region, cross-country differences in perceptions do not correlate with homicide rates, the principle objective indicator of insecurity. There is also a disconnect between perceptions of insecurity and the priority that leaders in each country in the region assign to security problems (Fig. 9.3 and IDB 2008, Chapter 10).

It is possible that the disconnect that we find between objective and subjective indicators, and between public opinion and the perceptions of leaders, is explained, at least in part, by adaptation. This is surely suggested by the fact that most of the countries where public concerns for insecurity are highest have only recently had

[*]This version: October 2010

C. Graham (✉)
The Brookings Institution, 1775 Massachusetts Avenue NW, Washington, DC 20036, USA
e-mail: CGRAHAM@brookings.edu

J.C. Chaparro
Department of Applied Economics, University of Minnesota, 231 Classroom Office Building, 1994 Buford Avenue, St. Paul, MN 55108, USA
e-mail: chap0441@umn.edu

D. Webb and E. Wills-Herrera (eds.), *Subjective Well-Being and Security*, Social Indicators Research Series 46, DOI 10.1007/978-94-007-2278-1_9, © Springer Science+Business Media B.V. 2012

	Region	Mugged	Stolen
na	North America	1.0	11.3
eap	Eastern Asia and Pacific	3.6	13.5
we	Western Europe	4.0	10.7
sa	South Asia	4.1	9.6
eca	Eastern Europe and Central Asia	4.9	11.8
mena	Middle East and North Africa	8.3	14.8
lac	Latin America and the Caribbean	12.3	19.5
ssa	Sub-Saharan Africa	13.0	24.3

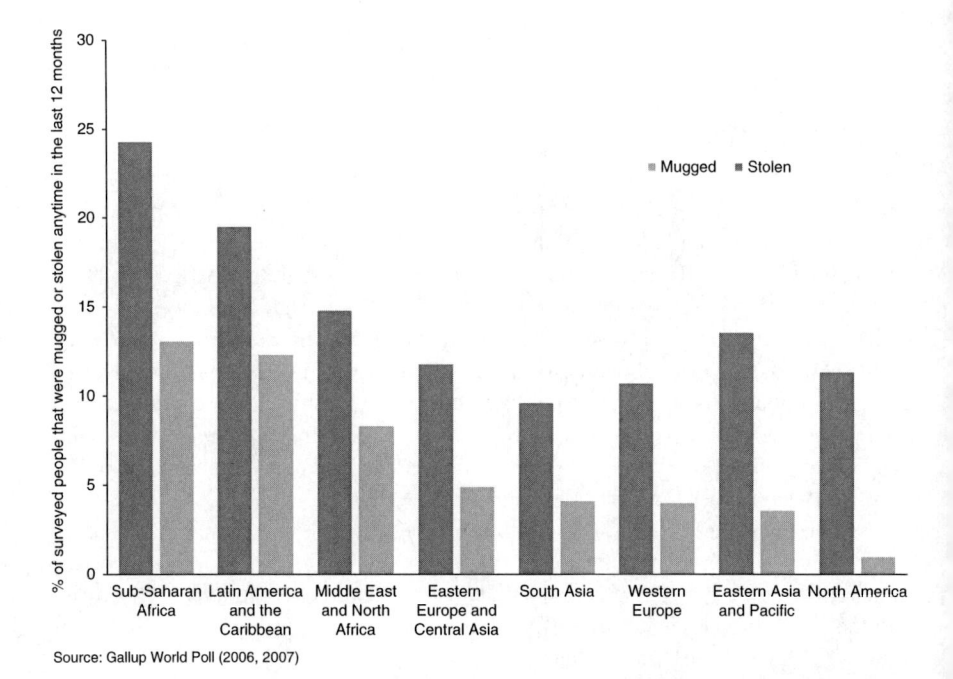

Source: Gallup World Poll (2006, 2007)

Fig. 9.1 Measures of victimization, by regions

increases in criminality, and those concerns are lower in those countries where the problem has persisted for longer periods of time. While this kind of adaptation may be a positive phenomenon from an individual psychological perspective, it may be an obstacle to mobilizing the public support that is necessary to implement the appropriate policies to combat crime.

One of the most common arguments used to generate public support for security measures is the high economic cost of crime, understood as the loss of production and income, as well as the increase of public costs that are associated with high crime levels. The IADB (Inter-American Development Bank) has been a leader in generating studies that attempt to measure these costs for Latin America (Londoño et al. 2000). Yet the effects of insecurity and crime on the well-being of societies are

	Region	Trust in the police	Feel safe walking at night
lac	Latin America and the Caribbean	49.7	47.9
eca	Eastern Europe and Central Asia	57.6	58.4
ssa	Sub-Saharan Africa	58.9	58.2
sa	South Asia	62.0	72.3
mena	Middle East and North Africa	65.2	70.2
eap	Eastern Asia and Pacific	76.0	72.2
we	Western Europe	80.0	74.8
na	North America	85.0	75.1

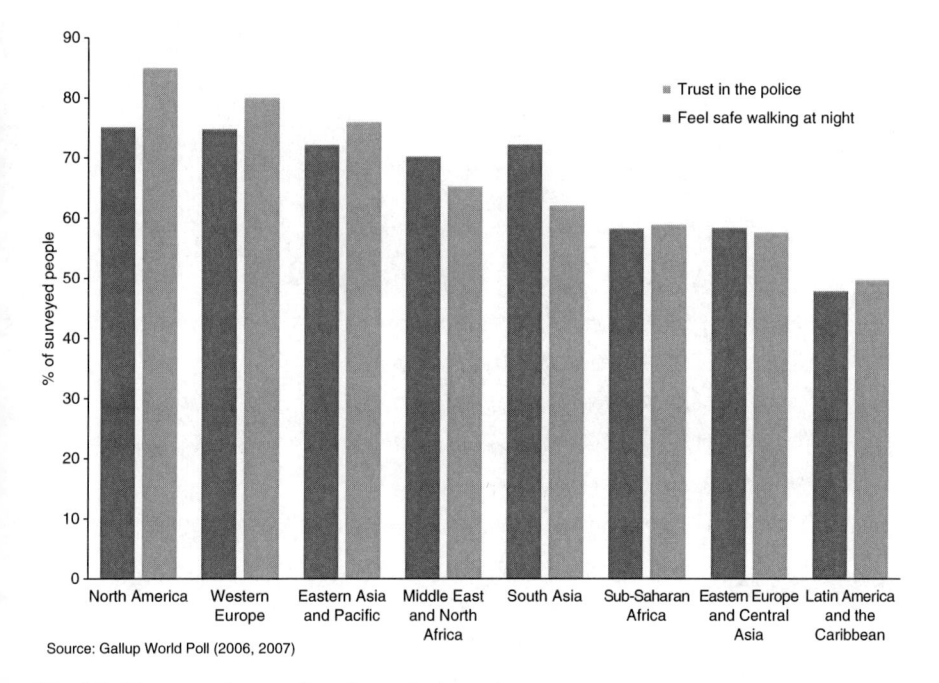

Fig. 9.2 Measures of perception of security, by regions

not limited to the economic costs. There can be much greater losses to individual well-being which stem from the physical and mental health costs, as well as on collective well-being due to changes in the way societies interact and function as a result of high levels of insecurity.

Our chapter explores how victimization and perceptions of insecurity affect well-being and health, as well as how adaptation mediates those effects. More specifically, it seeks to answer the following questions:

• What are the effects of victimization and insecurity on individual well-being? How do the well-being effects of crime and insecurity compare to those of other relevant variables, such as income and friendships?

Country	Percentage of people dissatisfied with crime levels	Violent crime considered one of top five problems by leaders	Homicide rate
Uruguay	62.1	13.3	5.0
Chile	54.7	38.5	5.3
Costa Rica	56.2	33.3	6.5
Argentina	61.2	11.1	6.8
Mexico	46.3	48.0	11.4
Panama	48.0	25.0	13.5
Nicaragua	41.2	0.0	15.1
Ecuador	45.3	11.1	16.2
Paraguay	48.7	9.1	20.7
Guatemala	44.5	33.3	24.0
Brazil	57.0	43.2	31.7
Venezuela	53.3	50.0	34.5
El Salvador	32.9	80.0	45.6
Colombia	43.7	66.7	79.7

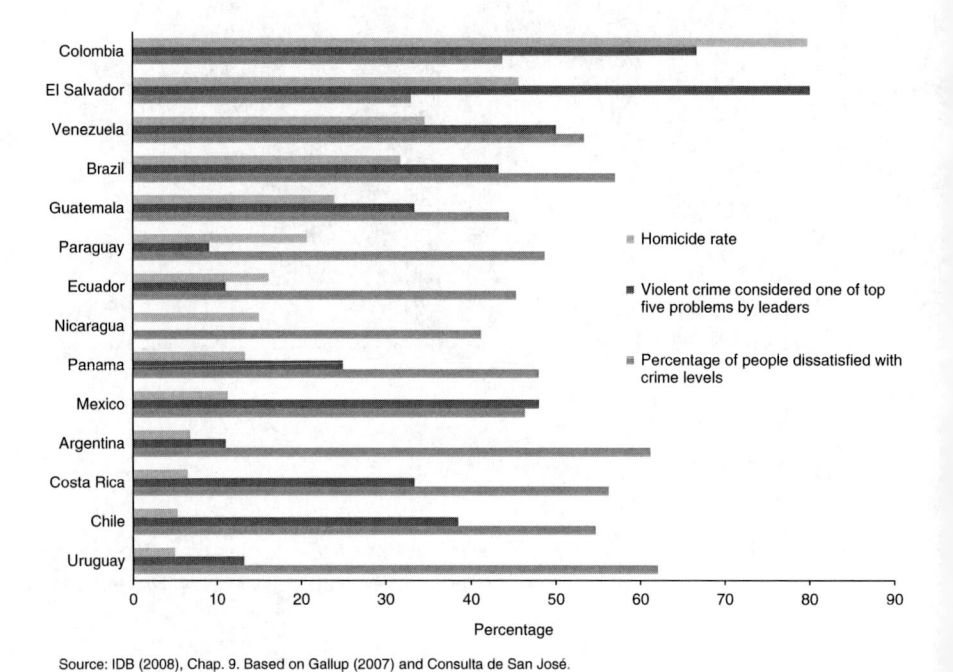

Source: IDB (2008), Chap. 9. Based on Gallup (2007) and Consulta de San José.

Fig. 9.3 Homicide rates and perceptions of people and leaders on security

- Victimization and insecurity also can affect well-being through health channels, such as mental health. Are the effects of these phenomena on health similar to those of well-being?

- Do the answers to the above questions vary for individuals who have adapted to insecurity and/or have a high probability of being crime victims? Does adaptation occur similarly across well-being and health arenas?

2 The Literature

Some of the most relevant studies to our queries come from the recent literature on the economics of happiness. A summary and a number of case studies for Latin America and the Caribbean come from a recent study of the IADB (2008) as well as from Graham and Lora (2009). The method and empirics underlying the study of subjective well-being and its determinants, based on surveys of public opinion, are discussed in detail in Van Praag and Ferrer-i-Carbonell (2007).

DiTella et al. (2008) conducted an initial exploration into the effects of victimization on anxiety and other positive and negative sentiments. Their results ran in the expected direction, with victimization having a positive correlation with anxiety and other negative sentiments and a negative correlation with positive sentiments like smiling. Earlier work by Schargrodsky et al. (2009) explored adaptive behaviors as crime rates increased in Argentina. They found that, when possible, the rich mimicked the behavior of the poor to avoid victimization, for example, by not wearing jewelry or carrying other valuables on the street, behaviors which had no negative spillover effects. Yet a second set of behaviors on the part of the rich – the purchase of private security and other protective mechanisms for their homes and other assets – resulted in negative spillover effects for less wealthy cohorts. Given the increase of private security and an increased risk in robbing[1] from the rich, criminals then shift their efforts and attention to the middle class and near poor, and victimization rates and robberies increase for these cohorts.

Related work by DiTella and Schargrodsky (2009), also based on panel data for Argentina, finds that victimization does not have a significant relationship with reported happiness, but it does result in changes in ideological position. Victims of crime are more likely to later declare that inequality is higher in Argentina, as well as to demand lower penalties for those who commit the same crime. The latter finding is explained by a sort of empathy effect in which criminals are seen as much as victims of an unjust economic system as they are as perpetrators of crime.

In research targeted more specifically on the role of adaptation, Graham (2009) shows how the well-being costs of phenomena such as crime, corruption, and ill health are mediated by norms and expectations. In other words, in places where high levels of crime and corruption are the norm, people adapt to these phenomena and suffer lower reported well-being costs when they occur, both because they already anticipate their occurrence and because they feel less stigmatized by them. The same occurs to various health-related conditions, such as obesity and smoking.

---

[1] A "robbery" is defined herein as the theft of personal property using force or threat of force.

The obese, for example, are typically less happy than others. But if they are in a reference group where obesity and/or smoking are the norm, then they suffer lower well-being costs as they feel less stigma from their conditions or behaviors. Powdthavee (2005), based on data for South Africa, finds that the effects of crime victimization vary a great deal depending on both the crime rate for the neighborhood where victims live in (with lower well-being costs reported in those where crime is more common), as well as the racial balance underlying victimization.

Graham posits that the ability to adapt to negative phenomena may be a good thing from an individual happiness/survival perspective but may result in lower aggregate welfare, as it allows societies to persist in bad equilibria. Understanding how these norms can be "tipped" is an objective of this research. Most recently, in a new study of happiness in Afghanistan, Graham and Chattopadhyay (2009) show that adaptation can reach extreme levels. Crime and corruption are so rampant in Afghanistan that victims there do not report lower happiness levels than nonvictims, unlike virtually everywhere that victimization has been studied. More generally, happiness levels (and having smiled the previous day) in Afghanistan are as high as the average for Latin America, suggesting a remarkable human capacity to adapt and retain natural levels of cheerfulness while in conditions of adversity and poverty that would be intolerable by most country's standards.

3   Data and Methods

In this chapter, we take advantage of a unique data set for Latin America, which combines data on happiness and crime victimization with detailed data on health status. The data are a subset of the Gallup World Poll for 2006, 2007, and 2008 for 24 countries in the region (most of these had more than 1 year of coverage). These data have been used widely in studies of the economics of happiness. One of the authors (Graham) has previously made extensive use of the Latinobarometro data to explore happiness in the region. The more recent studies based on Gallup data confirm her earlier findings, despite some modest differences in sampling and in the phrasing of the life satisfaction questions.[2] And, as noted, DiTella et al. (2008) have also used the Gallup data in an initial exploration of the well-being effects of crime in the region.

The Latin America subset of the Gallup Poll includes the EQ5D (Euro-Quality Five Dimensions) health index. This is an index of assessed health based on respondents'

---

[2] See Graham and Pettinato (2002). The Latinobarometro uses an open-ended happiness question, phrased simply as "generally speaking, how happy are you with your life?," with possible answers on a four point scale from not at all to very happy, similar to what is in the World Values and Eurobarometer surveys. The World Poll uses the Cantril best possible life question, where respondents are asked to imagine the best possible life and then to rank their life compared to that life on a 10 step ladder. While both questions are clearly good measures of life satisfaction, there are differences in particular, with how closely they correlate with income. The best possible life question is a more framed question and typically correlates more closely with income than do more open-ended happiness questions. For detail on these methodological differences and the debate they have generated, see Graham et al. (2010).

answers about whether they have extreme, moderate, or no problems with the following conditions: mobility, self-care, the usual acts (such as going to work and other daily activities), pain, and anxiety. The EQ5D has been used widely in Europe and the USA as a health self-assessment that tracks closely with objective indicators of health and as a way to value the relative well-being costs of different health conditions. Dolan pioneered its usage in the UK; Shaw and Combs implemented it in the USA, and most recently, Graham et al. (2010) used the EQ5D to value health conditions in Latin America, based on the Gallup data.[3] Our primary methodology in the study is the standard usage of regression analysis to study the determinants of reported well-being. The most orthodox approach is to rely on ordered logit regressions, as most of the variables that measure happiness are categorical rather than continuous. More recently, it has become common practice to also run OLS, POLS, COLS, and probit regressions on the same data. The results are very similar, and the latter methods allow more room for making inferences about cardinality as well as about the relative weights of the resulting coefficients. Van Praag and Ferrer-i-Carbonell (2007) discuss the merits and demerits of the various approaches in detail.

It is important to note that the coefficients that result from these sorts of estimations reflect statistical associations or correlations and cannot be interpreted in a causal manner due to endogeneity. The information that is reported by individuals can be biased by their inherent personality traits. For example, more optimistic individuals tend to report higher levels of life satisfaction and less insecurity than more pessimistic individuals. This can be corrected, to some extent, by the construction of an individual bias or "optimism" variable, which is calculated based on each respondent's responses to questions across several quality-of-life domains and the latent correlation between them – e.g., that which is not explained by socioeconomic and demographic traits. For detail on the method, see Graham and Lora (2009).

We are particularly interested in the links between victimization and insecurity on the one hand and mental health (as captured by anxiety variable) on the other. Graham et al. (2010) find that of all of the conditions in the EQ5D, anxiety has the strongest (negative) association with life satisfaction. While this finding must be tempered by the above stated endogeneity problem (more anxious people being more likely to report unhappiness or poor health), it highlights the very strong effects of mental health on well-being, relative to those of physical conditions like mobility problems.

There are, presumably, many ways to explore our adaptation hypothesis. Our first strategy involved a two-stage regression approach. In the first stage, we sought to predict individuals' probability of being victims of crime, based on a logit regression with three separate crime questions from the Gallup 2006–2008 surveys on the dependent variables. The three questions that we used were: Do you feel safe walking in your neighborhood at night? In the past 12 months, have you had anything stolen? In the past year, were you mugged? The independent variables included the usual vector of sociodemographic variables; income; a control for individual optimism, based on each respondent's assessments of his/her prospects of upward mobility

---

[3] See Dolan (1997), Shaw et al. (2005), and Graham et al. (2010).

(POUM) in the next 5 years,[4] country-level rule of law; GDP growth; country fixed effects; and an error term or residual. We then used the coefficient on the residual – e.g., the unexplained probability of being a crime victim as a proxy for living in a higher or lower crime norm area.

Our second-stage regressions had, respectively, life satisfaction and the EQ5D index as the dependent variables (in order to test the effects on both happiness and health), with the same sociodemographic variables and income as the independent, as well as each of our insecurity variables – safe walk, stolen, and mugged, respectively. We also included the corresponding insecurity residual among the independent variables. We ran the same second-stage regressions by separate gender, age, and income cohorts. The latter were defined as being above or below the median income for the respondent's country.[5]

4　Results

Our initial results provide support for our hypotheses that crime victimization would have negative effects on both happiness and health. The probability of being a crime victim is higher for the young, those without friends, the employed, those without concerns for food security (e.g., the nonpoor), those with lower levels of natural optimism, and, not surprisingly, those who live in a country with less rule of law. Perceptions of security (e.g., reporting to feel safe walking at night) were higher in the young, the employed, those in rural areas, the optimistic, and those in countries with better rule of law. We included POUM as a proxy for optimism, under the assumption that more optimistic people might be less likely to report crime and certainly less likely to perceive insecurity. Our results support that proposition, with those respondents with brighter prospects for the future less likely to report feeling insecure and/or to report being victimized (see Table 9.1).

Our second-stage regressions show that insecurity and crime victimization have negative and significant effects on both reported well-being and health, although are more consistent for the former. The links we find between crime victimization and well-being are confirmed by other studies (Di Tella et al. 2009; Powdthavee 2005) and not a particular surprise. The links between some kinds of victimization, perceptions of insecurity, and self-assessed health – as measured by the EQ5D index – are intuitive, but as far as we know, a fairly novel finding. Both crime victimization (being mugged) and perceptions of insecurity (not being able to walk safely in one's neighborhood) have significant negative effects on both happiness and health (see Table 9.2).

---

[4]POUM scores typically correlate closely with happiness and reflect innate optimism as well as realistic assessments for prospects for the future. We chose POUM rather than individual happiness as a control because the latter is the dependent variable in the second-stage regressions. In an additional specification, we used the principal component of several residuals as a control and got similar results. These latter results are available from the authors.

[5]See Technical Appendix A.1 for regression equation details.

Table 9.1 First step regressions

Dependent variables	(1) Do you feel safe walking alone at night in the city or area where you live? (Yes = 1) (Safe walk)	(2) Within the last 12 months: Have you had money or property stolen from you or another household member? (Yes = 1) (Stolen)	(3) Within the past 12 months: Have you been assaulted or mugged? (Yes = 1) (Mugged)	(4) Are there gangs in the area where you live? (Yes = 1) (Gangs)	(5) Is there illicit drug trafficking or drug sales in the area where you live? (Yes = 1) (Drugs)
Age (years)	0.0008*	−0.0067***	−0.0108***	−0.0056***	−0.0063***
	[0.0004]	[0.0006]	[0.0008]	[0.0011]	[0.0012]
Have friends	0.1452***	−0.1096***	−0.1835***	−0.0421	−0.0936*
	[0.0197]	[0.0240]	[0.0311]	[0.0512]	[0.0562]
Have employment	0.2751***	0.1640***	0.1427***	−0.0249	0.0984**
	[0.0144]	[0.0179]	[0.0244]	[0.0359]	[0.0393]
Live in urban area	−0.6713***	0.4045***	0.3582***	0.8049***	0.8640***
	[0.0153]	[0.0192]	[0.0253]	[0.0379]	[0.0414]
Does not have shortage of income to cover food costs	0.1269***	−0.3334***	−0.3269***	−0.2152***	−0.1507***
	[0.0185]	[0.0226]	[0.0308]	[0.0430]	[0.0473]
Does not have shortage of income to cover household costs	0.1164***	−0.2079***	−0.3739***	−0.0508	0.1392**
	[0.0202]	[0.0241]	[0.0316]	[0.0517]	[0.0571]
Prospects of Upward Mobility (POUM): Life situation expected in five years, 0 to 10 scale	0.0416***	−0.0012	−0.0180***	−0.0224***	−0.0170**
	[0.0031]	[0.0039]	[0.0053]	[0.0071]	[0.0077]
Constant term	−0.7322***	−1.5110***	−0.9774***	0.0272	0.1091
	[0.1103]	[0.1434]	[0.1725]	[0.1446]	[0.1528]
Number of observations	104419	106951	106984	14198	12594
Pseudo R Squared	0.109	0.0665	0.100	0.0580	0.0976

Standard errors in brackets
*** $p<0.01$, ** $p<0.05$, * $p<0.1$

Table 9.2a Second step: entire sample, dependent variable: life satisfaction

Dependent variable: life satisfaction, 0 to 10 scale	All the sample (without residuals)	All the sample (with residuals)	All the sample (without residuals)	All the sample (with residuals)	All the sample (without residuals)	All the sample (with residuals)	All the sample (without residuals)	All the sample (with residuals)	All the sample (without residuals)	All the sample (with residuals)
	(1)	(2)	(3)	(4)	(5)	(6)	(7)	(8)	(9)	(10)
Male	-0.1734*** [0.0353]	-0.1700*** [0.0374]	-0.1679*** [0.0349]	-0.1617*** [0.0370]	-0.1673*** [0.0349]	-0.1601*** [0.0370]	-0.1718*** [0.0359]	-0.1653*** [0.0380]	-0.1638*** [0.0380]	-0.1635*** [0.0400]
Age (years)	-0.0505*** [0.0055]	-0.0518*** [0.0059]	-0.0494*** [0.0054]	-0.0511*** [0.0058]	-0.0489*** [0.0054]	-0.0510*** [0.0058]	-0.0495*** [0.0056]	-0.0513*** [0.0060]	-0.0498*** [0.0059]	-0.0506*** [0.0063]
Age squared	0.0004*** [0.0001]	0.0005*** [0.0001]	0.0004*** [0.0001]	0.0004*** [0.0001]	0.0004*** [0.0001]	0.0004*** [0.0001]	0.0004*** [0.0001]	0.0004*** [0.0001]	0.0004*** [0.0001]	0.0004*** [0.0001]
Health score (EQ-5D)	1.2174*** [0.1314]	1.3094*** [0.1426]	1.2532*** [0.1307]	1.3417*** [0.1417]	1.2596*** [0.1307]	1.3524*** [0.1416]	1.2063*** [0.1342]	1.2820*** [0.1459]	1.1531*** [0.1426]	1.2715*** [0.1535]
Complete primary education	-0.0038 [0.0630]	0.0025 [0.0688]	0.0088 [0.0625]	0.0109 [0.0682]	0.0115 [0.0625]	0.0144 [0.0683]	0.0452 [0.0647]	0.0386 [0.0707]	0.0568 [0.0690]	0.0536 [0.0744]
Complete secondary education	0.0794 [0.0679]	0.0601 [0.0733]	0.0837 [0.0673]	0.0623 [0.0728]	0.0812 [0.0673]	0.0605 [0.0728]	0.1204* [0.0694]	0.0881 [0.0751]	0.1119 [0.0740]	0.0874 [0.0790]
Complete superior education	0.2512*** [0.0795]	0.2341*** [0.0858]	0.2653*** [0.0789]	0.2419*** [0.0852]	0.2581*** [0.0788]	0.2351*** [0.0851]	0.2748*** [0.0817]	0.2494*** [0.0879]	0.2674*** [0.0855]	0.2460*** [0.0913]
Married	-0.0208 [0.0441]	0.0101 [0.0464]	-0.0218 [0.0437]	0.0048 [0.0460]	-0.0243 [0.0437]	0.0036 [0.0461]	-0.0183 [0.0450]	0.0147 [0.0474]	-0.0182 [0.0472]	0.0184 [0.0495]
Divorced	-0.0495 [0.0783]	-0.0294 [0.0834]	-0.0635 [0.0777]	-0.0385 [0.0833]	-0.0634 [0.0780]	-0.0349 [0.0836]	-0.0662 [0.0799]	-0.0375 [0.0855]	-0.0667 [0.0842]	-0.0581 [0.0897]

	(1)	(2)	(3)	(4)	(5)	(6)	(7)	(8)	(9)	(10)
Widowed	0.0632 [0.0879]	0.1128 [0.0950]	0.0584 [0.0871]	0.0993 [0.0943]	0.0623 [0.0876]	0.1050 [0.0949]	0.0431 [0.0902]	0.0909 [0.0973]	0.0872 [0.0977]	0.1154 [0.1045]
Have one child	0.0108 [0.0451]	−0.0098 [0.0475]	0.0037 [0.0447]	−0.0167 [0.0472]	0.0046 [0.0449]	−0.0149 [0.0473]	0.0023 [0.0461]	−0.0133 [0.0485]	0.0125 [0.0487]	−0.0133 [0.0511]
Have two or more children	−0.0015 [0.0456]	−0.0101 [0.0483]	−0.0105 [0.0453]	−0.0149 [0.0480]	−0.0112 [0.0454]	−0.0152 [0.0482]	0.0036 [0.0465]	0.0074 [0.0492]	0.0188 [0.0493]	0.0157 [0.0521]
Consider religion to be important	0.2520*** [0.0419]	0.2287*** [0.0439]	0.2518*** [0.0415]	0.2322*** [0.0435]	0.2540*** [0.0416]	0.2321*** [0.0435]	0.2601*** [0.0425]	0.2348*** [0.0444]	0.2638*** [0.0453]	0.2349*** [0.0473]
Have friends	0.4274*** [0.0492]	0.4186*** [0.0534]	0.4324*** [0.0490]	0.4394*** [0.0533]	0.4318*** [0.0490]	0.4343*** [0.0533]	0.4373*** [0.0505]	0.4396*** [0.0546]	0.4332*** [0.0533]	0.4439*** [0.0574]
Have employment	0.0989*** [0.0369]	0.0508 [0.0397]	0.1052*** [0.0367]	0.0889** [0.0391]	0.1045*** [0.0367]	0.0893** [0.0391]	0.1066*** [0.0376]	0.0790** [0.0400]	0.1168*** [0.0399]	0.0896** [0.0423]
Household income (monthly per capita in PPP US$)	0.2256*** [0.0236]	0.2203*** [0.0253]	0.2238*** [0.0235]	0.2189*** [0.0252]	0.2243*** [0.0235]	0.2189*** [0.0253]	0.2278*** [0.0242]	0.2222*** [0.0258]	0.2378*** [0.0254]	0.2300*** [0.0270]
Live in urban area	−0.0110 [0.0375]	0.0491 [0.0411]	−0.0221 [0.0369]	−0.0117 [0.0397]	−0.0217 [0.0369]	−0.0088 [0.0395]	−0.0191 [0.0383]	0.0307 [0.0428]	−0.0277 [0.0402]	0.0040 [0.0449]
Access to running water service	0.0535 [0.0614]	−0.0029 [0.0665]	0.0476 [0.0612]	−0.0014 [0.0663]	0.0512 [0.0614]	0.0036 [0.0665]	0.0647 [0.0620]	0.0251 [0.0672]	0.0806 [0.0664]	0.0150 [0.0713]
Access to electricity service	0.3795*** [0.1085]	0.4495*** [0.1184]	0.3428*** [0.1089]	0.4070*** [0.1186]	0.3441*** [0.1087]	0.4117*** [0.1184]	0.3582*** [0.1116]	0.4077*** [0.1219]	0.3551*** [0.1161]	0.4218*** [0.1250]
Access to telephone service	0.1554*** [0.0407]	0.1719*** [0.0429]	0.1605*** [0.0404]	0.1730*** [0.0427]	0.1594*** [0.0404]	0.1682*** [0.0428]	0.1750*** [0.0415]	0.1758*** [0.0437]	0.1720*** [0.0441]	0.1834*** [0.0464]

(continued)

Table 9.2a (continued)

Dependent variable: life satisfaction, C to 10 scale	All the sample (without residuals) (1)	All the sample (with residuals) (2)	All the sample (without residuals) (3)	All the sample (with residuals) (4)	All the sample (without residuals) (5)	All the sample (with residuals) (6)	All the sample (without residuals) (7)	All the sample (with residuals) (8)	All the sample (without residuals) (9)	All the sample (with residuals) (10)
Asset index	0.1390*** [0.0157]	0.1406*** [0.0167]	0.1383*** [0.0156]	0.1405*** [0.0166]	0.1359*** [0.0156]	0.1381*** [0.0166]	0.1310*** [0.0161]	0.1315*** [0.0171]	0.1260*** [0.0169]	0.1251*** [0.0179]
Does not have shortage of income to cover food costs	0.4960*** [0.0411]	0.4852*** [0.0442]	0.4872*** [0.0408]	0.4914*** [0.0441]	0.4897*** [0.0409]	0.4846*** [0.0442]	0.5007*** [0.0417]	0.4963*** [0.0449]	0.4768*** [0.0445]	0.4813*** [0.0475]
Does not have shortage of income to cover household costs	0.2109*** [0.0519]	0.1676*** [0.0552]	0.2208*** [0.0515]	0.1920*** [0.0550]	0.2198*** [0.0517]	0.1793*** [0.0552]	0.2144*** [0.0527]	0.1869*** [0.0561]	0.2250*** [0.0564]	0.2127*** [0.0599]
Safe walk	**0.0984*** [0.0335]**	**0.5578*** [0.0789]**								
Safe walk residuals		**−1.0821*** [0.1731]**								
Stolen			**−0.0824** [0.0400]**	**−0.1346 [0.0971]**						
Stolen residuals				**0.0873 [0.1910]**						

9 The Linkages Between Insecurity, Health, and Well-Being in Latin America...

209

	1	2	3	4	5	6	7	8	9	10
Mugged					−0.0675 [0.0507]	−0.3915*** [0.1175]				
Mugged residuals						0.6292*** [0.2148]				
Gangs							−0.0606* [0.0343]	−0.3060*** [0.0863]		
Gangs residuals								0.5208*** [0.1865]		
Drugs									−0.0845** [0.0373]	−0.2484*** [0.0896]
Drugs residuals										0.3424* [0.1904]
Number of observations	11813	10521	11962	10644	11937	10624	11317	10107	10079	9070
Pseudo R Squared	0.0621	0.0621	0.0619	0.0613	0.0617	0.0613	0.0618	0.0610	0.0612	0.0605

Robust standard errors in brackets
*** p<0.01, ** p<0.05, * p<0.1

Table 9.2b Second step: entire sample, dependent variable: health score

Dependent variable: health score (EQ 5D)	All the sample (without residuals) (1)	All the sample (with residuals) (2)	All the sample (without residuals) (3)	All the sample (with residuals) (4)	All the sample (without residuals) (5)	All the sample (with residuals) (6)
Male	0.0516***	0.0482***	0.0512***	0.0478***	0.0454***	0.0413***
	[0.0071]	[0.0075]	[0.0071]	[0.0075]	[0.0071]	[0.0076]
Age (years)	−0.0036***	−0.0038***	−0.0037***	−0.0038***	−0.0036***	−0.0034***
	[0.0011]	[0.0012]	[0.0011]	[0.0012]	[0.0011]	[0.0012]
Age squared	−0.0000*	−0.0000	−0.0000*	−0.0000	−0.0000*	−0.0000*
	[0.0000]	[0.0000]	[0.0000]	[0.0000]	[0.0000]	[0.0000]
Complete primary education	0.0312***	0.0303***	0.0315***	0.0307***	0.0319***	0.0309***
	[0.0100]	[0.0109]	[0.0100]	[0.0109]	[0.0100]	[0.0110]
Complete secondary education	0.0451***	0.0396***	0.0480***	0.0426***	0.0468***	0.0400***
	[0.0115]	[0.0124]	[0.0115]	[0.0124]	[0.0116]	[0.0125]
Complete superior education	0.0418***	0.0428***	0.0465***	0.0471***	0.0436***	0.0432***
	[0.0149]	[0.0159]	[0.0148]	[0.0159]	[0.0150]	[0.0159]
Married	0.0051	0.0104	0.0052	0.0102	0.0058	0.0099
	[0.0088]	[0.0094]	[0.0088]	[0.0094]	[0.0089]	[0.0094]
Divorced	−0.0338**	−0.0280*	−0.0339**	−0.0283*	−0.0336**	−0.0289*
	[0.0142]	[0.0151]	[0.0142]	[0.0151]	[0.0144]	[0.0152]
Widowed	−0.0205	−0.0146	−0.0215	−0.0148	−0.0218	−0.0139
	[0.0152]	[0.0167]	[0.0152]	[0.0167]	[0.0154]	[0.0168]
Have one child	−0.0006	0.0026	−0.0002	0.0031	−0.0007	0.0020
	[0.0090]	[0.0096]	[0.0090]	[0.0096]	[0.0091]	[0.0097]
Have two or more children	−0.0051	−0.0106	−0.0037	−0.0089	−0.0044	−0.0105
	[0.0090]	[0.0095]	[0.0090]	[0.0095]	[0.0091]	[0.0096]
Consider religion to be important	0.0078	0.0080	0.0068	0.0074	0.0065	0.0072
	[0.0093]	[0.0097]	[0.0092]	[0.0097]	[0.0094]	[0.0098]
Have friends	0.0420***	0.0438***	0.0404***	0.0416***	0.0405***	0.0411***
	[0.0087]	[0.0093]	[0.0087]	[0.0093]	[0.0087]	[0.0094]
Have employment	0.0328***	0.0313***	0.0329***	0.0317***	0.0305***	0.0294***
	[0.0074]	[0.0078]	[0.0073]	[0.0078]	[0.0074]	[0.0079]
Household income (monthly per capita in PPP US$)	0.0155***	0.0163***	0.0157***	0.0166***	0.0147***	0.0155***
	[0.0042]	[0.0046]	[0.0042]	[0.0046]	[0.0043]	[0.0046]
Live in urban area	−0.0031	−0.0050	−0.0008	−0.0019	0.0021	0.0008
	[0.0073]	[0.0078]	[0.0073]	[0.0078]	[0.0074]	[0.0082]

(continued)

Table 9.2b (continued)

Dependent variable: health score (EQ 5D)	All the sample (without residuals) (1)	All the sample (with residuals) (2)	All the sample (without residuals) (3)	All the sample (with residuals) (4)	All the sample (without residuals) (5)	All the sample (with residuals) (6)
Access to running water service	−0.0211* [0.0116]	−0.0167 [0.0126]	−0.0239** [0.0116]	−0.0192 [0.0125]	−0.0235** [0.0118]	−0.0190 [0.0126]
Access to electricity service	−0.0011 [0.0187]	−0.0017 [0.0204]	−0.0046 [0.0187]	−0.0059 [0.0204]	−0.0015 [0.0189]	−0.0015 [0.0206]
Access to telephone service	0.0004 [0.0081]	−0.0017 [0.0086]	0.0022 [0.0081]	−0.0004 [0.0086]	0.0020 [0.0081]	0.0003 [0.0086]
Asset index	0.0065** [0.0031]	0.0069** [0.0033]	0.0075** [0.0031]	0.0078** [0.0033]	0.0067** [0.0031]	0.0073** [0.0033]
Does not have shortage of income to cover food costs	0.0929*** [0.0077]	0.0926*** [0.0084]	0.0911*** [0.0077]	0.0900*** [0.0084]	0.0932*** [0.0078]	0.0927*** [0.0084]
Does not have shortage of income to cover household costs	0.0201** [0.0090]	0.0229** [0.0098]	0.0210** [0.0090]	0.0226** [0.0097]	0.0221** [0.0091]	0.0250** [0.0098]
Mugged	**−0.0473*** [0.0098]**	**−0.0331 [0.0268]**				
Mugged residuals		**−0.0182 [0.0499]**				
Stolen			**−0.0661*** [0.0079]**	**−0.0702*** [0.0217]**		
Stolen residuals				**0.0212 [0.0434]**		
Safe walk					**0.0520*** [0.0067]**	**0.0477** [0.0188]**
Safe walk residuals						**0.0168 [0.0409]**
Constant term	1.1321*** [0.0626]	1.1194*** [0.0684]	1.0426*** [0.0469]	1.1096*** [0.0676]	1.1060*** [0.0627]	1.0763*** [0.0669]
Number of observations	12019	10643	12044	10663	11890	10539
Pseudo R Squared	0.195	0.186	0.200	0.191	0.197	0.190

Robust standard errors in brackets

*** $p<0.01$, ** $p<0.05$, * $p<0.1$

Our second baseline result is that as these phenomena become more common, individuals seem to adapt to them, a process which mitigates their negative effects. This result only holds for life satisfaction, and not for health. That is not surprising as it is likely that adapting to health shocks is more difficult than adapting to happiness drops. The mitigation effects in the life satisfaction arena – to the extent that is what we are capturing as opposed to unobserved variables that are also in the error term – are significant. As our residuals are likely capturing other unobservables, it is imprudent to attempt to attach relative weights to the coefficients; however, the sign on the residuals consistently runs in the opposite direction from the crime variables, and the magnitude of the coefficients is large (Table 9.2).

We first ran the regressions without including the residuals (Table 9.2a). The coefficients on our victimization variables are roughly the same – although slightly lower – when the residuals are not included. Including the residuals has no significant effects on our other covariates, suggesting that the residuals are not introducing random error into our specifications. Those respondents who have friends, for example, are less likely to be victimized, and having friends is also positively correlated with life satisfaction. When we include the residuals in the regression, the coefficient on having friends is essentially the same as when we do not, which, at the least, rules out the possibility that our proxy for a higher crime norm variable is picking up or diluting the friendships/network effects on life satisfaction.

Because the residuals are based on each individual's unexplained probability of being victimized, we posit that they are a better approximation of local-level crime rates than are national crime rates, which typically have a great deal of variance across cities and regions. Yet given that our residuals are likely also capturing any number of unobservables, we ran our second-stage life satisfaction regressions with national-level crime rate corresponding to each respondent (and clustering the standard errors), based on reported victimization in the sample, instead of our residuals. In this instance, the national-level victimization rates are correlated with lower levels of life satisfaction, suggesting that national-level rates and more local crime norms may operate differently. Another note of caution is that we are unable to control for country fixed effects when we include the national-level rates, so there may be many other country-level unobservables that are picked up by the national rates variables. Results are available from the authors.

Another plausible phenomenon that we are not able to capture with the Gallup data set, which is a cross-section across 2 years, is adaptation over time rather than to the level of crime at the moment. In another chapter, based on 10 years of Latinobarometro data, Soumya Chattopadhyay and Graham conducted a similar exercise in which we looked at the effects of victimization – and the unexplained probability of being victimized – on happiness across countries in Latin America. In this instance, we also included lagged victimization for 1 and 2 years. We found that being a victim a year ago was still negatively correlated with well-being, but being a victim 2 years before was positively correlated. This suggests that there is adaptation across time as well as to the overall level of crime.[6]

---

[6] We thank Rafael Di Tella for raising a question about why not using national rates of crime, as well as about levels versus over time effects. For the results, see Chap. 8 in Graham (2009).

The effects vary significantly across age and income cohorts (see Table 9.3a–c). The negative effects of victimization are, not surprisingly, worse for the life satisfaction of the elderly and the poor (more accurately, those respondents whose income is below the median), suggesting that crime has a regressive component. These groups are surely more vulnerable to crime, as they have less means to protect themselves from it. It is notable, for example, that the difference in the negative effects of victimization between the elderly and the young is much greater for being mugged than for having something stolen. Being mugged is a more direct and potentially violent experience than having something stolen, and one can imagine that the impact of this is greater for someone who is elderly and physically more vulnerable than for someone who is younger. Along the same vein, being mugged has negative and significant effects on women but not on men. In contrast, poorer and more vulnerable groups are less likely to be carrying valuables that are worth stealing (Table 9.3a–c).

The health effects of the perceptions of insecurity variables are similar but vary slightly across cohorts (Table 9.4a–c). The (positive) health effects of feeling safe walking in ones' neighborhood and the (negative) effects of being mugged or having something stolen, for example, are strongest for women, and the negative effects of having something stolen are the strongest for the elderly. One can imagine that the negative health effects of such experiences are worse for those cohorts that are more physically vulnerable than others (Table 9.4a–c). Adaptation, on the other hand, does not seem to occur in the health arena in the same way that it does in the happiness one.

It is, of course, possible that our residuals are merely picking up unobservable variables that have nothing to do with respondents' adaptation. Accepting that there is some error in what we are picking up, the consistency in the findings suggests there is something in what we are observing (or not observing) that mitigates the usual effects of these phenomena on reported happiness. The mitigation effects seem to be greater when the unexplained probabilities are higher – e.g., more common to the environment rather than explained by individual characteristics, which is suggestive of adaptation. This last finding, though, could be an artifact of construction: the residuals are greater when the unexplained probability of being a victim is greater precisely because we are able to explain less.

As a robustness check, we attempted an alternative specification, creating victimization propensities for each respondent and then testing how their actual victimization experience compares to those propensity scores. The gaps we find, in theory, should be equivalent to our unexplained probability residuals. Our results support our basic findings and results are available from the authors. Those respondents who report feeling safe in their neighborhood, for example, are significantly happier than those with similar characteristics but who do not report feeling safe. The coefficient on stolen is negative but insignificant, while that on mugged is negative and significant. This supports our above findings which suggest much stronger well-being effects for being mugged than for having something stolen, as the former is likely a more direct and unsettling experience [Results are available from the authors; for detail on the method, see Greene (2008)]. While the matching scores confirm the robustness of our victimization variables, however, they cannot fully resolve the question of the unobservables that our residuals are picking up.

Table 9.3a Second step: mugged, dependent variable: life satisfaction

Dependent variable: life satisfaction, 0 to 10 scale	All the sample (1)	Women (2)	Men (3)	15 to 35 Years old (4)	35 to 54 Years old (5)	55 to 74 Years old (6)	Income below the median (7)	Income above the median (8)
Male	−0.1601***			−0.1770***	−0.1779***	−0.0383	−0.1666***	−0.1572***
	[0.0370]			[0.0544]	[0.0646]	[0.0993]	[0.0552]	[0.0509]
Age (years)	−0.0510***	−0.0494***	−0.0521***	−0.1659***	−0.1094	−0.0056	−0.0590***	−0.0434***
	[0.0058]	[0.0076]	[0.0090]	[0.0449]	[0.0915]	[0.1868]	[0.0082]	[0.0083]
Age squared	0.0004***	0.0004***	0.0005***	0.0025***	0.0012	0.0001	0.0005***	0.0004***
	[0.0001]	[0.0001]	[0.0001]	[0.0009]	[0.0010]	[0.0015]	[0.0001]	[0.0001]
Health score (EQ-5D)	1.3524***	1.2129***	1.5468***	0.9308***	1.4317***	1.5349***	1.2672***	1.4533***
	[0.1416]	[0.1803]	[0.2305]	[0.2444]	[0.2581]	[0.2618]	[0.1957]	[0.2084]
Complete primary education	0.0144	0.0397	−0.0388	0.0895	−0.0920	−0.0442	0.0799	−0.1582
	[0.0683]	[0.0914]	[0.1030]	[0.1274]	[0.1215]	[0.1271]	[0.0831]	[0.1242]
Complete secondary education	0.0605	0.0585	0.0448	0.1622	−0.0573	0.0993	0.1473	−0.1275
	[0.0728]	[0.0977]	[0.1100]	[0.1295]	[0.1283]	[0.1550]	[0.0932]	[0.1257]
Complete superior education	0.2351***	0.2205*	0.2465*	0.3276**	0.1490	0.2020	0.3405***	0.0393
	[0.0851]	[0.1154]	[0.1283]	[0.1496]	[0.1456]	[0.1972]	[0.1301]	[0.1355]
Married	0.0036	0.0355	−0.1084	0.0125	0.0057	−0.1055	−0.0261	0.0284
	[0.0461]	[0.0609]	[0.0744]	[0.0633]	[0.0915]	[0.1492]	[0.0657]	[0.0658]
Divorced	−0.0349	−0.0577	−0.0046	−0.2278	−0.0712	0.1107	−0.1532	0.0602
	[0.0836]	[0.1052]	[0.1372]	[0.1711]	[0.1246]	[0.2071]	[0.1264]	[0.1137]
Widowed	0.1050	0.1667	−0.0867	0.0601	0.0671	0.0182	0.2080	−0.0435
	[0.0949]	[0.1100]	[0.1961]	[0.3919]	[0.1966]	[0.1691]	[0.1305]	[0.1393]
Have one child	−0.0149	−0.1271**	0.1371*	0.1361**	−0.1254	−0.2226	−0.0622	−0.0080
	[0.0473]	[0.0647]	[0.0703]	[0.0687]	[0.0809]	[0.1412]	[0.0771]	[0.0635]

Have two or more children	−0.0152 [0.0482]	−0.0408 [0.0648]	0.0090 [0.0734]	0.1226* [0.0719]	−0.0776 [0.0841]	−0.3831*** [0.1436]	−0.0680 [0.0709]	0.0525 [0.0717]
Consider religion to be important	0.2321*** [0.0435]	0.1618** [0.0632]	0.3117*** [0.0614]	0.3084*** [0.0603]	0.1445* [0.0795]	0.1271 [0.1309]	0.1934*** [0.0666]	0.2696*** [0.0590]
Have friends	0.4343*** [0.0533]	0.5118*** [0.0708]	0.3283*** [0.0820]	0.4418*** [0.0913]	0.3954*** [0.0847]	0.4149*** [0.1195]	0.3720*** [0.0673]	0.5015*** [0.0890]
Have employment	0.0893** [0.0391]	0.0261 [0.0532]	0.1841*** [0.0619]	0.0901 [0.0571]	0.1070 [0.0698]	0.1604 [0.1051]	0.0759 [0.0575]	0.0949* [0.0548]
Household income (monthly per capita in PPP US$)	0.2189*** [0.0253]	0.1887*** [0.0332]	0.2588*** [0.0387]	0.2416*** [0.0374]	0.2312*** [0.0446]	0.1207* [0.0673]	0.1766*** [0.0441]	0.2542*** [0.0475]
Live in urban area	−0.0088 [0.0395]	0.0129 [0.0537]	−0.0374 [0.0589]	0.0137 [0.0573]	0.0581 [0.0699]	−0.2047** [0.1037]	−0.0080 [0.0548]	−0.0043 [0.0586]
Access to running water service	0.0036 [0.0665]	−0.0058 [0.0893]	0.0154 [0.1009]	0.1040 [0.0961]	−0.0956 [0.1123]	−0.0244 [0.1871]	−0.0103 [0.0814]	0.0580 [0.1170]
Access to electricity service	0.4117*** [0.1184]	0.3630** [0.1598]	0.4985*** [0.1758]	0.4585** [0.1836]	0.3701** [0.1828]	0.2399 [0.3113]	0.2866** [0.1359]	0.7135*** [0.2525]
Access to telephone service	0.1682*** [0.0428]	0.1716*** [0.0575]	0.1689*** [0.0643]	0.1553** [0.0605]	0.1750** [0.0764]	0.2370* [0.1214]	0.2262*** [0.0622]	0.0896 [0.0606]
Asset index	0.1381*** [0.0166]	0.1533*** [0.0232]	0.1220*** [0.0243]	0.1342*** [0.0242]	0.1468*** [0.0299]	0.1530*** [0.0443]	0.1455*** [0.0257]	0.1326*** [0.0227]

(continued)

Table 9.3a (continued)

Dependent variable: life satisfaction, 0 to 10 scale	All the sample	Women	Men	15 to 35 Years old	35 to 54 Years old	55 to 74 Years old	Income below the median	Income above the median
	(1)	(2)	(3)	(4)	(5)	(6)	(7)	(8)
Does not have shortage of income to cover food costs	0.4846***	0.5515***	0.3727***	0.4397***	0.5302***	0.5960***	0.3704***	0.6427***
	[0.0442]	[0.0586]	[0.0683]	[0.0663]	[0.0738]	[0.1162]	[0.0569]	[0.0701]
Does not have shortage of income to cover household costs	0.1793***	0.0492	0.3616***	0.1653**	0.1255	0.2856*	0.1721**	0.1636*
	[0.0552]	[0.0752]	[0.0816]	[0.0837]	[0.0905]	[0.1543]	[0.0690]	[0.0922]
Mugged	**−0.3915***	**−0.4712***	**−0.2832**	**−0.4291***	**−0.4736***	**0.1735**	**−0.5800***	**−0.3023***
	[0.1175]	**[0.1551]**	**[0.1847]**	**[0.1455]**	**[0.2438]**	**[0.3779]**	**[0.1970]**	**[0.1493]**
Mugged residuals	**0.6292***	**0.8192***	**0.3555**	**0.7745***	**0.5278**	**−0.3601**	**0.9174***	**0.4886***
	[0.2148]	[0.2808]	[0.3408]	[0.2661]	[0.4429]	[0.6922]	[0.3600]	[0.2736]
Number of observations	10624	5892	4732	5094	3544	1652	5180	5444
Pseudo R Square	0.0613	0.0597	0.0664	0.0578	0.0635	0.0637	0.0510	0.0521

Robust standard errors in brackets
*** p<0.01, ** p<0.05, * p<0.1

Table 9.3b Second step: stolen, dependent variable: life satisfaction

Dependent variable: life satisfaction, 0 to 10 scale	All the sample (1)	Women (2)	Men (3)	15 to 35 Years old (4)	35 to 54 Years old (5)	55 to 74 Years old (6)	Income below the median (7)	Income above the median (8)
Male	-0.1617*** [0.0370]			-0.1804*** [0.0543]	-0.1789*** [0.0647]	-0.0379 [0.0990]	-0.1669*** [0.0551]	-0.1603*** [0.0509]
Age (years)	-0.0511*** [0.0058]	-0.0499*** [0.0076]	-0.0518*** [0.0090]	-0.1653*** [0.0447]	-0.1152 [0.0915]	0.0109 [0.1861]	-0.0584*** [0.0082]	-0.0442*** [0.0083]
Age squared	0.0004*** [0.0001]	0.0004*** [0.0001]	0.0005*** [0.0001]	0.0025*** [0.0009]	0.0013 [0.0010]	-0.0000 [0.0015]	0.0005*** [0.0001]	0.0004*** [0.0001]
Health score (EQ-5D)	1.3417*** [0.1417]	1.1985*** [0.1810]	1.5387*** [0.2304]	0.9124*** [0.2443]	1.4166*** [0.2592]	1.5247*** [0.2610]	1.2680*** [0.1955]	1.4361*** [0.2090]
Complete primary education	0.0109 [0.0682]	0.0378 [0.0914]	-0.0462 [0.1027]	0.0886 [0.1272]	-0.1063 [0.1215]	-0.0418 [0.1270]	0.0744 [0.0830]	-0.1612 [0.1240]
Complete secondary education	0.0623 [0.0728]	0.0614 [0.0979]	0.0436 [0.1094]	0.1615 [0.1293]	-0.0637 [0.1281]	0.1066 [0.1553]	0.1378 [0.0932]	-0.1148 [0.1256]
Complete superior education	0.2419*** [0.0852]	0.2295** [0.1157]	0.2502* [0.1280]	0.3302** [0.1496]	0.1474 [0.1454]	0.2183 [0.1968]	0.3429*** [0.1296]	0.0511 [0.1356]
Married	0.0048 [0.0460]	0.0360 [0.0608]	-0.1070 [0.0742]	0.0115 [0.0631]	0.0066 [0.0915]	-0.0981 [0.1494]	-0.0262 [0.0655]	0.0297 [0.0658]
Divorced	-0.0385 [0.0833]	-0.0648 [0.1049]	-0.0019 [0.1362]	-0.2297 [0.1696]	-0.0809 [0.1239]	0.1093 [0.2076]	-0.1689 [0.1256]	0.0653 [0.1137]
Widowed	0.0993 [0.0943]	0.1599 [0.1091]	-0.0874 [0.1956]	0.0520 [0.3907]	0.0473 [0.1926]	0.0306 [0.1689]	0.1944 [0.1292]	-0.0378 [0.1391]
Have one child	-0.0167 [0.0472]	-0.1274** [0.0648]	0.1383** [0.0698]	0.1385** [0.0686]	-0.1196 [0.0806]	-0.2514* [0.1409]	-0.0611 [0.0768]	-0.0110 [0.0633]
Have two or more children	-0.0149 [0.0480]	-0.0419 [0.0647]	0.0139 [0.0733]	0.1234* [0.0717]	-0.0784 [0.0841]	-0.3803*** [0.1424]	-0.0653 [0.0705]	0.0545 [0.0717]

(continued)

Table 9.3b (continued)

Dependent variable: life satisfaction, 0 to 10 scale	All the sample (1)	Women (2)	Men (3)	15 to 35 Years old (4)	35 to 54 Years old (5)	55 to 74 Years old (6)	Income below the median (7)	Income above the median (8)
Consider religion to be important	0.2322***	0.1620**	0.3124***	0.3082***	0.1441*	0.1261	0.1921***	0.2706***
	[0.0435]	[0.0631]	[0.0612]	[0.0604]	[0.0788]	[0.1305]	[0.0663]	[0.0590]
Have friends	0.4394***	0.5177***	0.3329***	0.4483***	0.4025***	0.4096***	0.3822***	0.5076***
	[0.0533]	[0.0707]	[0.0821]	[0.0911]	[0.0850]	[0.1192]	[0.0672]	[0.0890]
Have employment	0.0889**	0.0272	0.1788***	0.0886	0.1100	0.1521	0.0711	0.0976*
	[0.0391]	[0.0532]	[0.0620]	[0.0571]	[0.0700]	[0.1053]	[0.0574]	[0.0548]
Household income (monthly per capita in PPP US$)	0.2189***	0.1901***	0.2577***	0.2416***	0.2296***	0.1233*	0.1769***	0.2546***
	[0.0252]	[0.0332]	[0.0386]	[0.0374]	[0.0447]	[0.0673]	[0.0441]	[0.0474]
Live in urban area	−0.0117	0.0142	−0.0493	0.0175	0.0500	−0.2034*	−0.0263	0.0035
	[0.0397]	[0.0536]	[0.0596]	[0.0572]	[0.0711]	[0.1040]	[0.0550]	[0.0589]
Access to running water service	−0.0014	−0.0085	0.0098	0.1061	−0.1139	−0.0231	−0.0118	0.0430
	[0.0663]	[0.0893]	[0.1004]	[0.0958]	[0.1114]	[0.1867]	[0.0813]	[0.1160]
Access to electricity service	0.4070***	0.3504**	0.5065***	0.4539**	0.3695**	0.2302	0.2837**	0.7252***
	[0.1186]	[0.1595]	[0.1768]	[0.1846]	[0.1833]	[0.3130]	[0.1356]	[0.2534]
Access to telephone service	0.1730***	0.1756***	0.1749***	0.1649***	0.1784**	0.2220*	0.2283***	0.0988
	[0.0427]	[0.0575]	[0.0643]	[0.0604]	[0.0766]	[0.1205]	[0.0620]	[0.0606]
Asset index	0.1405***	0.1563***	0.1237***	0.1348***	0.1513***	0.1566***	0.1478***	0.1358***
	[0.0166]	[0.0232]	[0.0242]	[0.0241]	[0.0299]	[0.0439]	[0.0255]	[0.0227]
Does not have shortage of income to cover food costs	0.4914***	0.5570***	0.3823***	0.4492***	0.5355***	0.5875***	0.3877***	0.6405***
	[0.0441]	[0.0585]	[0.0684]	[0.0663]	[0.0738]	[0.1160]	[0.0567]	[0.0701]

Does not have shortage of income to cover household costs	0.1920***	0.0592	0.3750***	0.1798**	0.1436	0.2763*	0.1947***	0.1742*
	[0.0550]	[0.0749]	[0.0813]	[0.0837]	[0.0898]	[0.1530]	[0.0684]	[0.0922]
Stolen	**-0.1346**	**-0.2632****	**0.0343**	**-0.1703**	**-0.1563**	**0.0833**	**-0.0300**	**-0.2247***
	[0.0971]	**[0.1294]**	**[0.1486]**	**[0.1211]**	**[0.2072]**	**[0.3516]**	**[0.1590]**	**[0.1255]**
Stolen residuals	**0.0873**	**0.3394**	**-0.2473**	**0.2225**	**0.0544**	**-0.3549**	**-0.0244**	**0.1582**
	[0.1910]	[0.2513]	[0.2957]	[0.2372]	[0.4090]	[0.6887]	[0.3123]	[0.2465]
Number of observations	10644	5902	4742	5104	3547	1659	5192	5452
Pseudo R Squared	0.0613	0.0598	0.0664	0.0576	0.0638	0.0635	0.0506	0.0525

Robust standard errors in brackets
*** $p<0.01$, ** $p<0.05$, * $p<0.1$

Table 9.3c Second step: safe walk, dependent variable: life satisfaction

Dependent variable: life satisfaction, 0 to 10 scale	All the sample (1)	Women (2)	Men (3)	15 to 35 Years old (4)	35 To 54 Years old (5)	55 to 74 Years old (6)	Income below the median (7)	Income above the median (8)
Male	−0.1700***			−0.1864***	−0.1942***	−0.0149	−0.1707***	−0.1741***
	[0.0374]			[0.0546]	[0.0654]	[0.1006]	[0.0557]	[0.0515]
Age (years)	−0.0518***	−0.0508***	−0.0521***	−0.1711***	−0.1073	−0.0089	−0.0580***	−0.0458***
	[0.0059]	[0.0077]	[0.0092]	[0.0449]	[0.0921]	[0.1884]	[0.0083]	[0.0085]
Age squared	0.0005***	0.0004***	0.0005***	0.0026***	0.0012	0.0001	0.0005***	0.0004***
	[0.0001]	[0.0001]	[0.0001]	[0.0009]	[0.0010]	[0.0015]	[0.0001]	[0.0001]
Health score (EQ-5D)	1.3094***	1.1740***	1.4970***	0.8924***	1.4620***	1.3815***	1.1888***	1.4492***
	[0.1426]	[0.1806]	[0.2351]	[0.2470]	[0.2563]	[0.2641]	[0.1974]	[0.2098]
Complete primary education	0.0025	0.0191	−0.0392	0.1154	−0.1391	−0.0701	0.0669	−0.1722
	[0.0688]	[0.0921]	[0.1037]	[0.1280]	[0.1228]	[0.1281]	[0.0834]	[0.1256]
Complete secondary education	0.0601	0.0609	0.0380	0.1827	−0.0653	0.0981	0.1387	−0.1203
	[0.0733]	[0.0986]	[0.1107]	[0.1301]	[0.1294]	[0.1562]	[0.0939]	[0.1269]
Complete superior education	0.2341***	0.2204*	0.2430*	0.3433**	0.1549	0.1692	0.3150**	0.0508
	[0.0858]	[0.1166]	[0.1291]	[0.1502]	[0.1469]	[0.1990]	[0.1312]	[0.1369]
Married	0.0101	0.0437	−0.1044	0.0198	0.0079	−0.1084	−0.0351	0.0490
	[0.0464]	[0.0614]	[0.0748]	[0.0632]	[0.0924]	[0.1503]	[0.0660]	[0.0664]
Divorced	−0.0294	−0.0632	0.0178	−0.1979	−0.0771	0.0772	−0.1528	0.0731
	[0.0834]	[0.1055]	[0.1358]	[0.1685]	[0.1249]	[0.2105]	[0.1258]	[0.1138]
Widowed	0.1128	0.1832*	−0.1030	0.0394	0.1051	0.0236	0.2386*	−0.0525
	[0.0950]	[0.1097]	[0.2010]	[0.3947]	[0.1934]	[0.1721]	[0.1309]	[0.1397]
Have one child	−0.0098	−0.1266*	0.1487**	0.1402**	−0.1022	−0.2649*	−0.0704	−0.0017
	[0.0475]	[0.0654]	[0.0701]	[0.0688]	[0.0814]	[0.1418]	[0.0774]	[0.0638]
Have two or more children	−0.0101	−0.0348	0.0132	0.1258*	−0.0690	−0.3742***	−0.0718	0.0546
	[0.0483]	[0.0651]	[0.0735]	[0.0718]	[0.0848]	[0.1438]	[0.0712]	[0.0718]

	(1)	(2)	(3)	(4)	(5)	(6)	(7)	(8)
Consider religion to be important	0.2287***	0.1584**	0.3037***	0.3043***	0.1414*	0.0936	0.2013***	0.2549***
	[0.0439]	[0.0637]	[0.0620]	[0.0608]	[0.0797]	[0.1340]	[0.0669]	[0.0595]
Have friends	0.4186***	0.5033***	0.3030***	0.4333***	0.3676***	0.3739***	0.3593***	0.4811***
	[0.0534]	[0.0710]	[0.0821]	[0.0911]	[0.0850]	[0.1202]	[0.0675]	[0.0892]
Have employment	0.0508	-0.0048	0.1353**	0.0627	0.0555	0.0559	0.0254	0.0657
	[0.0397]	[0.0539]	[0.0630]	[0.0576]	[0.0710]	[0.1083]	[0.0581]	[0.0557]
Household income (monthly per capita in PPP US$)	0.2203***	0.1901***	0.2607***	0.2470***	0.2170***	0.1369**	0.1917***	0.2553***
	[0.0253]	[0.0331]	[0.0389]	[0.0371]	[0.0448]	[0.0689]	[0.0438]	[0.0478]
Live in urban area	0.0491	0.0650	0.0286	0.0487	0.1372*	0.0247	0.0488	0.0523
	[0.0411]	[0.0564]	[0.0608]	[0.0586]	[0.0742]	[0.1161]	[0.0579]	[0.0605]
Access to running water service	-0.0029	-0.0191	0.0167	0.1067	-0.1079	-0.0413	-0.0041	0.0261
	[0.0665]	[0.0895]	[0.1010]	[0.0964]	[0.1118]	[0.1863]	[0.0818]	[0.1165]
Access to electricity service	0.4495***	0.4082***	0.5332***	0.4658***	0.4214**	0.3734	0.3172**	0.7730***
	[0.1184]	[0.1579]	[0.1780]	[0.1828]	[0.1842]	[0.3261]	[0.1354]	[0.2535]
Access to telephone service	0.1719***	0.1821***	0.1615**	0.1550**	0.1835**	0.2492**	0.2336***	0.0903
	[0.0429]	[0.0579]	[0.0643]	[0.0607]	[0.0765]	[0.1224]	[0.0624]	[0.0609]
Asset index	0.1406***	0.1554***	0.1251***	0.1341***	0.1540***	0.1544***	0.1491***	0.1357***
	[0.0167]	[0.0234]	[0.0244]	[0.0242]	[0.0301]	[0.0446]	[0.0257]	[0.0229]
Does not have shortage of income to cover food costs	0.4852***	0.5633***	0.3565***	0.4483***	0.5298***	0.5310***	0.3762***	0.6398***
	[0.0442]	[0.0586]	[0.0684]	[0.0663]	[0.0737]	[0.1178]	[0.0567]	[0.0702]

(continued)

Table 9.3c (continued)

Dependent variable: life satisfaction, 0 to 10 scale	All the sample (1)	Women (2)	Men (3)	15 to 35 Years old (4)	35 To 54 Years old (5)	55 to 74 Years old (6)	Income below the median (7)	Income above the median (8)
Does not have shortage of income to cover household costs	0.1676*** [0.0552]	0.0438 [0.0752]	0.3390*** [0.0816]	0.1694** [0.0838]	0.1087 [0.0894]	0.1787 [0.1557]	0.1668** [0.0685]	0.1500 [0.0928]
Safe walk	**0.5578*** [0.0789]**	**0.4914*** [0.1045]**	**0.6450*** [0.1214]**	**0.3554*** [0.0967]**	**0.8443*** [0.1651]**	**1.6496*** [0.3589]**	**0.6393*** [0.1299]**	**0.5210*** [0.1028]**
Safe walk residuals	**−1.0821*** [0.1731]**	**−0.9295*** [0.2285]**	**−1.2667*** [0.2662]**	**−0.7163*** [0.2161]**	**−1.6605*** [0.3574]**	**−3.3551*** [0.7676]**	**−1.3118*** [0.2829]**	**−0.9486*** [0.2272]**
Number of observations	10521	5821	4700	5069	3507	1624	5133	5388
Pseudo R Squared	0.0621	0.0606	0.0671	0.0582	0.0655	0.0657	0.0517	0.0534

Robust standard errors in brackets

*** p<0.01, ** p<0.05, * p<0.1

9 The Linkages Between Insecurity, Health, and Well-Being in Latin America...

223

Table 9.4a Second step: mugged, dependent variable: health score

Dependent variable: health score (EQ 5D)	All the sample (1)	Women (2)	Men (3)	15 to 35 Years old (4)	35 to 54 Years old (5)	55 to 74 Years old (6)
Male	0.0482***			0.0333***	0.0692***	0.0472***
	[0.0075]			[0.0126]	[0.0128]	[0.0156]
Age (years)	−0.0038***	−0.0061***	−0.0005	−0.0158	−0.0030	−0.0134
	[0.0012]	[0.0015]	[0.0019]	[0.0104]	[0.0168]	[0.0318]
Age squared	−0.0000	0.0000	−0.0000**	0.0002	−0.0000	0.0001
	[0.0000]	[0.0000]	[0.0000]	[0.0002]	[0.0002]	[0.0002]
Complete primary education	0.0303***	0.0306**	0.0257	−0.0018	0.0322*	0.0168
	[0.0109]	[0.0140]	[0.0176]	[0.0233]	[0.0180]	[0.0193]
Complete secondary education	0.0396***	0.0448***	0.0270	0.0077	0.0490**	0.0443*
	[0.0124]	[0.0159]	[0.0200]	[0.0246]	[0.0203]	[0.0244]
Complete superior education	0.0428***	0.0510**	0.0279	0.0190	0.0267	0.0360
	[0.0159]	[0.0203]	[0.0257]	[0.0301]	[0.0249]	[0.0342]
Married	0.0104	0.0152	−0.0056	0.0179	−0.0071	−0.0270
	[0.0094]	[0.0117]	[0.0159]	[0.0146]	[0.0170]	[0.0245]
Divorced	−0.0280*	−0.0214	−0.0393	−0.0389	−0.0459**	−0.0682**
	[0.0151]	[0.0181]	[0.0273]	[0.0327]	[0.0227]	[0.0324]
Widowed	−0.0146	0.0010	−0.0458	0.0173	−0.0511	−0.0219
	[0.0167]	[0.0195]	[0.0332]	[0.0850]	[0.0321]	[0.0280]
Have one child	0.0026	0.0084	−0.0076	−0.0160	0.0218	−0.0028
	[0.0096]	[0.0122]	[0.0155]	[0.0167]	[0.0152]	[0.0212]
Have two or more children	−0.0106	−0.0120	−0.0128	−0.0324**	0.0008	−0.0077
	[0.0095]	[0.0122]	[0.0152]	[0.0163]	[0.0160]	[0.0214]
Consider religion to be important	0.0080	0.0303**	−0.0141	0.0178	−0.0149	0.0174
	[0.0097]	[0.0133]	[0.0144]	[0.0144]	[0.0173]	[0.0243]

(continued)

Table 9.4a (continued)

Dependent variable: health score (EQ 5D)	All the sample (1)	Women (2)	Men (3)	15 to 35 Years old (4)	35 to 54 Years old (5)	55 to 74 Years old (6)
Have friends	0.0438*** [0.0093]	0.0502*** [0.0117]	0.0315** [0.0154]	0.0485*** [0.0181]	0.0294** [0.0141]	0.0546*** [0.0184]
Have employment	0.0313*** [0.0078]	0.0177* [0.0101]	0.0499*** [0.0125]	−0.0044 [0.0129]	0.0476*** [0.0126]	0.0699*** [0.0169]
Household income (monthly per capita in PPP US$)	0.0163*** [0.0046]	0.0103* [0.0058]	0.0236*** [0.0074]	0.0109 [0.0076]	0.0183** [0.0080]	0.0265*** [0.0094]
Live in urban area	−0.0050 [0.0078]	−0.0001 [0.0099]	−0.0090 [0.0124]	0.0046 [0.0130]	−0.0036 [0.0130]	−0.0020 [0.0160]
Access to running water service	−0.0167 [0.0126]	−0.0291* [0.0165]	0.0012 [0.0193]	−0.0131 [0.0194]	−0.0309 [0.0214]	−0.0002 [0.0301]
Access to electricity service	−0.0017 [0.0204]	0.0035 [0.0276]	−0.0074 [0.0305]	0.0109 [0.0341]	0.0212 [0.0336]	−0.0322 [0.0441]
Access to telephone service	−0.0017 [0.0086]	0.0095 [0.0109]	−0.0167 [0.0138]	0.0224 [0.0145]	−0.0150 [0.0141]	−0.0521*** [0.0186]
Asset index	0.0069** [0.0033]	0.0041 [0.0043]	0.0112** [0.0051]	−0.0042 [0.0056]	0.0134** [0.0056]	0.0179*** [0.0067]
Does not have shortage of income to cover food costs	0.0926*** [0.0084]	0.1030*** [0.0105]	0.0746*** [0.0140]	0.1003*** [0.0139]	0.0921*** [0.0135]	0.0672*** [0.0181]
Does not have shortage of income to cover household costs	0.0229** [0.0098]	0.0111 [0.0125]	0.0459*** [0.0158]	0.0242 [0.0159]	0.0447*** [0.0155]	−0.0227 [0.0232]

Mugged	-0.0331	-0.0884**	0.0310	0.0024	-0.1234**	-0.1132
	[0.0268]	[0.0351]	[0.0406]	[0.0342]	[0.0541]	[0.0706]
Mugged residuals	-0.0182	0.0695	-0.1210	-0.1195*	0.1603	0.1848
	[0.0499]	[0.0647]	[0.0759]	[0.0639]	[0.1015]	[0.1273]
Constant term	1.1194***	1.2191***	1.0426***	1.4243***	0.8652**	1.2235
	[0.0684]	[0.0946]	[0.1010]	[0.1655]	[0.3780]	[1.0150]
Number of observations	10643	5906	4737	5105	3548	1656
Pseudo R Squared	0.186	0.211	0.153	0.115	0.164	0.170

Robust standard errors in brackets
*** p<0.01, ** p<0.05, * p<0.1

Table 9.4b Second step: stolen, dependent variable: health score

Dependent variable: health score (EQ 5D)	All the sample (1)	Women (2)	Men (3)	15 to 35 Years old (4)	35 to 54 Years old (5)	55 to 74 Years old (6)	Income below the median (7)	Income above the median (8)
Male	0.0478***			0.0316**	0.0707***	0.0462***	0.0430***	0.0512***
	[0.0075]			[0.0126]	[0.0128]	[0.0156]	[0.0104]	[0.0109]
Age (years)	−0.0038***	−0.0063***	−0.0004	−0.0135	−0.0032	−0.0142	−0.0047***	−0.0025
	[0.0012]	[0.0015]	[0.0019]	[0.0104]	[0.0168]	[0.0317]	[0.0016]	[0.0017]
Age squared	−0.0000	0.0000	−0.0000**	0.0002	−0.0000	0.0001	−0.0000	−0.0000
	[0.0000]	[0.0000]	[0.0000]	[0.0002]	[0.0002]	[0.0002]	[0.0000]	[0.0000]
Complete primary education	0.0307***	0.0310**	0.0260	0.0003	0.0319*	0.0166	0.0234*	0.0443**
	[0.0109]	[0.0139]	[0.0176]	[0.0233]	[0.0179]	[0.0192]	[0.0134]	[0.0189]
Complete secondary education	0.0426***	0.0484***	0.0288	0.0132	0.0497**	0.0485**	0.0227	0.0643***
	[0.0124]	[0.0159]	[0.0199]	[0.0246]	[0.0202]	[0.0244]	[0.0161]	[0.0202]
Complete superior education	0.0471***	0.0570***	0.0298	0.0256	0.0308	0.0381	0.0226	0.0656***
	[0.0159]	[0.0203]	[0.0257]	[0.0301]	[0.0248]	[0.0342]	[0.0247]	[0.0233]
Married	0.0102	0.0150	−0.0059	0.0169	−0.0056	−0.0271	0.0197	−0.0085
	[0.0094]	[0.0117]	[0.0159]	[0.0146]	[0.0169]	[0.0244]	[0.0124]	[0.0143]
Divorced	−0.0283*	−0.0220	−0.0392	−0.0394	−0.0467**	−0.0645**	−0.0402**	−0.0275
	[0.0151]	[0.0181]	[0.0272]	[0.0327]	[0.0225]	[0.0325]	[0.0201]	[0.0230]
Widowed	−0.0148	0.0008	−0.0464	0.0154	−0.0467	−0.0230	0.0253	−0.0704***
	[0.0167]	[0.0194]	[0.0332]	[0.0856]	[0.0316]	[0.0279]	[0.0215]	[0.0262]
Have one child	0.0031	0.0087	−0.0061	−0.0152	0.0234	−0.0026	−0.0000	0.0037
	[0.0096]	[0.0122]	[0.0155]	[0.0166]	[0.0152]	[0.0213]	[0.0143]	[0.0133]
Have two or more children	−0.0089	−0.0103	−0.0113	−0.0285*	0.0018	−0.0075	−0.0293**	0.0162
	[0.0095]	[0.0122]	[0.0152]	[0.0163]	[0.0159]	[0.0213]	[0.0133]	[0.0147]

Consider religion to be important	0.0074 [0.0097]	0.0285** [0.0133]	-0.0143 [0.0143]	0.0160 [0.0144]	-0.0136 [0.0171]	0.0171 [0.0242]	-0.0120 [0.0141]	0.0240* [0.0135]
Have friends	0.0416*** [0.0093]	0.0487*** [0.0117]	0.0290* [0.0154]	0.0452** [0.0181]	0.0286** [0.0140]	0.0534*** [0.0186]	0.0511*** [0.0117]	0.0246 [0.0156]
Have employment	0.0317*** [0.0078]	0.0191* [0.0101]	0.0497*** [0.0125]	-0.0050 [0.0129]	0.0466*** [0.0126]	0.0728*** [0.0169]	0.0256** [0.0107]	0.0394*** [0.0115]
Household income (monthly per capita in PPP US$)	0.0166*** [0.0046]	0.0110* [0.0058]	0.0236*** [0.0074]	0.0114 [0.0076]	0.0185** [0.0079]	0.0271*** [0.0094]	0.0134* [0.0071]	0.0211** [0.0101]
Live in urban area	-0.0019 [0.0078]	0.0026 [0.0100]	-0.0059 [0.0125]	0.0056 [0.0129]	0.0001 [0.0130]	0.0042 [0.0163]	-0.0100 [0.0105]	0.0077 [0.0118]
Access to running water service	-0.0192 [0.0125]	-0.0297* [0.0164]	-0.0039 [0.0193]	-0.0164 [0.0194]	-0.0348* [0.0211]	-0.0004 [0.0302]	-0.0043 [0.0145]	-0.0418* [0.0250]
Access to electricity service	-0.0059 [0.0204]	-0.0027 [0.0273]	-0.0084 [0.0305]	0.0042 [0.0341]	0.0190 [0.0334]	-0.0352 [0.0442]	0.0195 [0.0228]	-0.0898* [0.0468]
Access to telephone service	-0.0004 [0.0086]	0.0096 [0.0108]	-0.0142 [0.0139]	0.0261* [0.0144]	-0.0140 [0.0141]	-0.0514*** [0.0185]	0.0001 [0.0119]	-0.0033 [0.0124]
Asset index	0.0078** [0.0033]	0.0051 [0.0043]	0.0117** [0.0051]	-0.0033 [0.0055]	0.0145*** [0.0055]	0.0178*** [0.0067]	0.0102** [0.0048]	0.0055 [0.0046]
Does not have shortage of income to cover food costs	0.0900*** [0.0084]	0.1012*** [0.0105]	0.0708*** [0.0141]	0.0974*** [0.0140]	0.0897*** [0.0136]	0.0636*** [0.0183]	0.0856*** [0.0107]	0.0943*** [0.0135]
Does not have shortage of income to cover household costs	0.0226** [0.0097]	0.0103 [0.0123]	0.0454*** [0.0157]	0.0221 [0.0158]	0.0483*** [0.0153]	-0.0217 [0.0231]	0.0303*** [0.0117]	0.0077 [0.0170]

(continued)

Table 9.4b (continued)

Dependent variable: health score (EQ 5D)	All the sample (1)	Women (2)	Men (3)	15 to 35 Years old (4)	35 to 54 Years old (5)	55 to 74 Years old (6)	Income below the median (7)	Income above the median (8)
Stolen	**−0.0702*****	**−0.1036*****	**−0.0325**	**−0.0480***	**−0.1023****	**−0.1757*****	**−0.0847****	**−0.0591****
	[0.0217]	**[0.0277]**	**[0.0334]**	**[0.0279]**	**[0.0436]**	**[0.0631]**	**[0.0338]**	**[0.0280]**
Stolen residuals	**0.0212**	**0.0586**	**−0.0112**	**−0.0688**	**0.0855**	**0.3220*****	**0.0476**	**0.0055**
	[0.0434]	[0.0554]	[0.0669]	[0.0567]	[0.0865]	[0.1247]	[0.0673]	[0.0560]
Constant term	1.0313***	1.2263***	0.9503***	1.3592***	0.9087**	1.1933	1.0253***	1.0924***
	[0.0520]	[0.0945]	[0.0794]	[0.1497]	[0.3775]	[1.0110]	[0.0814]	[0.0951]
Number of observations	10663	5916	4747	5115	3551	1663	5205	5458
Pseudo R Squared	0.191	0.219	0.154	0.120	0.170	0.175	0.228	0.156

Robust standard errors in brackets
*** p<0.01, ** p<0.05, * p<0.1

Table 9.4c Second step: safe walk, dependent variable: health score

Dependent variable: health score (EQ 5D)	All the sample (1)	Women (2)	Men (3)	15 to 35 Years old (4)	35 to 54 Years old (5)	55 to 74 Years old (6)
Male	0.0413*** [0.0076]			0.0241* [0.0127]	0.0649*** [0.0129]	0.0437*** [0.0158]
Age (years)	−0.0034*** [0.0012]	−0.0061*** [0.0015]	0.0003 [0.0019]	−0.0156 [0.0103]	−0.0049 [0.0170]	−0.0188 [0.0319]
Age squared	−0.0000* [0.0000]	0.0000 [0.0000]	−0.0001*** [0.0000]	0.0002 [0.0002]	−0.0000 [0.0002]	0.0001 [0.0002]
Complete primary education	0.0309*** [0.0110]	0.0324** [0.0141]	0.0250 [0.0175]	−0.0041 [0.0233]	0.0344* [0.0181]	0.0183 [0.0194]
Complete secondary education	0.0400*** [0.0125]	0.0458*** [0.0161]	0.0278 [0.0198]	0.0084 [0.0245]	0.0483** [0.0204]	0.0481* [0.0246]
Complete superior education	0.0432*** [0.0159]	0.0531*** [0.0205]	0.0262 [0.0255]	0.0192 [0.0300]	0.0275 [0.0250]	0.0335 [0.0343]
Married	0.0099 [0.0094]	0.0135 [0.0118]	−0.0056 [0.0158]	0.0176 [0.0145]	−0.0075 [0.0172]	−0.0306 [0.0247]
Divorced	−0.0289* [0.0152]	−0.0244 [0.0183]	−0.0363 [0.0272]	−0.0396 [0.0329]	−0.0477** [0.0227]	−0.0654** [0.0331]
Widowed	−0.0139 [0.0168]	−0.0003 [0.0196]	−0.0473 [0.0334]	0.0054 [0.0852]	−0.0503 [0.0322]	−0.0217 [0.0282]
Have one child	0.0020 [0.0097]	0.0075 [0.0124]	−0.0070 [0.0154]	−0.0162 [0.0166]	0.0223 [0.0153]	−0.0097 [0.0215]
Have two or more children	−0.0105 [0.0096]	−0.0113 [0.0124]	−0.0130 [0.0151]	−0.0289* [0.0163]	−0.0026 [0.0161]	−0.0075 [0.0216]

(continued)

Table 9.4c (continued)

Dependent variable: health score (EQ 5D)	All the sample (1)	Women (2)	Men (3)	15 to 35 Years old (4)	35 to 54 Years old (5)	55 to 74 Years old (6)
Consider religion to be important	0.0072 [0.0098]	0.0279** [0.0135]	-0.0133 [0.0143]	0.0154 [0.0145]	-0.0140 [0.0174]	0.0202 [0.0248]
Have friends	0.0411*** [0.0094]	0.0489*** [0.0119]	0.0267* [0.0154]	0.0430** [0.0181]	0.0293** [0.0142]	0.0568*** [0.0186]
Have employment	0.0294*** [0.0079]	0.0126 [0.0102]	0.0508*** [0.0126]	-0.0062 [0.0130]	0.0478*** [0.0128]	0.0641*** [0.0174]
Household income (monthly per capita in PPP US$)	0.0155*** [0.0046]	0.0091 [0.0059]	0.0233*** [0.0074]	0.0101 [0.0077]	0.0168** [0.0080]	0.0253*** [0.0094]
Live in urban area	0.0008 [0.0082]	0.0082 [0.0105]	-0.0063 [0.0129]	0.0080 [0.0133]	0.0011 [0.0138]	0.0020 [0.0183]
Access to running water service	-0.0190 [0.0126]	-0.0329** [0.0167]	-0.0002 [0.0193]	-0.0158 [0.0194]	-0.0354* [0.0215]	-0.0015 [0.0307]
Access to electricity service	-0.0015 [0.0206]	0.0035 [0.0281]	-0.0067 [0.0301]	0.0070 [0.0345]	0.0218 [0.0338]	-0.0223 [0.0444]
Access to telephone service	0.0003 [0.0086]	0.0131 [0.0109]	-0.0164 [0.0138]	0.0231 [0.0144]	-0.0117 [0.0141]	-0.0484** [0.0188]
Asset index	0.0073** [0.0033]	0.0042 [0.0043]	0.0120** [0.0051]	-0.0045 [0.0055]	0.0147*** [0.0056]	0.0191*** [0.0067]
Does not have shortage of income to cover food costs	0.0927*** [0.0084]	0.1050*** [0.0105]	0.0721*** [0.0139]	0.0969*** [0.0139]	0.0975*** [0.0135]	0.0709*** [0.0182]
Does not have shortage of income to cover household costs	0.0250** [0.0098]	0.0146 [0.0126]	0.0466*** [0.0156]	0.0258 [0.0159]	0.0493*** [0.0154]	-0.0185 [0.0234]

Safe walk	**0.0477****	**0.0813*****	**0.0060**	**0.0490***	**0.0472**	**0.0348**
	[0.0188]	**[0.0240]**	**[0.0293]**	**[0.0251]**	**[0.0362]**	**[0.0553]**
Safe walk residuals	0.0168	−0.0505	0.1110*	0.0284	0.0118	0.0720
	[0.0409]	[0.0520]	[0.0637]	[0.0554]	[0.0784]	[0.1180]
Constant term	1.0763***	1.2287***	0.9224***	1.3568***	1.1038***	1.3938
	[0.0669]	[0.0945]	[0.0969]	[0.1635]	[0.3889]	[1.0139]
Number of observations	10539	5834	4705	5080	3511	1627
Pseudo R Squared	0.190	0.212	0.162	0.119	0.169	0.175

Robust standard errors in brackets

*** p<0.01, ** p<0.05, * p<0.1

4.1 Split Sample Results

As an additional test of our hypothesis that individuals adapt – at least in part – to higher crime norms, we split our sample into two sets of country clusters. The first was those above and below the median homicide rate for the region, with the split serving as a proxy for major differences in crime levels across the two groups. The second split was based on the percent of respondents in each country that answered the question "safe walking alone at night in one's neighborhood" positively. Again we split the sample into those countries that were above and below the median; in this case, the median response was 48%.

The countries that were below the regional median homicide rate were Mexico, Costa Rica, Argentina, Chile, the Dominican Republic, Jamaica, Nicaragua, Panama, Peru, Trinidad and Tobago, and Uruguay. Venezuela, Brazil, Bolivia, Colombia, Ecuador, El Salvador, Guatemala, Guyana, Honduras, and Paraguay were above the median. Our results only partially support our hypothesis: the well-being effects (as measured by our life satisfaction variable) of being a crime victim (as gauged by our mugged variable) were insignificant in countries with *lower* homicide rates. In contrast, the residual (and the potential mitigating effects that it is picking up) was significant; in other words, being mugged in a country with a higher crime probability was a less negative experience. Being mugged had significant and negative effects on well-being in the high-homicide rate countries, and the coefficient on the residuals was positive and significant (see Table 9.5). There were no significant differences in the health effects of being a crime victim across these two samples, however.

We also got similar results with the sample split into those countries where most respondents felt safe walking alone at night and those that did not; again, we get mixed support for our hypothesis. The general direction of the findings run in the same direction as those reported for the full sample, but we do not find any difference between the subsamples. The countries below the median response (e.g., those where respondents feel less secure) are Venezuela, Brazil, Argentina, Bolivia, Chile, the Dominican Republic, Ecuador, El Salvador, Haiti, Paraguay, Trinidad and Tobago, and Uruguay. Those above the median are Mexico, Costa Rica, Colombia, Guatemala, Honduras, Jamaica, Nicaragua, Panama, and Peru. Note that security *perceptions* across countries do not correlate closely with objective indicators – at least with homicide rates. The effect of being mugged on life satisfaction was roughly similar in the sample of countries where respondents generally felt more safe or secure with those in countries where they did not (Table 9.6). Again, our residuals ran in the opposite direction of our coefficients on victimization. And, as above, the difference in the effects was much more important for life satisfaction than it was for health status, as measured by the EQ5D.

4.2 Societal-Level Effects: Friends and Institutions

We also explored the potential society-wide effects of crime victimization and perceptions of insecurity. We looked at the impact of crime victimization on friendships,

Table 9.5 Second step: sample split by homocide rate, dependent variable: life satisfaction

Dependent variable: life satisfaction, 0 to 10 scale	All countries in the sample (1)	Countries with low homocide rate (below the region median) (2)	Countries with high homocide rate (above the region median) (3)
Male	−0.1601***	−0.0752	−0.2452***
	[0.0370]	[0.0528]	[0.0523]
Age (years)	−0.0510***	−0.0489***	−0.0554***
	[0.0058]	[0.0081]	[0.0085]
Age squared	0.0004***	0.0004***	0.0005***
	[0.0001]	[0.0001]	[0.0001]
Health score (EQ-5D)	1.3524***	1.1844***	1.5398***
	[0.1416]	[0.1861]	[0.2175]
Complete primary education	0.0144	0.1323	−0.0561
	[0.0683]	[0.1043]	[0.0910]
Complete secondary education	0.0605	0.1453	0.0090
	[0.0728]	[0.1091]	[0.0984]
Complete superior education	0.2351***	0.2443**	0.2756**
	[0.0851]	[0.1246]	[0.1183]
Married	0.0036	0.0563	−0.0344
	[0.0461]	[0.0677]	[0.0636]
Divorced	−0.0349	−0.0205	−0.0186
	[0.0836]	[0.1129]	[0.1257]
Widowed	0.1050	0.2047	0.0285
	[0.0949]	[0.1327]	[0.1376]
Have one child	−0.0149	0.0335	−0.0586
	[0.0473]	[0.0682]	[0.0666]
Have two or more children	−0.0152	0.0488	−0.0762
	[0.0482]	[0.0710]	[0.0666]

(continued)

Table 9.5 (continued)

Dependent variable: life satisfaction, 0 to 10 scale	All countries in the sample (1)	Countries with low homocide rate (below the region median) (2)	Countries with high homocide rate (above the region median) (3)
Consider religion to be important	0.2321*** [0.0435]	0.2724*** [0.0556]	0.1790** [0.0706]
Have friends	0.4343*** [0.0533]	0.5343*** [0.0813]	0.3638*** [0.0708]
Have employment	0.0893** [0.0391]	0.0760 [0.0560]	0.1018* [0.0550]
Household income (monthly per capita in PPP US$)	0.2189*** [0.0253]	0.2339*** [0.0393]	0.2058*** [0.0332]
Live in urban area	−0.0088 [0.0395]	0.0008 [0.0585]	−0.0143 [0.0540]
Access to running water service	0.0036 [0.0665]	0.0515 [0.1046]	−0.0195 [0.0870]
Access to electricity service	0.4117*** [0.1184]	0.2339 [0.1914]	0.5415*** [0.1516]
Access to telephone service	0.1682*** [0.0428]	0.1641*** [0.0576]	0.1800*** [0.0648]
Asset index	0.1381*** [0.0166]	0.1465*** [0.0244]	0.1272*** [0.0229]
Does not have shortage of income to cover food costs	0.4846*** [0.0442]	0.5201*** [0.0625]	0.4508*** [0.0633]

Does not have shortage of income to cover household costs	0.1793*** [0.0552]	0.2023*** [0.0772]	0.1580** [0.0797]
Mugged	**-0.3915*** [0.1175]**	**-0.2541** [0.1570]	**-0.5378*** [0.1781]**
Mugged residuals	**0.6292*** [0.2148]**	**0.5441*** [0.2814]	**0.7560** [0.3307]**
Number of observations	10624	5399	5225
Pseudo R Squared	0.0613	0.0666	0.0530

Robust standard errors in brackets
*** p<0.01, ** p<0.05, * p<0.1

Table 9.6 Second step: sample split by security perceptions, dependent variable: life satisfaction

Dependent variable: life satisfaction, 0 to 10 scale	All countries in the sample (1)	Countries with low security perceptions (% of people feeling safe is below the region median) (2)	Countries with high security perceptions (% of people feeling safe is below the region median) (3)
Male	−0.1601***	−0.2064***	−0.1098*
	[0.0370]	[0.0488]	[0.0567]
Age (years)	−0.0510***	−0.0578***	−0.0464***
	[0.0058]	[0.0076]	[0.0092]
Age squared	0.0004***	0.0005***	0.0004***
	[0.0001]	[0.0001]	[0.0001]
Health score (EQ-5D)	1.3524***	1.5524***	1.1601***
	[0.1416]	[0.1866]	[0.2198]
Complete primary education	0.0144	−0.0828	0.1040
	[0.0683]	[0.0903]	[0.1038]
Complete secondary education	0.0605	−0.0866	0.2048*
	[0.0728]	[0.0974]	[0.1103]
Complete superior education	0.2351***	0.1654	0.2950**
	[0.0851]	[0.1151]	[0.1277]
Married	0.0036	0.0304	−0.0019
	[0.0461]	[0.0622]	[0.0686]
Divorced	−0.0349	0.0289	−0.1368
	[0.0836]	[0.1113]	[0.1276]
Widowed	0.1050	−0.0171	0.3791**
	[0.0949]	[0.1176]	[0.1698]

Have one child	-0.0149 [0.0473]	-0.0245 [0.0639]	-0.0016 [0.0714]
Have two or more children	-0.0152 [0.0482]	-0.0308 [0.0647]	0.0052 [0.0731]
Consider religion to be important	0.2321*** [0.0435]	0.1640*** [0.0587]	0.3181*** [0.0658]
Have friends	0.4343*** [0.0533]	0.3764*** [0.0663]	0.5467*** [0.0908]
Have employment	0.0893** [0.0391]	0.1105** [0.0520]	0.0633 [0.0594]
Household income (monthly per capita in PPP US$)	0.2189*** [0.0253]	0.2534*** [0.0342]	0.1937*** [0.0373]
Live in urban area	-0.0088 [0.0395]	-0.0283 [0.0541]	0.0061 [0.0580]
Access to running water service	0.0036 [0.0665]	0.0863 [0.0862]	-0.0942 [0.1049]
Access to electricity service	0.4117*** [0.1184]	-0.0677 [0.1769]	0.5932*** [0.1516]
Access to telephone service	0.1682*** [0.0428]	0.1771*** [0.0591]	0.1485** [0.0619]

(continued)

Table 9.6 (continued)

Dependent variable: life satisfaction, 0 to 10 scale	All countries in the sample	Countries with low security perceptions (% of people feeling safe is below the region median)	Countries with high security perceptions (% of people feeling safe is below the region median)
	(1)	(2)	(3)
Asset index	0.1381***	0.0990***	0.1879***
	[0.0166]	[0.0218]	[0.0259]
Does not have shortage of income to cover food costs	0.4846***	0.5121***	0.4453***
	[0.0442]	[0.0588]	[0.0675]
Does not have shortage of income to cover household costs	0.1793***	0.1691**	0.1784**
	[0.0552]	[0.0762]	[0.0796]
Mugged	**−0.3915***	**−0.4497***	**−0.3389**
	[0.1175]	**[0.1667]**	**[0.1666]**
Mugged residuals	**0.6292***	**0.6942**	**0.5608***
	[0.2148]	**[0.3068]**	**[0.3012]**
Number of observations	10624	5972	4652
Pseudo R Squared	0.0613	0.0503	0.0675

Robust standard errors in brackets

*** p<0.01, ** p<0.05, * p<0.1

based on a question in the Gallup Poll that asks respondents whether they have friends or family that they can rely on in times of need. In earlier work using this variable, Eduardo Lora and colleagues found that having friends is the second most important variable to reported happiness for respondents in the region, after food security. Having friends is more important to the life satisfaction of the rich than of the poor.[7] In the absence of institutionalized safety nets in most of the region, it makes sense that friends and family are an important source of economic support, particularly for the poor, in addition to the obvious social support that these ties provide.

In this case, we replaced life satisfaction as the dependent variable with our friends variable in our second-stage regression. We found that crime victimization – in this case, mugging[8] – was negatively correlated with having friends. The correlation was slightly stronger for the middle aged and for those whose income is below the median. The income results suggest that more vulnerable groups who lack friendships experience worse well-being effects from being victimized (Table 9.7).

We also explored the effects of victimization on confidence in public institutions. We focused on respondents' responses to questions about confidence in three kinds of institutions: the police, the judiciary system, and the national government. As above, we replaced life satisfaction as the dependent variable in our second-stage regressions with each of these three variables, respectively. Being a crime victim – in this instance, mugged – was negatively and significantly correlated with confidence in the police and with confidence in the national government, but insignificant in the case of the judiciary. The link between victimization and confidence in the police is a direct and obvious one, and not surprisingly, more so than with attitudes about the judiciary. It may also affect general attitudes about the government more so than those in a more removed and less obvious institution like the judiciary, at least for the average respondent (see Table 9.8). As in our other regressions, our unexplained probability of victimization worked in the opposite direction, mitigating the negative effects. One can imagine that where higher crime rates are the norm, confidence in these kinds of institutions is already low, and an instance of victimization is less significant for that confidence, in the same way that it has lower effects on life satisfaction. Despite this mitigation, crime victimization has significant and negative effects on confidence in institutions in the region, demonstrating yet another cost related to the high rates of insecurity in the region.

We also posited that exposure to the media could play a mediating role on the well-being effects of crime victimization. These effects presumably could run in two directions: one would be in heightening insecurity by highlighting the existence of crime and the dangers surrounding it. The other would be to lower the stigma attached to crime victimization by making it seem a more "normal" event. We included an access to the Internet variable in our second-stage regressions with both life and health satisfactions as the dependent variables, but our results were insignificant.

---

[7] IDB (2008).

[8] A "mugging" is defined herein as an attack usually involving robbery.

Table 9.7 Second step: mugged, dependent variable: having friends

Dependent variable: having friends (0,1)	All the sample (1)	Women (2)	Men (3)	15 to 35 Years old (4)	35 to 54 Years old (5)	55 to 74 Years old (6)	Income below the median (7)	Income above the median (8)
Male	−0.0080			−0.0163	0.1254	−0.2982**	0.0144	−0.0451
	[0.0637]			[0.1072]	[0.1026]	[0.1478]	[0.0842]	[0.0992]
Age (years)	−0.0866***	−0.0985***	−0.0738***	−0.1576*	−0.3075**	−0.2319	−0.0877***	−0.0921***
	[0.0102]	[0.0141]	[0.0151]	[0.0873]	[0.1378]	[0.2896]	[0.0130]	[0.0169]
Age squared	0.0008***	0.0009***	0.0006***	0.0022	0.0034**	0.0018	0.0008***	0.0008***
	[0.0001]	[0.0002]	[0.0002]	[0.0017]	[0.0016]	[0.0023]	[0.0001]	[0.0002]
Health score (EQ-5D)	0.8990***	1.0065***	0.7683**	0.8892**	0.6789**	1.2050***	1.2154***	0.4196
	[0.1869]	[0.2328]	[0.3205]	[0.3886]	[0.3045]	[0.3608]	[0.2386]	[0.3137]
Complete primary education	0.0158	0.0654	−0.0546	0.2007	−0.1325	0.2583	0.0226	0.0703
	[0.0869]	[0.1129]	[0.1379]	[0.1625]	[0.1423]	[0.1801]	[0.1055]	[0.1588]
Complete secondary education	0.1628	0.2803**	0.0024	0.3799**	0.0362	0.2367	0.1735	0.1900
	[0.1041]	[0.1372]	[0.1622]	[0.1809]	[0.1685]	[0.2364]	[0.1340]	[0.1736]
Complete superior education	0.3626***	0.6222***	0.0787	0.5974**	0.3372	0.5533	0.4233**	0.3734*
	[0.1405]	[0.1940]	[0.2091]	[0.2451]	[0.2178]	[0.3366]	[0.2139]	[0.2107]
Married	−0.1914**	−0.1540	−0.2523**	−0.1825	−0.1229	−0.0550	−0.1651*	−0.2465*
	[0.0788]	[0.1044]	[0.1246]	[0.1170]	[0.1359]	[0.2082]	[0.0997]	[0.1316]
Divorced	−0.1464	0.0668	−0.4774**	0.0531	−0.0168	−0.0800	−0.0436	−0.2672
	[0.1277]	[0.1629]	[0.2076]	[0.2923]	[0.1853]	[0.2904]	[0.1672]	[0.2016]
Widowed	−0.1740	−0.0813	−0.4933**	−1.0017*	−0.3005	−0.1201	−0.0994	−0.3115
	[0.1416]	[0.1772]	[0.2470]	[0.5468]	[0.2534]	[0.2447]	[0.1789]	[0.2350]
Have one child	0.1379*	0.0741	0.2323*	0.0452	0.2959**	0.1633	0.0930	0.1975
	[0.0821]	[0.1096]	[0.1267]	[0.1420]	[0.1277]	[0.2078]	[0.1138]	[0.1273]

Have two or more children	0.0666	0.0621	0.0565	0.0940	0.1069	0.0774	0.0545	0.0840
	[0.0801]	[0.1078]	[0.1213]	[0.1431]	[0.1243]	[0.1998]	[0.1055]	[0.1368]
Consider religion to be important	0.2405***	0.3270***	0.1519	0.2683**	0.1166	0.3490*	0.3425***	0.1415
	[0.0808]	[0.1148]	[0.1140]	[0.1231]	[0.1374]	[0.2047]	[0.1066]	[0.1261]
Have employment	−0.0837	−0.2183**	0.0402	−0.0270	0.0149	−0.2415	−0.2051**	0.0775
	[0.0658]	[0.0886]	[0.1001]	[0.1102]	[0.1051]	[0.1586]	[0.0857]	[0.1033]
Household income (monthly per capita in PPP US$)	0.2122***	0.1934***	0.2443***	0.2392***	0.1845***	0.2434***	0.2692***	0.0786
	[0.0387]	[0.0512]	[0.0600]	[0.0648]	[0.0615]	[0.0905]	[0.0554]	[0.0965]
Live in urban area	−0.1306*	−0.1330	−0.1077	−0.1083	−0.0080	−0.2839	−0.1933**	−0.0263
	[0.0669]	[0.0883]	[0.1027]	[0.1107]	[0.1113]	[0.1967]	[0.0864]	[0.1082]
Access to running water service	−0.0250	−0.0216	−0.0259	0.0995	−0.1354	−0.0737	0.0317	−0.1447
	[0.0954]	[0.1284]	[0.1427]	[0.1450]	[0.1519]	[0.2469]	[0.1107]	[0.2008]
Access to electricity service	−0.0951	0.0183	−0.2349	−0.2858	−0.1757	0.5165	−0.3447*	0.7398**
	[0.1562]	[0.2173]	[0.2262]	[0.2364]	[0.2572]	[0.3887]	[0.1821]	[0.3169]
Access to telephone service	0.0679	0.1055	0.0069	−0.0291	0.1123	0.0358	0.0767	−0.0146
	[0.0720]	[0.0951]	[0.1116]	[0.1242]	[0.1136]	[0.1715]	[0.0968]	[0.1136]
Asset index	0.1646***	0.1592***	0.1685***	0.2310***	0.1179***	0.1004	0.1947***	0.1332***
	[0.0284]	[0.0386]	[0.0421]	[0.0483]	[0.0447]	[0.0662]	[0.0387]	[0.0425]
Does not have shortage of income to cover food costs	0.2982***	0.2278**	0.4034***	0.3159***	0.2006*	0.4290**	0.1688*	0.4962***
	[0.0692]	[0.0907]	[0.1084]	[0.1185]	[0.1106]	[0.1855]	[0.0871]	[0.1141]

(continued)

Table 9.7 (continued)

Dependent variable: having friends (0,1)	All the sample (1)	Women (2)	Men (3)	15 to 35 Years old (4)	35 to 54 Years old (5)	55 to 74 Years old (6)	Income below the median (7)	Income above the median (8)
Does not have shortage of income to cover household costs	0.1146 [0.0769]	0.0990 [0.1015]	0.1146 [0.1195]	0.1181 [0.1262]	0.0214 [0.1259]	−0.0658 [0.2240]	0.0459 [0.0937]	0.2353* [0.1364]
Mugged	**−2.0791*** [0.2539]	**−2.3337*** [0.3877]	**−1.8694*** [0.3362]	**−1.3882*** [0.2183]	**−3.8554*** [0.9237]	**−4.2165** [3.9138]	**−2.5714*** [0.4911]	**−1.6733*** [0.2642]
Mugged residuals	**3.9817*** [0.5022]	**4.3970*** [0.7639]	**3.6936*** [0.6682]	**2.8866*** [0.4378]	**7.2950*** [1.7952]	**7.7709** [7.5325]	**4.9948*** [0.9710]	**3.1494*** [0.5157]
Constant term	−0.1293 [0.5814]	−0.3241 [0.6743]	−0.7122 [0.8139]	1.3335 [1.4830]	3.2922 [3.1155]	2.5927 [9.2803]	−0.3194 [0.8164]	0.6318 [0.9392]
Number of observations	10643	5906	4737	5105	3548	1652	5191	5450
Pseudo R Squared	0.0975	0.0996	0.105	0.102	0.0801	0.105	0.0931	0.0842

Robust standard errors in brackets

*** $p<0.01$, ** $p<0.05$, * $p<0.1$

Table 9.8 Second step: mugged, dependent varibales: confidence in the police, the judiciary and the nat. government

	Dependent variable: confidence in the police (1,0)	Dependent variable: confidence in the judiciary system (1,0)	Dependent variable: confidence in the national government (1,0)
	(1)	(2)	(3)
Male	0.0115 [0.0446]	0.0657 [0.0490]	0.1066** [0.0458]
Age (years)	0.0229*** [0.0070]	−0.0104 [0.0077]	0.0095 [0.0072]
Age squared	−0.0001 [0.0001]	0.0001 [0.0001]	−0.0000 [0.0001]
Health score (EQ-5D)	1.0142*** [0.1579]	0.6494*** [0.1749]	0.5297*** [0.1638]
Complete primary education	−0.2967*** [0.0722]	−0.2812*** [0.0746]	−0.2332*** [0.0717]
Complete secondary education	−0.4646*** [0.0799]	−0.6228*** [0.0852]	−0.4827*** [0.0801]
Complete superior education	−0.4511*** [0.0985]	−0.7193*** [0.1080]	−0.3813*** [0.1003]
Married	−0.0099 [0.0550]	−0.0807 [0.0605]	0.1128** [0.0567]
Divorced	−0.0772 [0.0952]	−0.0222 [0.1057]	−0.0519 [0.0992]
Widowed	0.0607 [0.1147]	0.2196* [0.1195]	0.1983* [0.1153]
Have one child	0.0175 [0.0569]	0.1082* [0.0630]	−0.0183 [0.0583]
Have two or more children	−0.0077 [0.0579]	0.1269** [0.0644]	−0.0032 [0.0593]
Consider religion to be important	0.3871*** [0.0579]	0.4034*** [0.0673]	0.2498*** [0.0600]
Have friends	0.2777*** [0.0599]	0.2280*** [0.0679]	0.2304*** [0.0621]
Have employment	0.0255 [0.0466]	−0.0476 [0.0513]	0.0357 [0.0481]
Household income (monthly per capita in PPP US$)	−0.0182 [0.0284]	−0.0302 [0.0313]	−0.0533* [0.0292]
Live in urban area	−0.2185*** [0.0467]	−0.2793*** [0.0510]	−0.1500*** [0.0479]
Access to running water service	0.1452* [0.0771]	−0.0338 [0.0813]	−0.0358 [0.0782]
Access to electricity service	0.1926 [0.1251]	0.1945 [0.1339]	0.1004 [0.1249]

(continued)

Table 9.8 (continued)

	Dependent variable: confidence in the police (1,0)	Dependent variable: confidence in the judiciary system (1,0)	Dependent variable: confidence in the national government (1,0)
	(1)	(2)	(3)
Access to telephone service	−0.0610 [0.0511]	−0.0294 [0.0565]	0.0813 [0.0524]
Asset index	−0.0382** [0.0194]	−0.0631*** [0.0214]	−0.0809*** [0.0200]
Does not have shortage of income to cover food costs	0.1219** [0.0519]	0.1250** [0.0573]	0.1381*** [0.0535]
Does not have shortage of income to cover household costs	0.0005 [0.0613]	0.0629 [0.0679]	0.0046 [0.0628]
Mugged	**−0.9446*** [0.1439]**	**−0.1708 [0.1569]**	**−0.5497*** [0.1465]**
Mugged residuals	**0.7020*** [0.2630]**	**−0.2472 [0.2854]**	**0.2748 [0.2676]**
Constant term	−1.9798*** [0.3459]	−0.0361 [0.3727]	−1.7204*** [0.4360]
Number of observations	10308	10146	10199
Pseudo R Squared	0.0530	0.0832	0.0732

Robust standard errors in brackets
*** p<0.01, ** p<0.05, * p<0.1

4.3   Estimating the Costs: Income Equivalents for Crime Victimization

As a means to get at the cost of victimization relative to other experiences, we calculated the income equivalents. As is standard practice, we calculated the marginal effects of changes in our relevant variables on well-being while holding the obvious sociodemographic variables constant.[9]

Our results on most of the standard variables are very similar to those that have been found by Lora et al. for Latin America, also based on Gallup data. Friendships and food are the most important variables to well-being. Education and marriage are important, but the least so in relative terms. We also added a variable for suffering moderate pain, based on the EQ5D questions, and find that the effects are quite significant: almost four times of the monthly median income. The effects of feeling insecure

---

[9]For equation details, see Technical Appendix A.2.

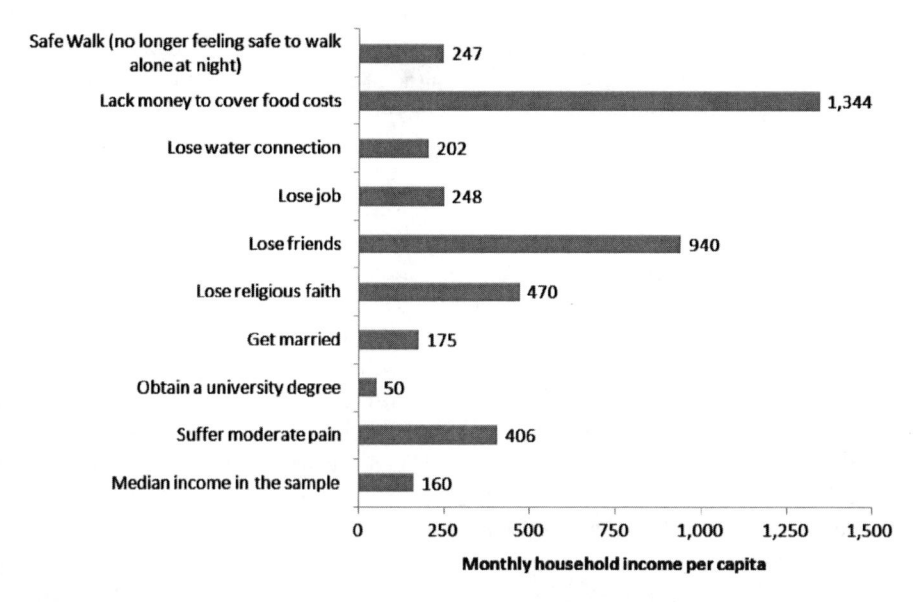

Fig. 9.4 Amount of income needed to maintain individual's initial level of satisfaction when faced with change

were also notable. Respondents would need one-and-a-half-times the median income to compensate for feeling insecure, roughly on par with what they would need if they lost their job. The negative effects of insecurity are greater than the positive effects of marriage, but lesser than those of losing friends or having insufficient income to cover food (see Fig. 9.4; Results are available from the authors).

5   Conclusions

In this chapter, we explored the welfare effects of the high levels of crime in Latin America on a large sample of respondents from the region. We measured the effects on both reported happiness and on health status, as measured by the EQ5D index, which is based on self-assessments of health across a range of physical and emotional conditions which correlate very closely with health status as assessed by a number of objective indicators.

Our baseline hypothesis was that crime victimization would have negative effects on both happiness and health. At the same time, we also posited that some of those effects would be mitigated by people's ability to adapt to those phenomena as they become more common. Our priors were that adaptation would most likely mitigate the happiness effects of victimization more than the health effects and that the ability to adapt would vary across cohorts.

Our results support our basic hypothesis. Crime victimization had significant and negative effects on both happiness and health. The effects of victimization also varied across cohorts, with things like mugging – which is typically a more threatening and physical experience than having something stolen – having stronger effects for more vulnerable groups, such as women and the elderly, or at times for groups for whom they are rare – such as the wealthy – and likely produce more stigma. The coefficients were typically quite a bit higher for happiness than for health, although the general direction of the findings is similar. There were some modest differences across the cohorts.

At the same time, we also found evidence of adaptation. Our victimization residuals – which were based on the unexplained probability of being victimized as a proxy for adaptation – ran in the opposite direction of our victimization variables, suggesting that a higher unexplained probability of victimization – e.g., a higher crime norm – mitigates the effects of victimization. This occurred much more in the happiness than in the health arena, suggesting that it is more difficult to adapt in the health arena, where the effects of victimization can result in permanent conditions.

It is possible that our residuals are merely picking up other unobservable variables that have nothing to do with our respondents' ability to adapt. Still, the consistency in the direction of the findings suggests something in what we are observing (or not observing) mitigates the usual effects of these phenomena on well-being. Some of what we find could, of course, be an artifact of construction: the residuals are greater when the unexplained probability of being a victim is greater precisely because we are able to explain less. In a next stage of this research, we will attempt to develop alternative specifications to get around this problem.

We also explored the society-wide costs of insecurity. In this case, we replaced life satisfaction as the dependent variable with our friends variable in our second-stage regressions. We found that crime victimization – in this case, mugging – was negatively correlated with having friends, a variable which is very important to the well-being of respondents in the region. The correlation was stronger, however, for the middle aged and for those whose income is below the median. The income results suggest that vulnerable groups who lack friendships experience worse well-being costs from being victimized. Victimization also had negative effects on confidence in public institutions – the police and national governments – for all of our cohorts. This seems to be a vicious cycle of sorts, in which institutions are weak and then crime victimization undermines already weak confidence in those institutions. The region's crime rates not only affect individual well-being but societal well-being as well.

Finally, we attempted to provide an order of magnitude estimate of these costs by calculating income equivalence values for crime victimization for our cohorts of respondents. Respondents would need one-and-a-half times the median monthly income to make up for not feeling safe walking in their neighborhood, an amount equivalent to the effect of losing one's job, greater than that for losing access to water, but less than that of suffering moderate pain or losing one's friends.

Our results are an initial exploration into a new area of research and should be treated as such. They provide a new means of measuring the well-being and health effects of victimization and insecurity. Not surprisingly, these phenomena have negative effects on both, effects which vary somewhat across age, gender, and income cohorts. Respondents seem to adapt to these things when they are more common, at least in the happiness arena. Adapting to the health effects seems more difficult. Despite the presence of adaptation, the well-being of both individuals and society suffer greatly due to high levels of crime in the region.

Acknowledgments The authors acknowledge helpful comments and inputs from Rafael Di Tella, Eduardo Lora, Jorge Srur, and Gustavo Beliz.

6 Technical Appendix

6.1 Cost of Victimization

The basic first stage equation was:

$$\text{Victimization ij} = a + b\, y_{ij} + c\, age_{ij} + d\, age_{ij}^2 + e\ fs_{ij} + g\, H_{ij} + \varepsilon \qquad (6.1)$$

Victimization is a zero-1 variable capturing the probability of being mugged, having something stolen, or perceiving insecurity (based on safe walk), respectively. The independent variables are income, age and age squared, a vector of other socio-demographic traits, a measure of health status, a measure of respondents' optimism as proxied by their POUM score (as discussed above), and an error term which captures the unexplained probability of being victimized. We also included country fixed effects in the first specification and measures for GDP growth and for rule of law in a second. The results are essentially the same with both specifications. The residuals reported in all of the tables are based on the specification with country fixed effects.

The second-stage base equation was

$$LS_{ij} = a + b\, y_{ij} + c\, age_{ij} + d\, age_{ij}^2 + e\, fs_{ij} + g\, H_{ij} + h\, L_{ij} + v_{ij} + v_{ij}\varepsilon \qquad (6.2)$$

The dependent variables are, respectively, life satisfaction and assessed health status (based on the EQ5D index), and the independent variables are the usual controls, plus a dummy variable for victimization (one of each of our three victimization variables) and then the unexplained probability of being victimized for that same respondent. We repeated the same equations for the split samples as well as with each of the five separate health conditions as dependent variables.

Appendix A Propensity score matching results

Safe walk (positive and significat treatment effect)

A. Average treatment effect on the treated (swalk = 1)

Variable	Sample	Treated	Controls	Difference	S.E.	T-stat	
wp16	ATT	5.8706	5.7404	0.1302	0.0523	2.49	

B. Bootstrap of treatment effect (100 iterations)

Variable	Reps	Observed	Bias	Std. Err.	[95% Conf.	Interval]	
_bs_1	100	0.1302	−0.0147	0.0568	0.0175	0.2430	(N)
					0.0219	0.2350	(P)
					0.0434	0.2430	(BC)

Stolen (treatment effect is not significant)

A. Average treatment effect on the treated (stolen = 1)

Variable	Sample	Treated	Controls	Difference	S.E.	T-stat	
wp16	ATT	5.7581	5.8179	−0.0599	0.0634	-0.94	

B. Bootstrap of treatment effect (100 iterations)

Variable	Reps	Observed	Bias	Std. Err.	[95% Conf.	Interval]	
_bs_1	100	−0.060	−0.029	0.069	−0.196	0.077	(N)
					−0.239	0.037	(P)
					−0.198	0.098	(BC)

Mugged (negative and significant treatment effect)

A. Average treatment effect on the treated (mugged = 1)

Variable	Sample	Treated	Controls	Difference	S.E.	T-stat	
wp16	ATT	5.6719	5.8579	−0.1860	0.0761	−2.44	

B. Bootstrap of treatment effect (100 iterations)

Variable	Reps	Observed	Bias	Std. Err.	[95% Conf.	Interval]	
_bs_1	100	−0.186	0.065	0.078	−0.340	−0.032	(N)
					−0.256	0.074	(P)
					−0.298	−0.110	(BC)

Appendix B Income equivalence calculations

Marginal Effects, All the sample (n = 11813)

variable		dy/dx	Std. Err.	z	P>|z|	[95%	C.I.]	X	Delta X	(B1 * Delta X)	Delta ln(y) = (B1 * Delta X) / B2	New ln(y) = Initial ln(y) + Delta ln(y)	Monthly Household Income per Capita , US$	
sex*|		−0.013417	0.0028	−4.88	0	−0.019	−0.008	0.4426			Initial income:	5.1	160	Median income in the sample
age |		−0.003923	0.0004	−9.05	0	−0.005	−0.003	39.043						
age2 |		0.000034	0	7.23	0	3E-05	4E-05	1810						
EQ_index |		0.094633	0.0104	9.08	0	0.0742	0.1151	0.9118	−0.173	−0.01636	0.93	6.0	406	Suffer moderate pain
educac~1*|		−0.000296	0.0049	−0.06	0.952	−0.01	0.0093	0.3979						
educac~2*|		0.006202	0.0053	1.16	0.244	−0.004	0.0166	0.3436						
educac~3*|		0.020203	0.0066	3.06	0.002	0.0073	0.0332	0.1139	1	0.02020	−1.15	3.9	50	Obtain a university degree
married*|		−0.001618	0.0034	−0.47	0.638	−0.008	0.0051	0.5568	1	−0.00162	0.09	5.2	175	Get married
divorced*|		−0.003816	0.006	−0.64	0.524	−0.016	0.0079	0.0654						
widow*|		0.004969	0.007	0.71	0.477	−0.009	0.0186	0.0554						
onechild*|		0.000844	0.0035	0.24	0.81	−0.006	0.0077	0.2575						
morech~n*|		−0.000116	0.0035	−0.03	0.974	−0.007	0.0068	0.3558						
religimp*|		0.018914	0.0031	6.16	0	0.0129	0.0249	0.8254	−1	−0.01891	1.08	6.2	470	Lose religious faith
friends*|		0.031088	0.0034	9.2	0	0.0245	0.0377	0.8468	−1	−0.03109	1.77	6.8	940	Lose friends
job*|		0.007711	0.0029	2.66	0.008	0.002	0.0134	0.429	−1	−0.00771	0.44	5.5	248	Lose job
ln_ipc~p |		0.017538	0.0019	9.36	0	0.0139	0.0212	5.0736						

Marginal Effects, All the
sample (n = 11813)

zone*|	−0.000859	0.0029	−0.29	0.769	−0.007	0.0049	0.6109					
water*|	0.004126	0.0047	0.88	0.38	−0.005	0.0133	0.8938	−1	−0.00413	0.24	5.3	202	Lose water connection
electr~y*|	0.027256	0.0071	3.82	0	0.0133	0.0412	0.9639					
teleph~e*|	0.012085	0.0032	3.8	0	0.0059	0.0183	0.4874					
assets		0.010808	0.0013	8.63	0	0.0084	0.0133	−0.032					
food*|	0.037359	0.0031	12.09	0	0.0313	0.0434	0.6363	−1	−0.03736	2.13	7.2	1,344	Lack money to cover food costs
shelter*|	0.015941	0.0038	4.18	0	0.0085	0.0234	0.8168					
swalk*|	0.007658	0.0026	2.93	0.003	0.0025	0.0128	0.4749	−1	−0.00766	0.44	5.5	247	Safe Walk (no longer feeling safe to walk alone at night)

Appendix C Life satisfaction regressions with national average victimization rates

Dependent variable: life satisfaction	All the sample (with national average victimization rates)		
	(1)	(2)	(3)
Variables	LAC_swalk_AVG	LAC_stolen_AVG	LAC_mugged_AVG
sex	-0.1489***	-0.1363***	-0.1098***
age	-0.0453***	-0.0452***	-0.0434***
age2	0.0004***	0.0004***	0.0003***
EQ_index	1.1197***	1.1849***	1.2465***
educacion1	-0.0184	-0.0203	-0.0658
educacion2	-0.0550	-0.0173	-0.1224*
educacion3	0.0196	0.1017	-0.0355
married	-0.0048	0.0060	-0.0132
divorced	-0.0222	-0.0257	-0.0481
widow	0.0594	0.0643	0.0380
onechild	-0.0112	-0.0052	0.0102
morechildren	-0.0386	-0.0238	-0.0247
religimp	0.2727***	0.2452***	0.2743***
friends	0.4655***	0.4689***	0.4860***
job	0.1135***	0.1058***	0.0856**
ln_ipcf_ppp	0.2370***	0.2311***	0.2281***
zone	-0.0209	-0.0489	-0.0494
water	0.1684***	0.2088***	0.2230***
electricity	0.4625***	0.4020***	0.3050***
telephone	0.2989***	0.2780***	0.2742***
assets	0.1735***	0.1622***	0.1747***
food	0.5367***	0.5204***	0.5230***
shelter	0.1330***	0.1357***	0.1158**
swalk	**0.1068***		
avg_swalk_country	**2.7307***		
stolen		**-0.0974**	
avg_stolen_country		**-4.3081***	
mugged			**-0.0759**
avg_mugged_country			**-3.0027***
Observations	11813	11962	11937
N	11813	11962	11937
r2_p	0.0500	0.0498	0.0482

Robust standard errors in brackets
*** p<0.01, ** p<0.05, * p<0.1

6.2 Cost of Insecurity

We used our safe walk variable as our insecurity variable, in the following equation:

$$
\begin{aligned}
LS_{ij} = a &+ b_1 gender_{ij} + b_2 age_{ij} + b_3 age_{ij}^2 + b_4 health\ index_{ij} + b_5 education_{ij} a \\
&+ b_6 marital\ status_{ij} + b_7\ family\ size_{ij} + b_8\ religous\ beliefs_{ij} + b_9 friends_{ij} \\
&+ b_{10} employment\ status_{ij} + b_{11}\ y_{ij} + b_{12} utilities_{ij} + b_{13} rural\ /\ urban\ area_{ij} \\
&+ b_{14} food\ security_{ij} + b_{15} housing\ security_{ij} + b_{16} safe\ walk_{ij} + v_i + \varepsilon_{ij}
\end{aligned}
\tag{6.3}
$$

References

Di Tella, R., & Shargrodsky, E. (2009). *Happiness, ideology, and crime in an individual panel in six argentine cities*. Cambridge: Mimeo, Harvard Business School.

Di Tella, R., Galiani, S., & Schargrodsky, E. (2006, November). *Crime distribution and victim behavior during a crime wave*. (Inter-American Development Bank, IDB Working Paper #112), Washington, D.C.

Di Tella, R., Ñopo, H., & MacCulloch, R. (2008). *Happiness and beliefs in criminal environments*. (Inter-American Development Bank, Research Department Working Papers WP-662), Washington, D.C.

Dolan, P. (1997). Modeling valuations for health care. *Medical Care, 11*, 1095–1108.

Graham, C. (2008). Happiness and health: Lessons – and questions – for public policy. *Health Affairs, 27*(1), 72–87.

Graham, C. (2009). *Happiness around the world: The paradox of happy peasants and miserable millionaires*. Oxford: Oxford University Press.

Graham, C., & Lora, E. (Eds.). (2009). *Paradox and perception: Measuring quality of life in Latin America*. Washington, DC: The Brookings Institution Press and the Inter-American Development Bank.

Graham, C., & Pettinto, S. (2002). *Happiness and hardship: Opportunity and insecurity in new market economies*. Washington, DC: The Brookings Institution Press.

Graham, C., & Chattopadhyay, S. (2009). Well-being and public attitudes in Afghanistan: Insights from the economics of happiness. *World Economics*, Vol. 10, No.3, July-September.

Graham, C., Chattopadhyay, S., & Picon, M. (2010). The Easterlin Paradox re-visited: Why both sides of the debate may be correct. In E. Diener, J. Helliwell, & D. Kahneman (Eds.), *International differences in well-being* (pp. 247–288). Oxford: Oxford University Press.

Graham, C., Higuera, L., & Lora, E. (2010). Which health conditions make you happy? Insights from new data from Latin America. *Health Affairs*. DOI 10.1002/hec.1682

Greene, W. (2008). *Econometric analysis* (6th ed.). Upper Saddle River: Pearson Prentice Hall.

Higuera, L. (2008). *LAPOP 2008 – Survey result's report* (Inter-American Development Bank, Research Department Working Papers WP-669).

Inter-American Development Bank. (2008). *Beyond facts: Understanding quality of life*. Cambridge: David Rockefeller Center for Latin American Studies, Harvard University Press.

Londoño, J. L, Gaviria, A., & Guerrero, R. (Eds.) (2000). *Asalto al desarrollo: Violencia en América Latina*. Inter-American Development Bank. Red de Centros de Investigación. Washington, D.C.

Powdthavee, N. (2005). Unhappiness and crime: Evidence from South Africa. *Economica, 72*, 531–547.

Shaw, J., Johnson, J., & Coons, S. (2005). U.S. valuation of the EQ-5D health states: Development and testing of the DI valuation model. *Medical Care, 43*(3), 203–220.

Van Praag, B., & Ferrer-i-Carbonell, A. (2007). *Happiness quantified: A satisfaction calculus approach*. New York: Oxford University Press.

Chapter 10
Satisfaction with Present Safety and Future Security as Components of Personal Well-Being Among Young People: Relationships with Other Psychosocial Constructs

Mònica González, Ferran Casas, Cristina Figuer, Sara Malo, and Ferran Viñas

1 Introduction

A review of the literature conducted by Cummins (1996) found that 22% of the definitions considered when identifying quality of life domains included the construct of 'safety'. Subsequently this domain, which included other constructs such as security, personal control, privacy, independence, autonomy, competence, knowledge of rights and residential stability, became one of seven to form the basis of his Comprehensive Quality of Life Scale (ComQol).

With the advent of the Personal Wellbeing Index (PWI) (Cummins et al. 2003), the construct of safety was preserved and included alongside the dimension of security. Respondents are required to express their satisfaction with present safety ('How satisfied are you with how safe you feel?') and future security ('How satisfied are you with your future security?') by contrast with other well-known instruments for measuring subjective or psychological well-being which are currently being used with adolescents and young person samples which do not include any explicit component on safety or security (for instance, Diener et al.'s *Satisfaction With Life Scale*, SWLS 1985; and Seligson et al.'s *Brief Multidimensional Student's Life Satisfaction Scale*, BMSLSS 2003).

The correlation between present safety and future security was observed to be 0.72 in data collected ($N=2,000$) from research using the 2010 Australian Unity Wellbeing Index,[1] meaning they are highly related constructs. However, the two are clearly distinguishable and suffer unequal variation if we take into account macro

---

[1] The Australian Unity regularly measures how satisfied Australians are with their lives and life in Australia. The PWI forms part of the Australian Unity Well-being Index.

M. González (✉) • F. Casas • C. Figuer • S. Malo • F. Viñas
Quality of Life Research Institute, University of Girona, M-20. Campus Montilivi, 17071 Girona, Spain
e-mail: monica.gonzalez@udg.edu

D. Webb and E. Wills-Herrera (eds.), *Subjective Well-Being and Security*,   253
Social Indicators Research Series 46, DOI 10.1007/978-94-007-2278-1_10,
© Springer Science+Business Media B.V. 2012

social events such as terrorist attacks, which affect present safety, or the global economic crisis, which affects future security. This kind of report was first compiled in 2001, and data have been gathered each year since to enable systematic comparisons over time.

The two aspects seem to be related to and moderated by different psychological and psychosocial constructs. What these are and the scope of such relationships have not been established, but a certain consensus does exist in considering the general concept of security to be central to personal well-being. According to Maslow (1970), the preoccupation with security reflects the need to maintain safety, which involves longing for protection, surety and survival, these being the prerequisites for normal life. From this perspective, insecurity can be defined, following Jacobson (1991, quoted in Bar-Tal and Jacobson 1998, page 61) as 'a cognitive response of appraisal formulation to a perceived danger in the environment by which a person perceives himself/herself to be threatened'. We still know little about the relationship between satisfaction with present safety and future security and other psychosocial constructs closely related to personal well-being, such as self-concept, freedom of choice and control over one's own life and values, among others, or the overall sense of meaning found in one's own life. Consequently this study goes some way to bridging the gap in knowledge.

When attempting to determine what the aforementioned psychosocial-related constructs might be, we already know that satisfaction with both present safety and future security are closely related to the other life domains included in the PWI, or they would not constitute a single dimension after principal component analysis (see, for instance, the work by Lau et al. 2005). We also know something about analysing these two items separately from the others in relation to their effect on the more general construct of satisfaction with life as a whole, also known as overall life satisfaction (OLS) (see, for instance, report no. 23 on the Australian Unity Wellbeing Index 2010). Another example of their relevance can be found in the work conducted by Tomyn and Cummins (2011), this time on a sample of 351 students aged between 12 and 20 who were administered the Personal Wellbeing Index – School Children Version (PWI-SC). It was observed that both present safety and future security, and particularly the former, were significant predictors of OLS. Neither present safety nor future security was among the predictors with the highest weight, these being life achievements and standard of living.

A review of the literature on security and quality of life reveals, among other things, that the majority of research has been conducted using adult samples – meaning further research is needed with adolescents and young people – and that the financial dimension often stands out most. Examples of this are fear of losing one's job, situations of unemployment (especially when long-term) and also facing high economic demands with only scarce resources (see, for instance the work by Veenhoven 2005; Böhnke 2008). Security in this respect refers more to social security at the macro social level rather than security as an aspect of personal well-being, that is to say, to the perceptions and evaluations of people regarding their own life. An exception can be found in reports based on the Australian Unity Wellbeing Index. Specifically, the 2006 report (Australian Unity of Wellbeing

Index 2006) was devoted to analysing the well-being of Australians in general but with a strong emphasis on income security. The authors found income security to be one of the most powerful determinants of well-being and suggested that policies aimed at increasing income security would likely raise the well-being of the population.

Another exception is the work by La Guardia et al. (2000), who link security (specifically, security of attachment[2]) to well-being in adults by means of self-determination theory. Thus, satisfying needs (in terms of autonomy, competence and relatedness) was expected to relate to greater security of attachment and to enhance well-being. Results showed that security of attachment and basic satisfaction of psychological needs have substantial shared variance when predicting well-being and that each variable also makes a unique contribution to it. This suggests the interest of including both relational and personal dimensions when exploring personal well-being and its links to perceptions of security. A third exception is given by Wills et al. (2011), who study the relationships between perceptions of insecurity (personal, political, economical and communitarian) with some of the items of the PWI (excluding satisfaction with present safety and future security). They conclude that personal well-being is influenced by the previously mentioned perceptions of insecurity and that these perceptions are influenced by social connections and life experiences.

With regard to security in terms of personal safety, another important branch of research studies the relationships between perceptions of security and crime or robbery statistics in a certain location and the discrepancies and concordances among them. This has occasionally been studied by showing young people maps on which they were asked to locate what they thought were unsafe points in North American cities (see, for instance, work by Pamela Wridt et al. at http://www.umapthecommunity.org/). Remarkably, there is very little spatial correlation between reported crime and the risks identified by young people (Wridt 2010). This type of research is thought to be very helpful for local authorities to better plan police actions so as to increase perceptions of security among younger citizens.

Without any doubt, both evaluations of (1) one's own economic circumstances (economic security) and (2) fear of crime or robbery, or even terrorism, are closely related to personal well-being and quality of life and deserve the attention of the scientific community. However, we still have a very limited knowledge regarding perceptions of security in general, that is, unlinked to specific aspects such as the economy, crime or the political regime in force at a particular time. Some papers demonstrate that security does not exist in isolation from an individual's perceptions and can therefore not be considered only in political, social and economic terms, but rather as a psychological phenomenon related to the general process of belief formation (Bar-Tal and Jacobson 1998). To this we would also add the need to adopt a

---

[2] Attachment is a psychological concept which was first defined by Bowlby (1999) with reference to an intensive and long-term bonding which develops and consolidates between two people, through their reciprocal interaction with the aim of providing protection and security.

psychosocial perspective[3]; psychological processes do not occur separately from social relationships, being framed in particular social contexts. When considering an approach to well-being, and after noting that there is a lack of research on that issue, we come to realise that our understanding of how people evaluate their own security, or in other words, the degree of satisfaction they have with their security and the factors linked to this evaluation, is extremely restricted.

Of the few published papers we have identified on satisfaction with security, the one by Yiengprugsawan et al. (2010) shows that for a sample of 87,134 university students in Thailand (mean age approximately 29), the predictors that contributed most to OLS using PWI-8 (which includes satisfaction with spirituality or religious beliefs) are standard of living (β=0.196), security for the future (β=0.171) and life achievements (β=0.152), whilst community belongingness (β=0.015) and present safety (β=0.058) are among those which contribute the least. In a recent paper by Casas et al. (2011) on samples of 12- to 16-year-old adolescents from 3 countries (Brazil N=1,588, Spain N=2,900 and Chile N=843), the predictors that contributed most to OLS using PWI-7 were standard of living (β=0.192), present safety (β=0.179) and life achievements (β=0.131), whereas satisfaction with groups of people you belong to (β=0.058) and satisfaction with health (β=0.063) were among those which contributed the least. Different cultural understandings of safety and security might offer an explanation for such differences. In the method section, further comments on this issue will be provided.

In this study we are going to explore the hypothesis that, in addition to perceptions of economic security and security against crime, which have been already widely studied, the following factors might have a contribution to present safety and future security, as measured through the PWI, on behalf of adolescents and young people 15–24 year old:

- Inner personal security or security with self-concept
- Spiritual security
- Security of choice and control
- Security related to values aspired to

As far as we know, neither of those factors have been studied in relation to perceptions of security, at least measured through the PWI. However, a connection among them could be hypothesised if we take into account their relevance to explaining personal well-being. At the same time, we expect to find positive connections between perceptions of security (present safety and future security) and those items measuring well-being (the rest of the items included in the PWI and considered in respect to OLS).

As indicators of inner personal security or security with self-concept, we are going to use 4 components from García and Musitu's (1999) AF5 multidimensional

---

[3] The psychosocial perspective can be understood as the confluence between psychological and social factors and helps to explain, for instance, the influence of others in the way we perceive and evaluate things happening around us.

scale on self-concept.[4] We depart from the assumption that having a high self-concept provides the person with security as it is generally accompanied with feelings of self-competence and capability. Self-concept is also among the strongest and most consistent positive predictors of personal well-being (Diener 1994; Diener and Lucas 2000) both in childhood and adolescence (Dew and Huebner 1994; Huebner 1991; Huebner and Alderman 1993). Among the diverse scales available to evaluate self-concept, we have chosen the AF5 scale because it has been developed specifically for the Spanish context and has application in both the clinical and research fields. The connection between attachment and self-concept is well established in the literature (see, for instance, Bowlby 1999) as perceptions of secure relationships with other people are considered to be necessary in order to construct a good self-evaluation. Because the AF5 includes some items which evaluate the bond with close people (friends, family and teachers), security of attachment will not be studied using a specific scale.

With regard to the second factor, spiritual security, the frequent appearance in the scientific literature of purpose in life or sense of meaning regarding one's own life in relation to spirituality leads us to assume that people are less likely to feel spiritual security when they have no clear idea of what they are living for. Purpose in life or sense of meaning regarding one's own life is considered, in coherence with that assumption, important for personal well-being, as it is deemed to provide life with direction and meaning. This is true to the extent that it has already been included in some scales measuring psychological well-being, particularly those formulated within the context of the eudaemonic tradition of well-being (see for instance, Ryff's scale 1989a, b). However, many of the scales that have been used to date to evaluate such constructs have major weaknesses, particularly problems of construct validity. More generally, an additional problem pointed out for many scales is that they make explicit references to God, whereas some religions (e.g. Buddhism) and spiritual traditions (e.g. new age traditions) do not accept that God in a 'creator' sense exists (Casas et al. 2009b).

Furthermore, purpose in life has been studied on only a few occasions and almost never with young people or adolescents, meaning that further attention and development is needed with this population. The relationships between sense of meaning, evaluated through a single-item scale on overall sense of meaning in one's own life and other elements conforming personal well-being such as satisfaction with spirituality and religion, have been explored with two samples of young people (adolescents aged 12–17 and young adults from 18 to 35) (Casas et al. 2009b).

In the above study, the item relating to overall sense of meaning in one's own life – which was called the 'Existential Sense of Meaning Scale' (ESMS) – showed positive, significant and fairly high correlations with the four well-being scales used (Cummins et al.'s Personal Wellbeing Index 2003; Diener et al.'s Satisfaction With

---

[4] From Rosenberg's work in 1979, there is agreement among the scientific community that self-concept refers to the self-evaluations that people make about different areas of their lives.

Life Scale 1985; a single-item scale on overall satisfaction, and Fordyce's single-item scale on happiness 1988). Moreover, it seemed that the ESMS contributed even more than happiness to overall life satisfaction (at least, as measured through Fordyce's scale). As far as we know, there are no existing studies that explore the relationship between the ESMS and perceptions of security. Because we hypothesise that spiritual security is part of one's general perceptions of security, we are going to use the single-item ESMS as an indicator of spiritual security. This way, some contribution to the existing gap within well-being studies on this issue is expected to be made.

We also hypothesise that security of election and control may help to explain people's perceptions of security because the more people have the feeling that things happening around them are under their control, the more secure they might feel. Moreover, perception of control has for many years been considered a strong predictor of personal well-being during both childhood and adolescence (Huebner 2004), with many studies having shown it to play a crucial role as a protective factor in many diverse situations and social roles (Cohen and Edwards 1989; quoted in Lacković-Grgin et al. 2001). Interest in studying this area is therefore on the increase (Strickland 1989; quoted in Leone and Burns 2000). Many models have been formulated to try to explain the effects of the presence or absence of perception of control. Among these, one of the most influential has been Rotter's (1966) differentiation between external and internal perceptions of *locus* of reinforcement.

From the work conducted by Rotter, we find that people who perceive causal relationships between their own behaviour and its consequences hold internal control beliefs, whereas those perceiving consequences to be random or unpredictable and the result of luck hold external control beliefs. Internal control beliefs can be measured through the degree of freedom the individual perceives to have in his or her life in general. This was the focus of a 2007 report by Javaloy on well-being and happiness among young Spanish people. In this study it was observed that those with high scores for happiness where the ones who believed they had freedom of choice and control in how their lives were developing, and also those expressing higher self-acceptance and self-esteem.

The fourth factor we associate with perceptions of security in this study is the feeling of security related to values aspired to, that is, specific values both adolescents and young people would like to be appreciated for when they become adults (for instance, sympathy or solidarity). The rationale of assuming a connection between aspirational values in the future and perceptions of security is that giving importance to some values (projected towards the future in the case of our study) can be perceived as an inversion towards assuring a good future in terms of having satisfying social relationships, having enough material goods or having the ability to obtain desirable things. In fact, some authors (Csikzentmihalyi 1997; Diener and Fujita 1995; Diener et al. 1997) have argued for the inclusion of values, particularly as a basis for exploring personal well-being in cross-cultural studies. It is noticeable that security has been studied more as a value than as an evaluation in terms of satisfaction (one noteworthy exception is the PWI, as we have already commented). For example, Schwartz' *circumplex theory of human values* (1992) is a case to point.

Another example can be found in Murkherjee's (1989) four-dimension classification of values, which includes the category of security in the life of humans. These dimensions are: survival of the species (comprising suicide rate, length of life, infant mortality rate and self-rated health), security in the life span of humans (families at risk, violent crime rate and environmental toxins index), material prosperity for well-being (per capita personal income, unemployment rate, poverty rate and percentage of household with one or more persons per room) and mental progress to unfold potentials (percentage having spent 4 or more years at college).

In order to explore values, some researchers have developed models using lists of values appreciated at present. This is the case with Struch et al. (2002), who use the prompt 'As a guiding principle in my life, this value is...' to introduce a list of 56 values. Other studies, embedded within the eudaemonic tradition of studies of well-being aim to explore the relationships between the pursuit of specific goals and well-being (see, for example, Kasser and Ryan 1996). Values are then understood as aspirations for the future and related to life objectives.

Another way of exploring values among young people closely linked to the previously mentioned eudaemonic tradition is by asking them to what extent they would like to be appreciated for some specific quality when they become adults. In previous studies we have explored the relationships between future aspirational values (specifically: intelligence, technical skills, social skills, knowledge of computers, profession, sensitivity, pleasantness, money, power and knowledge of the world) and self-esteem, perception of control and perception of social support with an emphasis on the concordances and discrepancies of values between children and their parents (Casas et al. 2005, 2007a). We have also conducted an international study on this issue in five different countries (Casas et al. 2003). In both studies results suggest that values aspired to can be considered a well-being-related construct. The connection between aspirational values and perceptions of security has not been explored yet. This chapter aims to make some contribution in exploring the potential connection between them, which is theoretically expected to exist.

This study focuses on Spanish students of post-compulsory secondary education (15- to 24-year-olds), and has the following objectives: (1) to analyse the relationships between satisfaction with present safety and future security and the items conforming the Catalan adaptation of Cummins et al.'s (2003) PWI-7 (satisfaction with health, standard of living, life achievements, groups of people you belong to and relationships with other people) and the OLS scale (for overall satisfaction); (2) to explore the relationships between present safety and future security and other psychosocial constructs such as self-concept, overall sense of meaning found in own life (ESMS), freedom of choice and control over own life, and values aspired to in the future which we have used as indicators of inner personal security or security with self-concept, spiritual security, security of choice and control and security related to values aspired to, respectively and (3) to identify potential gender differences and similarities between the above variables and relationships.

2   Method

2.1   Procedure and Sample

Data were obtained from 16 secondary schools[5] in the province of Girona, located
in the Autonomous Region of Catalonia (northeast Spain), in 2008. Schools and
number of classes were randomly selected to fulfil a quota for each age group, and
all steps were taken to comply with ethical guidelines for administering questionnaires to young people.

The school director, parents associations and teachers were asked for their cooperation and approval; following this, participants were informed of the confidentiality
of the data and were asked to participate. Questionnaires were administered to the
whole group in their regular classroom, with one of their usual teachers and at least
one researcher present during administration in order to clarify any issues that arose.

In Spain, compulsory education lasts from 6 to 16, following which there are two
pathways into post-compulsory education (from 16 to 18): either academic upper-
secondary education (*Bachillerato*) or intermediate specific vocational training.
Participants in our study were enrolled on the two pathways of official post-secondary
education, and our sample therefore excludes those not following official post-
compulsory education. 581 males and 823 females ($N=1,404$) responded to the
questionnaire.

The age range was 15–24 ($M=16.86$, SD$=1.068$). 94.1% of participants were
aged 18 or younger. Some of the participants were still under 16 because they were
born at the end of the year and completed the questionnaire before their sixteenth
birthday. Others are over 19 because they began a pathway in post-secondary education well after the age of 16 or because they have needed more time to complete this
pathway. The rationale for selecting this age range was that there is lack of scientific
studies on the issue of perceptions of security and its link to personal well-being
both in the adolescent and youth years.

2.2   Description of the Variables

The variables included in the questionnaire and analysed in this study are:

Personal Wellbeing Index (PWI) (Cummins et al. 2003)

Participants were asked to what extent they felt satisfied with different aspects of
their lives at the time of responding to the questionnaire. The 7-item version of

---

[5] In Spain, upper-secondary education (*Bachillerato*) is offered in secondary schools as well as
intermediate specific vocational training. For this reason, all participants in this study were
recruited from secondary schools.

PWI was used in this study, comprising the following domains: 'Satisfaction with health', 'Satisfaction with standard of living', 'Satisfaction with life achievements', 'Satisfaction with personal security', 'Satisfaction with groups of people you belong to', 'Satisfaction with security about the future' and 'Satisfaction with relationships with other people'. The original English version of the PWI domains and their back-translation from Castilian-Spanish into English has already been developed in Casas et al. (2008).

One of the items of the original scale refers to 'Satisfaction with feeling part of the community'. This item could not be used in Spain, because the concept of 'community' has changed completely in the modern Spanish urban world. In the urban world, 'community' denotes the 'cluster of owners of apartments in the same building'. For this reason, it has been substituted by the item on 'Satisfaction with groups of people you belong to'. Besides, the original item on 'Satisfaction with personal relationships' has been substituted by 'Satisfaction with relationships with other people', after piloting the scale and in order to improve the comprehension of respondents. Finally and as explained in the translation issues section, the original item on 'Satisfaction with future security' has been substituted by 'Satisfaction with security about the future' whilst 'Satisfaction with personal safety' has been substituted by 'Satisfaction with personal security'. In both cases, changes were necessary due to the different understanding of what security and safety refers to in the Spanish and English languages.

In this study we have used the Catalan adaptation of the 2008 Spanish version because Catalan is the official language within the educational system in the region. This same version has been used in previous research with non-adult populations in Spain with good respondent understanding. The Cronbach alpha for this study is 0.78, which lies between 0.70 and 0.85 (the interval defined by the authors of the scale in Australia and overseas, Cummins et al. 2003).

The 8-item version (including satisfaction with spiritual beliefs or religion) of the PWI has not been applied in this study as the additional item has been shown to be problematic when used with samples of both 12- to 17-year-old adolescents and young adults enrolled at university (18- to 35-year-olds). This is due to the fact that it seems to have different meanings for them (Casas et al. 2009b). Thus, it is doubtful, at least among adolescents, whether uniting religion and spirituality in a single item makes a clear enough statement, in terms of referring to a life domain. In addition, understanding of this abstract topic may differ during the life cycle, so that adolescents' and youngsters' points of view on it may differ from adults'.

All the items of the PWI were measured using 11-point 0–10 scales (0 = *Completely dissatisfied* and 10 = *Completely satisfied*), following Cummins and Gullone's (2000) recommendations. The index is obtained by calculating the mean of the items and converting the result to a 0–100 scale. Two of the items comprising the index, specifically satisfaction with personal safety (satisfaction with personal security in the Spanish-Catalan version) and satisfaction with security for the future (satisfaction with the security about the future in the Spanish-Catalan version), are also analysed separately in relation to the rest of the explored variables.

Overall Life Satisfaction (OLS)

Participants were asked to express their satisfaction with their life as a whole, alternatively referred to as overall life satisfaction (OLS). The item was again measured using an 11-point 0–10 scale where 0 = *Completely dissatisfied* and 10 = *Completely satisfied*.

Self-concept (García and Musitu 1999)

Participants were encouraged to respond to García and Musitu's AF5 multidimensional scale (1999) using an 11-point scale, 0 meaning *Never* and 10 *Always*. The version used in this chapter comprises 24 items across four dimensions: *academic self-concept* ('I am a good student', 'My teachers consider me a hard working student', 'I work a lot in class', 'I do well with my schoolwork', 'My teachers love me', 'My teachers consider me an intelligent and hardworking student'); *family self-concept* ('My parents love me', 'My parents trust me', 'I am happy at home', 'My family would help me with any kind of problem'; 'I am criticised a lot at home' and 'My family is disappointed with me'); *physical self-concept* ('I like myself physically', 'I am good at sports', 'I am an attractive person', 'Others look for me to do sports activities', 'I take care of myself physically' and 'I consider myself elegant') and *social self-concept* ('I make friends easily', 'It is very difficult for me to make friends', 'I am a friendly person', 'I have a lot of friends', 'My friends love me' and 'It is difficult for me to talk to strangers'). The Cronbach alpha is 0.84 (academic self-concept, 0.86; family self-concept, 0.82; physical self-concept, 0.76 and social self-concept, 0.74), which is higher than expected according to the results of the authors of the scale (0.81).

Overall Sense of Meaning in Own Life (ESMS) (Casas et al. 2009b)

A single-item scale assessing 'Overall sense of meaning found in own life', which we call the 'Existential Sense of Meaning Scale' (ESMS), was included in the questionnaire. It was also measured using an 11-point scale. The scaling of this item ranges from 0 = *devoid of meaning* to 10 = *full of meaning*. In order to contextualise what we were referring to, we included a previous explanation. The exact wording of the question was 'Some thinkers consider that people are freely able to give a global sense of meaning to their overall life, from birth to death. To what extent do you agree that up to now you have been able to give an overall sense of meaning to your life in a scale ranging from *devoid* to *full of meaning*?'

Freedom of Choice and Control over Own Life (Javaloy 2007)

Javaloy's single-item scale was used to measure perception of control. The exact wording of the question was as follows: 'Some people have the feeling that they have complete freedom of choice and control over their own lives, whereas other people feel that they do not have real control over what happens to them. Please respond to this scale, where 0 means *None* and 10 *A lot* to indicate the degree of freedom of choice and control you think you have over the way your life develops'.

Values Aspired To in the Future (Casas et al. 2004; Coenders et al. 2005)

A closed-ended list was used to explore the values participants aspired to in the future, specifically at the age of 21. Similar lists have been used previously in other research to identify the structure of these aspirations shared by parents and their children (Casas et al. 2003). For the purposes of this study, the list comprises 21 values all measured using an 11-point scale, with $0 = None$ and $10 = A$ *lot*. The items are as follows: 'Intelligence', 'Technical abilities', 'Abilities with people', 'Willpower', 'Profession', 'Family', 'Optimism', 'Sympathy', 'Money', 'Power', 'Sense of humour', 'Image', 'Coherence', 'Solidarity', 'Tolerance', 'Sense of meaning in life', 'Enjoying life', 'Humanity', 'Spiritual richness', 'Personality' and 'Kindness'.

2.3   Data Analysis

The analyses carried out in this study are structured as follows. First, the mean and standard deviations of each variable are calculated and potential differences by gender identified through the T-student statistical test. Second, each studied variable is correlated with the items on satisfaction with present safety and future security using the bivariate Pearson statistical test. The same procedure is applied to males and females separately. Three regression models are then developed (one for the whole sample, one for males and one for females), taking satisfaction with present safety and future security as dependent variables and the other items from each of the described scales as independent variables. Three more regression models are then calculated, this time considering only those variables entering each partial regression model as predictors of safety and security. An aggregate measure of the PWI has only been used for descriptive purposes in the first part of the results section but not to calculate these regression models as it would have necessarily included the items on present safety and future security. Finally, in order to verify whether the structure of the self-concept scale presented in this study follows the authors' approach, a Principal Component Analysis (PCA) is also performed.

2.4   Translation Issues

Some translation issues exist with regard to the language used in this article which, after being analysed together with a native English translator, appear to be very relevant to the interpretation of the results. A simple translation and back-translation of the wording of the two core items analysed hides the cultural and linguistic background of the issue.

Table 10.1 The original English version of the PWI domains on present safety and future security and their back-translation from Catalan

Original English	Catalan translation	Back-translation into English
How satisfied are you with...	*Actualment, fins a quin punt et trobes satisfet o satisfeta amb...*	*At present, to what extent do you feel satisfied with...*
How safe you feel?	el segur o segura que et sents?	How safe you feel?
Your future security?	la seguretat pel teu futur?	Your future security?

In Catalan, 'safety' and 'security' have the same translation, '*seguretat*'. The same is true for Spanish: there are not two different words with the different connotations they have in English. However, when using 'safe' together with the verb 'feel' in the Catalan or Spanish cultural context, there is a strong connotation that the question refers to a feeling, independently of any objective circumstances. Therefore, a Catalan or Spanish speaker may emphasise different things than an English-speaking respondent when answering the same question. Specifically, they will not always emphasise the physical connotation that 'safety' has in English because they may also be referring to a 'psychological' security as a present feeling (Table 10.1).

By contrast, when referring to the 'future', the question is no longer limited to feelings, because it in fact asks for a 'subjective evaluation' of both 'objective and subjective' conditions of future security, although with some strong connotations – both in Catalan and Spanish – related to material living conditions (employment, income, housing, social security and so on) as opposed to the psychosocial living conditions that may also be considered by some respondents (i.e. supportive networks, personal autonomy).

The inclusion of 'future' in the second item also emphasises the temporal dimension, because the first item is clearly restricted to the present. That said, the temporal dimension is most probably the same in the three languages. As 'safety' can be considered to be included in 'security', many of our results and conclusions will refer only to 'security', because no real conclusions on 'safety' can be reached from our wording of the question in the Catalan language.

3 Results

3.1 Personal Wellbeing Index

The mean scores obtained for each of the 7 items comprising the PWI are as follows: *satisfaction with health* ($M=7.76$, SD$=1.96$, $N=1,401$), *satisfaction with standard of living* ($M=7.90$, SD$=1.70$, $N=1,399$), *satisfaction with life achievements* ($M=7.34$, SD$=1.82$, $N=1,390$), *satisfaction with personal safety* ($M=6.73$, SD$=2.23$, $N=1,387$), *satisfaction with groups of people you belong to* ($M=8.20$, SD$=1.92$, $N=1,386$), *satisfaction with security about the future* ($M=6.40$, SD$=2.23$, $N=1,390$) and *satisfaction with relationships with other people* ($M=7.77$, SD$=1.88$,

Table 10.2 Mean difference between males and females for PWI scale items and the whole index

PWI items	Males		Females		Mean difference
	Mean	SD	Mean	SD	
Satisfaction with health	**7.97**	1.85	7.62	2.03	$t(1,310,872) = 3.439$ $p = .001$
Satisfaction with standard of living	**8.03**	1.56	7.81	1.79	$t(1,337,846) = 2.437$ $p = .015$
Satisfaction with life achievements	7.30	1.78	7.36	1.85	$p = .575$
Satisfaction with personal safety	**7.09**	1.96	6.47	2.37	$t(1,352,129) = 5.378$ $p < .0005$
Satisfaction with groups of people you belong to	8.13	1.87	8.25	1.95	$p = .238$
Satisfaction with security about the future	**6.61**	2.15	6.25	2.28	$t(1,388) = 2.947$ $p = .003$
Satisfaction with relationships with other people	7.68	1.92	7.84	1.85	$p = .139$
PWI	**75.7**	12.2	73.7	13.2	$t(1,327) = 2.73$ $p = .006$

Significant differences are highlighted in **bold**

Table 10.3 Pearson correlations for Personal Wellbeing Index items and OLS and *satisfaction with present safety* and *future security*

PWI items	Satisfaction with present safety		Satisfaction with future security	
	r	Significance	r	Significance
Satisfaction with health	.281	$p < .0005$	.236	$p < .0005$
Satisfaction with standard of living	.332	$p < .0005$	.344	$p < .0005$
Satisfaction with life achievements	.456	$p < .0005$	.387	$p < .0005$
Satisfaction with groups of people you belong to	.278	$p < .0005$	.302	$p < .0005$
Satisfaction with relationships with other people	.362	$p < .0005$	.365	$p < .0005$
OLS	.477	$p < .0005$	.414	$p < .0005$

$N = 1,384$). Both *satisfaction with personal safety* (which we have called *present safety* in the following analysis) and *satisfaction with security for future* (which we have called *future security*) are the only ones with mean scores under 7, the mean for *present safety* being higher than that of *future security*. The mean for the index is 74.56 (SD = 12.8) on a scale from 0 to 100.

Table 10.2 displays the mean scores for males and females for each of the items in the PWI. Significant differences are observed for *satisfaction with health, satisfaction with standard of living, satisfaction with personal safety (present safety)* and *satisfaction with security for future (future security)*. In all cases, the mean scores are higher for males. Males' result for the PWI is higher than females'.

The correlation between *present safety* and *future security* is moderate, $r = 0.486$ ($p < 0.0005$). Table 10.3 shows that *satisfaction with present safety* correlates most with *satisfaction with life achievements* and least with *satisfaction with groups of*

Table 10.4 Pearson correlations for Personal Wellbeing Index items and OLS and *satisfaction with present safety* and *future security* in the case of males and females separately

	Satisfaction with present safety		Satisfaction with future security	
	r	Significance	r	Significance
Males' PWI items				
Satisfaction with health	.318	$p < .0005$	.217	$p < .0005$
Satisfaction with standard of living	.332	$p < .0005$	.334	$p < .0005$
Satisfaction with life achievements	.449	$p < .0005$	.408	$p < .0005$
Satisfaction with groups of people you belong to	.329	$p < .0005$	.337	$p < .0005$
Satisfaction with relationships with other people	.370	$p < .0005$	.404	$p < .0005$
OLS	.457	$p < .0005$	.414	$p < .0005$
Females' PWI items				
Satisfaction with health	.247	$p < .0005$	.239	$p < .0005$
Satisfaction with standard of living	.325	$p < .0005$	.345	$p < .0005$
Satisfaction with life achievements	.473	$p < .0005$	.377	$p < .0005$
Satisfaction with groups of people you belong to	.262	$p < .0005$	.286	$p < .0005$
Satisfaction with relationships with other people	.379	$p < .0005$	.346	$p < .0005$
OLS	.490	$p < .0005$	.411	$p < .0005$

people you belong to. With regard to *satisfaction with future security*, the highest correlation is also for *satisfaction with life achievements* and the lowest *satisfaction with health*. By comparison with *present safety*, *satisfaction with future security* correlates more with *satisfaction with standard of living, groups of people you belong to* and *relationships with other people*.

There is a moderate correlation between the OLS and items referring to *satisfaction with both present safety and future security*. In terms of gender (Table 10.4), when comparing whether correlations are higher for *present* or *future security*, responses by females and males display very similar patterns, with the exception of *satisfaction with relationships with other people*, which is higher for females in the present, the opposite of the males' response. Correlations between *present safety* and *future security* and the OLS are moderate for both genders, being slightly higher for females for *present safety* and higher for males for *future security*.

The most important items for predicting *satisfaction with present safety* are *satisfaction with future security* and *satisfaction with life achievements,* whilst the one which best predicts *satisfaction with future security* is *satisfaction with present safety* followed by *satisfaction with relationships with other people* (Table 10.5).

The same models have been calculated considering males and females separately (Table 10.6). In relation to *present safety*, the males' model includes five items and

Table 10.5 Regression models for predicting *satisfaction with present safety* and *future security* (dependent variables) (using PWI items for both)

	Satisfaction with present safety		Satisfaction with future security	
	34.5%		32.4%	
	$F_{4,1328} = 174.012$		$F_{5,1328} = 126.686$	
Explained variance	$p < .0005$	β	$p < .0005$	β
Significant items in the model[a]	Satisfaction with future security	+.318	Satisfaction with present safety	+.321
	Satisfaction with life achievements	+.254	Satisfaction with relationships with other people	+.131
	Satisfaction with relationships with other people	+.131	Satisfaction with standard of living	+.131
	Satisfaction with health	+.096	Satisfaction with life achievements	+.118
			Satisfaction with groups of people you belong to	+.090

[a]Items are ordered according to the beta score. The + symbol shows the direction of the relationship

the females' only three. *Satisfaction with life achievements* is the strongest predictor for males and *satisfaction with future security* for females. With regard to *future security*, the strongest predictor for both genders is *satisfaction with present safety*, followed by *satisfaction with life achievements* for males and *satisfaction with standard of living* for females.

3.2 Overall Life Satisfaction

The mean score obtained for this item is 7.66 (SD = 1.754, $N = 1,400$), with no statistically significant differences between males and females. Correlations between this item and *satisfaction with present safety* and *future security* are statistically significant ($r = 0.477, p < 0.0005$ and $r = 0.414, p < 0.0005$, respectively). Correlations for males are $r = 0.457, p < 0.0005$ (*present safety*) and $r = 0.414, p < 0.0005$ (*future security*). Correlations for females are $r = 0.490, p < 0.0005$ (*present safety*) and $r = 0.411, p < 0.0005$ (*future security*). OLS acts as a strong predictor of both *satisfaction with present safety* and *future security* (Table 10.7), the beta score being higher for the former than for the latter. However, the explained variance is not very high for either *present safety* or *future security*.

The same regression models have been calculated for males and females separately (Table 10.8). The beta score is fairly similar for males and females for both *present safety* and *future security*, it being lower for *future security*.

Table 10.6 Regression models for predicting *satisfaction with present safety* and *future security* (dependent variables) among males and females (using PWI variables for both)

	Satisfaction with present safety males		Satisfaction with present safety females	
	30.9%		38.1%	
Explained variance	$F_{5,547}=48.498$ $p<.0005$	β	$F_{3,780}=159.678$ $p<.0005$	β
Significant items in the model[a]	Satisfaction with life achievements	+.249	Satisfaction with future security	+.360
	Satisfaction with future security	+.203	Satisfaction with life achievements	+.285
	Satisfaction with health	+.133	Satisfaction with relationships with other people	+.154
	Satisfaction with groups of people you belong to	+.115		
	Satisfaction with relationships with other people	+.099		
	Satisfaction with future security males		Satisfaction with future security females	
	30.3%		33.9%	
Explained variance	$F_{5,547}=47.062$ $p<.0005$	β	$F_{5,780}=79.522$ $p<.0005$	β
Significant items in the model[a]	Satisfaction with present safety	+.199	Satisfaction with present safety	+.380
	Satisfaction with life achievements	+.184	Satisfaction with standard of living	+.141
	Satisfaction with relationships with other people	+.164	Satisfaction with relationships with other people	+.106
	Satisfaction with standard of living	+.121	Satisfaction with groups of people you belong to	+.081
	Satisfaction with groups of people you belong to	+.117	Satisfaction with life achievements	+.078

[a]Items are ordered according to the beta score. The+symbol shows the direction of the relationship

Table 10.7 Regression models for predicting *satisfaction with present safety* and *future security* (dependent variables) (using the OLS item for both)

	Satisfaction with present safety		Satisfaction with future security	
	22.7%		17.1%	
Explained variance	$F_{1,1384}=407.216$ $p<.0005$	β	$F_{1,1387}=285.947$ $p<.0005$	β
Significant items in the model[a]	OLS	+.477	OLS	+.414

[a]The+symbol shows the direction of the relationship

Table 10.8 Regression models for predicting *satisfaction with present safety* and *future security* (dependent variables) among males and females (using OLS item for both)

	Satisfaction with present safety males		Satisfaction with present safety females	
	20.9%		24.0%	
	$F_{1,573} = 150.971$		$F_{1,810} = 255.957$	
Explained variance	$p < .0005$	β	$p < .0005$	β
Significant items in the model[a]	OLS	+.457	OLS	+.490
	Satisfaction with future security males		Satisfaction with future security females	
	17.2%		16.9%	
	$F_{1,575} = 118.895$		$F_{1,811} = 164.389$	
Explained variance	$p < .0005$	β	$p < .0005$	β
Significant items in the model[a]	OLS	+.414	OLS	+.411

[a]The + symbol shows the direction of the relationship

Table 10.9 Mean difference between males and females for self-concept dimensions

	Males		Females		
	Mean	SD	Mean	SD	Mean difference
Academic self-concept	−0.21025	1.00085	**0.14556**	0.97384	$t(1,208) = -6.178, p < .0005$
Family self-concept	−0.07568	0.93143	**0.05240**	1.04226	$t(1,208) = -2.194, p = .028$
Physical self-concept	**0.41604**	0.95806	−0.28803	0.92474	$t(1,208) = 12.830, p < .0005$
Social self-concept	−0.11544	0.97857	**0.07992**	1.00752	$t(1,208) = -3.355, p = .001$

Significant differences are highlighted in **bold**

3.3   Self-concept

A Principal Component Analysis with Varimax rotation was carried out with items from García and Musitu's (1999) AF5 self-concept scale. According to the authors' model, four dimensions explain 54.87% of the total variance. These dimensions are: *academic self-concept* (16.37% of the variance), *family self-concept* (14.02% of the variance), *physical self-concept* (12.63% of the variance) and *social self-concept* (11.84% of the variance).

Gender differences are detected in relation to these four dimensions (Table 10.9). The mean for *academic self-concept* is higher for females than males, as is the case with *family* and *social self-concept*. By contrast, *physical self-concept* is higher for males.

Once the aforementioned dimensions had been calculated, correlations with both *present safety* and *future security* were explored. They are given below (Table 10.10).

As displayed in Table 10.10, correlations range between 0.135 and 0.328 for *present safety* and between 0.134 and 0.239 for *future security*. The highest correlations for *present*

Table 10.10 Pearson correlations for self-concept dimensions and satisfaction with *present safety* and *future security*

	Satisfaction with present safety		Satisfaction with future security	
Self-concept dimensions	r	Significance	r	Significance
Academic self-concept	.135	p<.0005	.233	p<.0005
Family self-concept	.174	p<.0005	.234	p<.0005
Physical self-concept	.328	p<.0005	.239	p<.0005
Social self-concept	.231	p<.0005	.134	p<.0005

Table 10.11 Pearson correlations for self-concept dimensions and *satisfaction with present safety* and *future security* in the case of males and females separately

	Satisfaction with present safety		Satisfaction with future security	
	r	Significance	r	Significance
Males' self-concept dimensions				
Academic self-concept	.139	p=.002	.293	p<.0005
Family self-concept	.222	p<.0005	.252	p<.0005
Physical self-concept	.349	p<.0005	.213	p<.0005
Social self-concept	.263	p<.0005	.144	p=.001
Females' self-concept dimensions				
Academic self-concept	.181	p<.0005	.227	p<.0005
Family self-concept	.166	p<.0005	.235	p<.0005
Physical self-concept	.274	p<.0005	.233	p<.0005
Social self-concept	.242	p<.0005	.144	p<.0005

safety are *physical* and *social self-concept,* in that order, whilst the highest for *future security* is also *physical self-concept* but with *family self-concept* in second position.

In Table 10.11 these same correlations have been computed taking males and females separately. Males' correlations range from 0.139 to 0.349 for *present safety* and from 0.144 to 0.293 for *future security*. In the case of females, they range from 0.166 to 0.274 for *present safety* and from 0.144 to 0.235 for *future security*. For both genders, the highest correlation in the present is with *physical self-concept,* whilst for the future it is with *academic self-concept* (for males) and *family self-concept* (for females).

Following this analysis, different regression models were calculated taking *satisfaction with present safety* and *satisfaction with future security* as dependent variables and the four self-concept dimensions as independent variables (Table 10.12).

All four self-concept dimensions contribute to explaining both *satisfaction with present safety* and *with future security*. The explained variance is slightly higher in the case of *present safety*. The contribution of each dimension differs for each satisfaction domain. Thus, *physical* and *social self-concept* have a higher contribution for *present safety* whilst for *future security* it is *physical* and *family self-concept*.

Some gender differences appear when these same regression models are computed taking gender into account (Table 10.13). In the case of *present safety*, the highest contributing variables for males are *physical* and *social self-concept*

Table 10.12 Regression models for predicting *satisfaction with present safety* and *future security* (dependent variables) (using self-concept dimensions for both)

	Satisfaction with present safety		Satisfaction with future security	
	20.8%		18.5%	
	$F_{4,1199} = 78.673$		$F_{4,1200} = 67.980$	
Explained variance	$p < .0005$	β	$p < .0005$	β
Significant items in the model[a]	Physical self-concept	+.327	Physical self-concept	+.241
	Social self-concept	+.228	Family self-concept	+.236
	Family self-concept	+.175	Academic self-concept	+.235
	Academic self-concept	+.135	Social self-concept	+.132

[a]Items are ordered according to the beta score. The + symbol shows the direction of the relationship

Table 10.13 Regression models for predicting satisfaction with *present safety* and *future security* (dependent variables) among males and females (using self-concept dimensions for both)

	Satisfaction with present safety males		Satisfaction with present safety females	
	22.3%		19.5%	
	$F_{4,489} = 34.733$		$F_{4,709} = 42.563$	
Explained variance	$p < .0005$	β	$p < .0005$	β
Significant items in the model[a]	Physical self-concept	+.301	Physical self-concept	+.270
	Social self-concept	+.211	Family self-concept	+.257
	Family self-concept	+.193	Academic self-concept	+.181
	Academic self-concept	+.139	Social self-concept	+.156
	Satisfaction with future security males		Satisfaction with future security females	
	19.7%		18.3%	
	$F_{4,493} = 29.976$		$F_{4,706} = 39.227$	
Explained variance	$p < .0005$	β	$p < .0005$	β
Significant items in the model[a]	Academic self-concept	+.291	Family self-concept	+.251
	Family self-concept	+.230	Academic self-concept	+.215
	Physical self-concept	+.174	Physical self-concept	+.221
	Social self-concept	+.117	Social self-concept	+.163

[a]Items are ordered according to the beta score. The + symbol shows the direction of the relationship

whilst for females they are *physical* and *family self-concept. Academic* and *family self-concept* are the most relevant predictors of *future security* for both females and males. However, the order is not exactly the same in terms of the beta scores.

3.4 Sense of Meaning in Life

The mean obtained for this item is 7.27 (SD=1.66, N=1,372) on a scale from 0 to 10, with no statistically significant mean difference between genders. Moderate

Table 10.14 Regression models for predicting *satisfaction with present safety* and *future security* (dependent variables) (using the ESMS item for both)

	Satisfaction with present safety		Satisfaction with future security	
	12.6%		10.5%	
	$F_{1,1355} = 196.044$		$F_{1,1358} = 159.991$	
Explained variance	$p < .0005$	β	$p < .0005$	β
Significant items in the model[a]	ESMS	+.356	ESMS	+.325

[a]Items are ordered according to the beta score. The + symbol shows the direction of the relationship

Table 10.15 Regression models for predicting *satisfaction with present safety* and *future security* (dependent variables) among males and females (using the ESMS item for both)

	Satisfaction with present safety males		Satisfaction with present safety females	
	12.6%		13.9%	
	$F_{1,555} = 79.916$		$F_{1,799} = 129.321$	
Explained variance	$p < .0005$	β	$p < .0005$	β
Significant items in the model[a]	ESMS	+.355	ESMS	+.373
	Satisfaction with future security males		Satisfaction with future security females	
	10.7%		10.9%	
	$F_{1,557} = 66.512$		$F_{1,800} = 97.318$	
Explained variance	$p < .0005$	β	$p < .0005$	β
Significant items in the model[a]	ESMS	+.327	ESMS	+.330

[a]The + symbol shows the direction of the relationship

correlations are observed between the *sense of meaning in life* item and *satisfaction with present safety* and *future security*, the former being higher than the latter ($r = 0.356$, $p < 0.0005$ *versus* $r = 0.325$, $p < 0.0005$). Correlations are slightly higher for females than males both for *satisfaction with present safety* ($r = 0.373$, $p < 0.0005$ *versus* $r = 0.355$, $p < 0.0005$) and *future security* ($r = 0.330$, $p < 0.0005$ *versus* $r = 0.327$, $p < 0.0005$). The item *sense of meaning in life* is a good predictor of *satisfaction with present safety*, as it is for *satisfaction with future security* (Table 10.14). However, the percentage of explained variance is low in both cases.

When these same regression models are calculated considering genders separately, we observe that the results are quite similar for males and females (Table 10.15).

3.5 Freedom of Choice and Control over Own Life

The mean obtained for this item is 6.89 (SD = 1.62, N = 1,386), the males' mean (M = 7.02, SD = 1.72) being statistically higher, t (1384) = 2.523, p = 0.012, than the females' (M = 6.80, SD = 1.55). Correlations between *freedom of choice and control*

Table 10.16 Regression models for predicting *satisfaction with present safety* and *future security* (dependent variables) (using the *freedom of choice and control over own life* item for both)

	Satisfaction with present safety		Satisfaction with future security	
	6.4%		3.8%	
Explained variance	$F_{1,1369}=94.217$ $p<.0005$	β	$F_{1,1373}=53.928$ $p<.0005$	β
Significant items in the model[a]	Freedom of choice and control over own life	+.254	Freedom of choice and control over own life	+.194

[a]The + symbol shows the direction of the relationship

Table 10.17 Regression models for predicting *satisfaction with present safety* and *future security* (dependent variables) among males and females (using the *freedom of choice and control over own life* item for both)

	Satisfaction with present safety males		Satisfaction with future security females	
	6.7%		5.9%	
Explained variance	$F_{1,563}=40.160$ $p<.0005$	β	$F_{1,805}=50.793$ $p<.0005$	β
Significant items in the model[a]	Freedom of choice and control over own life	+.258	Freedom of choice and control over own life	+.244
	Satisfaction with future security males		Satisfaction with future security females	
	3.5%		3.8%	
Explained variance	$F_{1,566}=20.422$ $p<.0005$	β	$F_{1,806}=31.517$ $p<.0005$	β
Significant items in the model[a]	Freedom of choice and control over own life	+.187	Freedom of choice and control over own life	+.194

[a]The + symbol shows the direction of the relationship

over own life and *satisfaction with present safety* and *future security* are as follows: $r=0.254$, $p<0.0005$ (*present safety*) and $r=0.194$ $p<0.0005$ (*future security*). Correlations for males are: $r=0.258$, $p<0.0005$ (*present safety*) and $r=0.187$, $p<0.0005$ (*future security*). Correlations for females are: $r=0.244$, $p<0.0005$ (*present safety*) and $r=0.194$, $p<0.0005$ (*future security*). For both genders, correlations for *future security* are lower than those for *present safety*.

Freedom of choice and control over own life is a moderate predictor of *satisfaction with present safety* or *satisfaction with future security* (Table 10.16). The explained variance is very low in both cases, especially for females (Table 10.17).

3.6   Values Aspired to for the Future

The individual mean scores for the 21 values explored in this study are displayed in Table 10.18. Among those values with the lowest mean scores, we find *money,*

Table 10.18 Mean difference between males and females in values aspired to for the future

	Whole sample		Males		Females		Mean difference
	Mean	SD	Mean	SD	Mean	SD	
Value given to intelligence	7.40	1.61	7.49	1.591	7.34	1.630	$p=.099$
Value given to technical abilities	7.70	1.56	7.79	1.541	7.63	1.576	$p=.054$
Value given to abilities with people	8.01	1.42	7.88	1.467	**8.10**	1.381	$t(1,395)=-2.928$ $p=.003$
Value given to willpower	8.24	1.52	8.10	1.556	**8.35**	1.492	$t(1,386)=-3.048$ $p=.002$
Value given to profession	7.83	1.84	**8.01**	1.687	7.70	1.939	$t(1,329,550)=3.170$ $p=.002$
Value given to family	8.15	1.97	7.90	2.013	**8.33**	1.966	$t(1,390)=-3.992$ $p<.0005$
Value given to optimism	7.86	1.80	7.58	1.891	**8.06**	1.705	$t(1,144,819)=-4.887$ $p<.0005$
Value given to sympathy	8.42	1.52	8.23	1.653	**8.55**	1.401	$t(1,100,638)=-3.809$ $p<.0005$
Value given to money	4.61	3.12	**5.07**	3.104	4.29	3.085	$t(1,388)=4.639$ $p<.0005$
Value given to power	4.70	3.00	**5.24**	2.973	4.32	2.963	$t(1,374)=5.652$ $p<.0005$
Value given to sense of humour	7.89	1.77	7.96	1.904	7.84	1.676	$p=.207$
Value given to image	6.73	2.49	**6.97**	2.357	6.56	2.573	$t(1,300,350)=3.082$ $p=.002$
Value given to coherence	7.46	1.73	7.48	1.707	7.44	1.747	$p=.679$
Value given to solidarity	7.75	1.86	7.40	2.122	**8.00**	1.609	$t(1,014,384)=-5.719$ $p<.0005$
Value given to tolerance	7.47	1.86	7.27	1.990	**7.61**	1.754	$t(1,138,001)=-3.321$ $p=.001$

Value given to sense of meaning in life	7.84	1.75	7.65	1.783	**7.97**	1.722	$t(1,197,612)=-5.587$ $p=.001$
Value given to enjoying life	8.18	1.77	7.86	1.946	**8.41**	1.598	$t(1,074,767)=-2.928$ $p<.0005$
Value given to humanity	7.81	1.82	7.58	1.968	**7.98**	1.691	$t(1,112,512)=-3.984$ $p<.0005$
Value given to spiritual richness	6.46	2.66	6.14	2.872	**6.70**	2.469	$t(1,101,753)=-3.779$ $p<.0005$
Value given to personality	8.57	1.45	8.36	1.512	**8.72**	1.393	$t(1,175,689)=-4.411$ $p<.0005$
Value given to kindness	8.41	1.49	8.19	1.683	**8.56**	1.319	$t(1,040,037)=-4.339$ $p<.0005$

Significant differences are highlighted in **bold**

Table 10.19 Pearson correlations for values aspired to in the future and *satisfaction with present safety* and *future security*

Values aspired to in the future	Satisfaction with present safety		Satisfaction with future security	
	r	Significance	r	Significance
Value given to intelligence	.097	$p<.0005$	.116	$p<.0005$
Value given to technical abilities	.140	$p<.0005$	.137	$p<.0005$
Value given to abilities with people	.164	$p<.0005$	.134	$p<.0005$
Value given to willpower	.154	$p<.0005$	.137	$p<.0005$
Value given to profession	.177	$p<.0005$	.176	$p<.0005$
Value given to family	.133	$p<.0005$	.183	$p<.0005$
Value given to optimism	.239	$p<.0005$	.201	$p<.0005$
Value given to sympathy	.203	$p<.0005$	.170	$p<.0005$
Value given to money	.098	$p<.0005$	.121	$p<.0005$
Value given to power	.126	$p<.0005$	.124	$p<.0005$
Value given to sense of humour	.201	$p<.0005$	.183	$p<.0005$
Value given to image	.142	$p<.0005$	.158	$p<.0005$
Value given to coherence	.200	$p<.0005$	.116	$p<.0005$
Value given to solidarity	.100	$p<.0005$	.083	$p=.002$
Value given to tolerance	.134	$p<.0005$	.092	$p=.001$
Value given to sense of meaning in life	.206	$p<.0005$	.164	$p<.0005$
Value given to enjoying life	.259	$p<.0005$	.237	$p<.0005$
Value given to humanity	.181	$p<.0005$	.175	$p<.0005$
Value given to spiritual richness	.093	$p=.001$	.075	$p=.006$
Value given to personality	.135	$p<.0005$	.122	$p<.0005$
Value given to kindness	.098	$p<.0005$	.124	$p<.0005$

power (both below 5), *image* and *spiritual richness* (both below 7). Table 10.18 displays the mean scores found for males and females for these 21 values. Females' are statistically higher than males' for *abilities with people, willpower, family, optimism, sympathy, solidarity, tolerance, sense of meaning in life, enjoying life, humanity, spiritual richness, personality and kindness,* whilst males' are higher for *profession, money, power* and *image*.

All correlations between values aspired to in the future and both *present safety* and *future security* are statistically significant and range from low to moderate scores (Table 10.19). The highest correlations (above 0.2) for *satisfaction with present safety* correspond to *optimism, sense of humour, coherence, sense of meaning in life* and *enjoying life*. Only two values obtain a correlation above 0.2 in the case of *future security: optimism* and *enjoying life*. Correlations for *future security* are lower than those for *present safety*. This is true for all values with the exception of *intelligence, family, money, image* and *kindness*.

We observe that all correlations are statistically significant when divided according to gender, except for the relationship between *spiritual richness* and *future security* in the case of males (Table 10.20) and between *money* and *present safety* in the

Table 10.20 Pearson correlations for values aspired to in the future and *satisfaction with present safety* and *future security* in the case of males

Males' values	Satisfaction with present safety		Satisfaction with future security	
	r	Significance	r	Significance
Value given to intelligence	.084	$p = .044$	.165	$p < .0005$
Value given to technical abilities	.187	$p < .0005$	.210	$p < .0005$
Value given to abilities with people	.206	$p < .0005$	.191	$p < .0005$
Value given to willpower	.172	$p < .0005$	.166	$p < .0005$
Value given to profession	.201	$p < .0005$	.156	$p < .0005$
Value given to family	.193	$p < .0005$	.222	$p < .0005$
Value given to optimism	.291	$p < .0005$	.285	$p < .0005$
Value given to sympathy	.244	$p < .0005$	.169	$p < .0005$
Value given to money	.180	$p < .0005$	.130	$p = .002$
Value given to power	.170	$p < .0005$	.115	$p = .006$
Value given to sense of humour	.258	$p < .0005$	.220	$p < .0005$
Value given to image	.164	$p < .0005$	.135	$p = .001$
Value given to coherence	.212	$p < .0005$	.116	$p = .006$
Value given to solidarity	.145	$p = .001$	.108	$p = .010$
Value given to tolerance	.146	$p < .0005$	.107	$p = .010$
Value given to sense of meaning in life	.196	$p < .0005$	.185	$p < .0005$
Value given to enjoying life	.282	$p < .0005$	.263	$p < .0005$
Value given to humanity	.137	$p = .001$	.143	$p = .001$
Value given to spiritual richness	.092	$p = .029$	.078	$p = .063$
Value given to personality	.152	$p < .0005$	.148	$p < .0005$
Value given to kindness	.152	$p < .0005$	.107	$p = .011$

case of females (Table 10.21). The highest correlations (above 0.2) for males in relation to *present safety* correspond (in this order) to *optimism, enjoying life, sense of humour, sympathy, abilities with people and profession,* whilst for *future security* they are *optimism, enjoying life, family and technical abilities.*

When it comes to females, the highest correlations with *present safety* are found for (in this order) *enjoying life, optimism* and *humanity, sense of meaning in life* and *sympathy,* whilst for the future only two correlations are above 0.2, *enjoying life* and *humanity* (Table 10.20).

Finally, regression models were calculated to predict *satisfaction with* both *present safety* and *future security* using values as independent variables (Table 10.22). Following the same procedure with the previous variables analysed, the same regression model was developed considering genders separately (Table 10.22).

Only 9 of the 21 values aspired to that were considered in this study have entered the regression models. Some of them are common for both *present safety* and *future security,* for instance, *enjoying life, optimism* and *profession,* whilst others are specifically for *present safety* (*sense of humour, sympathy* and *power*) or *future security* (*image, solidarity* and *family*). However, beta scores and percentage of explained

Table 10.21 Pearson correlations for values aspired to in the future and *satisfaction with present safety* and *future security* in the case of females

Females' values	Satisfaction with present safety		Satisfaction with future security	
	r	Significance	r	Significance
Value given to intelligence	.097	$p=.006$	.080	$p=.023$
Value given to technical abilities	.105	$p=.003$	.083	$p=.018$
Value given to abilities with people	.160	$p<.0005$	.107	$p=.002$
Value given to willpower	.169	$p<.0005$	.130	$p<.0005$
Value given to profession	.151	$p<.0005$	.179	$p<.0005$
Value given to family	.126	$p<.0005$	.173	$p<.0005$
Value given to optimism	.246	$p<.0005$	.164	$p<.0005$
Value given to sympathy	.213	$p<.0005$	.190	$p<.0005$
Value given to money	.025	$p=.473$	.101	$p=.004$
Value given to power	.071	$p=.043$	.113	$p=.001$
Value given to sense of humour	.163	$p<.0005$	.153	$p<.0005$
Value given to image	.117	$p=.001$	.164	$p<.0005$
Value given to coherence	.196	$p<.0005$	.116	$p=.001$
Value given to solidarity	.112	$p=.001$	.089	$p=.012$
Value given to tolerance	.152	$p<.0005$	.095	$p=.007$
Value given to sense of meaning in life	.240	$p<.0005$	.166	$p<.0005$
Value given to enjoying life	.297	$p<.0005$	.247	$p<.0005$
Value given to humanity	.246	$p<.0005$	.220	$p<.0005$
Value given to spiritual richness	.122	$p=.001$	.088	$p=.013$
Value given to personality	.158	$p<.0005$	.122	$p=.001$
Value given to kindness	.095	$p=.007$	.160	$p<.0005$

Table 10.22 Regression models for predicting *satisfaction with present safety* and *future security* (dependent variables) (using values aspired to in the future for both)

	Satisfaction with present safety		Satisfaction with future security	
	9.9%		8.6%	
	$F_{6,1266}=23.066$		$F_{6,1269}=19.871$	
Explained variance	$p<.0005$	β	$p<.0005$	β
Significant items in the model[a]	Value given to enjoying life	+.170	Value given to enjoying life	+.167
	Value given to optimism	+.101	Value given to profession	+.096
	Value given to profession	+.094	Value given to image	+.070
	Value given to sense of humour	+.084	Value given to solidarity	−.068
	Value given to sympathy	−.081	Value given to optimism	+.067
	Value given to power	+.057	Value given to family	+.063

[a]The + and − symbols show the direction of the relationship

Table 10.23 Regression models for predicting *satisfaction with present safety* and *future security* (dependent variables) among males and females (using the values aspired to in the future for both)

	Satisfaction with present safety males		Satisfaction with present safety females	
	11.1%		12.5%	
	$F_{3,514} = 21.264$		$F_{5,751} = 21.254$	
Explained variance	$p < .0005$	β	$p < .0005$	β
Significant items in the model[a]	Value given to optimism	+.194	Value given to enjoying life	+.275
	Value given to enjoying life	+.141	Value given to kindness	−.184
	Value given to power	+.119	Value given to humanity	+.126
			Value given to willpower	+.085
			Value given to profession	+.078
	Satisfaction with future security males		Satisfaction with future security females	
	10.2%		9.5%	
	$F_{3,517} = 19.477$		$F_{3,751} = 26.034$	
Explained variance	$p < .0005$	β	$p < .0005$	β
Significant items in the model[a]	Value given to optimism	+.170	Value given to enjoying life	+.229
	Value given to technical abilities	+.134	Value given to profession	+.114
	Value given to enjoying life	+.108	Value given to image	+.088

[a]The + symbol shows the direction of the relationship

variance are generally quite low. It must also be highlighted that the value given to *sympathy* contributes negatively to explaining *present safety*, as is the case with *solidarity* and *future security*.

Values acting as predictors of *satisfaction with present safety* and *future security* differ considerably between males and females with the exception of *enjoying life* (Table 10.23), which is the only value appearing in the four different regression models.

3.7   Participants' Satisfaction with Present Safety and Future Security

The last phase of data analysis is concerned with calculating a new regression model using all of the variables that entered each of the previously discussed regression models. Thus, items which were excluded from previous models have not been

Table 10.24 Regression models for predicting *satisfaction with present safety* and *future security* (dependent variables) (using all scores entering into previous regression models)

	Satisfaction with present safety		Satisfaction with future security	
	41.3%		37.9%	
	$F_{8,1087} = 95.091$		$F_{9,1078} = 73.030$	
Explained variance	$p < .0005$	β	$p < .0005$	β
Significant items in the model[a]	Satisfaction with future security	+.274	Satisfaction with present safety	+.295
	Satisfaction with life achievements	+.233	Satisfaction with relationships with other people	+.184
	OLS	+.177	Academic self-concept	+.127
	Physical self-concept	+.165	OLS	+.120
	Social self-concept	+.118	Satisfaction with groups of people you belong to	+.103
	Value given to optimism	+.082	Social self-concept	−.102
	Value given to family	−.064	Family self-concept	+.095
	Academic self-concept	−.062	Satisfaction with standard of living	+.085
			Value given to image	+.074

[a]The + and − symbols show the direction of the relationship

considered in this section of the results. Five of the items from the PWI (excluding *present safety* and *future security*), the item *overall life satisfaction* (OLS), the four dimensions of self-concept (*physical, social, academic* and *family*), the item *overall sense of meaning in own life* (ESMS), the item *freedom of choice and control over own life* and 9 out of the 21 values aspired to in the future (*enjoying life, optimism, profession, sense of humour, sympathy, power, image, solidarity* and *family*) have been considered as independent variables to predict *present safety* and *future security*. In addition to this, *present safety* has also been explored as a predictor of *future security* and *future security* as a predictor of *present safety*.

Only eight of all of the aforementioned items contribute to explaining *present safety* and nine to explaining *future security*. These are displayed in Table 10.24. Interestingly, predictors of *present safety* differ from those of *future security* with the exception of OLS, *academic self-concept* and *social self-concept* (with a positive contribution to *present safety* and a negative contribution to *future security*).

Males' predictors of *present safety* are identical to females' with the exception of *optimism*, which only appears in the males' model (Table 10.25). Some of the predictors of *future security* are common for males and females, specifically OLS, *academic self-concept, satisfaction with relationships with other people, satisfaction with present safety, family self-concept* and *satisfaction with groups of people you belong to*. However, some others are specific to males (*sympathy, optimism* and *satisfaction with life achievements*) and others to females (*image, satisfaction with standard of living* and *social self-concept*).

Table 10.25 Regression models for predicting *satisfaction with present safety* and *future security* (dependent variables) among males and females (using all scores entering into previous regression models)

	Satisfaction with present safety males		Satisfaction with present safety females	
	38.6%		42.5%	
	$F_{6,438} = 45.195$		$F_{5,648} = 95.103$	
Explained variance	$p < .0005$	β	$p < .0005$	β
Significant items in the model[a]	Satisfaction with life achievements	+.251	Satisfaction with future security	+.323
	Physical self-concept	+.206	OLS	+.192
	OLS	+.152	Satisfaction with life achievements	+.208
	Value given to optimism	+.116	Social self-concept	+.139
	Satisfaction with future security	+.139	Physical self-concept	+.104
	Social self-concept	+.124		
	Satisfaction with future security males		Satisfaction with future security females	
	36.6%		40.0%	
	$F_{9,438} = 27.474$		$F_{9,648} = 47.423$	
Explained variance	$p < .0005$	β	$p < .0005$	β
Significant items in the model[a]	OLS	+.174	Satisfaction with present safety	+.343
	Academic self-concept	+.173	Satisfaction with relationships with other people	+.175
	Value given to sympathy	+.157	Academic self-concept	+.105
	Satisfaction with relationships with other people	+.142	Value given to image	+.097
	Satisfaction with present safety	+.134	Satisfaction with groups of people you belong to	+.096
	Family self-concept	+.131	Family self-concept	+.095
	Value given to optimism	+.127	Satisfaction with standard of living	+.082
	Satisfaction with life achievements	+.123	OLS	+.086
	Satisfaction with groups of people you belong to	+.104	Social self-concept	−.075

[a]The + symbol shows the direction of the relationship

4   Discussion

Our sample of 15- to 24-year-olds achieved a mean score of 74.56 on a scale of 0–100 for the PWI, which is almost identical to normative data for the Australian adult population (Cummins et al. 2005: $Mean = 74.65$, $SD = 12.63$), and higher than the 12- to 16-year-old adolescent Spanish samples studied in 2003: $Mean = 73.74$, $SD = 15.30$, and 2006: $Mean = 74.52$, $SD = 14.77$ (Casas et al. 2009b). The disparity in age between the sample in this study and the ones in previous studies may be the reason for such differences. Contrary to another study carried out with an Australian population in which gender differences only emerge at 26–35 years of age (Australian Unity Wellbeing Index 2010), in ours, differences in favour of males are detected when calculating the aggregate PWI measure. Our results also contradict another study in which the school version of the PWI is used with a sample of 12- to 20-year-old students. In this last case, females' scores were higher than males' (Tomyn and Cummins 2011). As the participants in our study are older, the reasons for such differences are unclear and require further research.

Those PWI items that obtained lower mean scores (under 7 on an 11-point scale) are satisfaction with present safety and future security, the mean for present safety ($M = 6.73$) being higher than that of future security ($M = 6.40$). Similar results for future security were also found in the 2010 research conducted on Australian adults for the Australian Unity Wellbeing Index (2010). Future security is found to be among the least satisfactory of life domains, along with community connection (in our study the equivalent item has been 'Satisfaction with the groups you belong to'). By contrast with our results, however, present safety has the second highest mean after standard of living in the aforementioned study using the Australian Unity of Wellbeing Index. When comparing these results with those of another study carried out on 266 Spanish families (Casas et al. 2008), we see that the scores of both 12- to 16-year-old adolescents and those of their parents regarding satisfaction with present safety and future security are among the lowest for all of the items in the PWI (future security obtains lower mean scores than present safety). The same result has also been detected in two different samples of adolescents ($N = 2,591$ and $N = 4,878$) and another of parents ($N = 861$) collected in Spain between 2003 and 2006 (Casas et al. 2009a).

These observations suggest that the importance given to present safety and future security might be better explained by cultural differences rather than attributable to different ways of thinking among generations (see translation issues section), although in neither country are participants highly satisfied with the security they expect to have in the future. To what extent a particular country's political and economic situation in the present might influence people's evaluations of security in the future is an area that requires more in-depth study.

Mean scores for satisfaction with health, standard of living and future security are statistically higher for males than for females. In a previous study on a sample of 1,297 Catalan adolescents (Casas et al. 2009a), gender differences were also identified with regard to satisfaction with relationships with other people (the mean was higher for girls) and present safety (the mean was higher for boys). Further in-depth research is needed to determine why so many differences exist between samples coming from the same cultural context in relation to males' and females' evaluations of present safety and future security.

The correlation between present safety and future security is only moderate by comparison with the findings of the 2010 Australian Unity Wellbeing Index report (in this case the correlation was 0.72, whilst ours is 0.486). The most important predictors of satisfaction with present safety, when only considering the rest of the items in the PWI are satisfaction with future security and satisfaction with life achievements, whilst in the case of satisfaction with future security, they are satisfaction with present safety and satisfaction with relationships with other people. Confidence in the future has to do with the evaluation students of post-compulsory secondary education make on how things are going at present. Simultaneously, evaluation of the present situation in terms of security is also made, departing from future evaluations. Later in this section we refer to a very well-known factor to explain personality, named optimism, which is understood as the general tendency to evaluate things in a more or less positive manner, which may be the explanation for both results.

Responses of students of post-compulsory secondary education in our study suggest that they see social relations as an inversion towards feeling secure in the future, as it is life achievements in the present. These results are coherent with the fact that among the aspirational values considered most important for the future, we have found in different data collection to be sympathy and kindness (Coenders et al. 2005; Casas et al. 2007a, b). We have also seen that both aspirational values are perceived by adolescents and young people as key to establishing social relations. Satisfaction with life achievements is the strongest predictor of present safety for both males and females, whilst in the case of future security, the most important predictor for both genders is satisfaction with present safety.

As both present safety and future security items belong to the PWI and are expected to contribute to the unique explained variance when a PCA is performed, their correlation with the PWI is high. When observing which of the other PWI items are most related to present safety and future security, we see that in both cases satisfaction with life achievements has the highest correlation (for both males and females). What young people have achieved seems to be very much the basis for their evaluation of satisfaction with security, probably as this enhances the feeling that if some desirable objective has already been achieved, so can others at a later date.

This would seem to reinforce our hypothesis that self-concept is an important factor to consider when it comes to evaluations regarding security. Interestingly, when these same correlations are calculated by gender, we see that males and females share very similar response patterns, with the exception of satisfaction with relationships with other people, which is lower for females in relation to future security, whilst the contrary is true for males. We have seen in previous research how important it is for adolescent girls and young women to perceive a high level of support from other people, especially from friends (Casas et al. 2007a, b).

OLS contributes moderately to both present safety and future security, the beta score being slightly higher for the former than the latter. The fact that this beta score is the highest of any of the regression models we calculated reinforces the idea that evaluations of security are strongly connected to personal well-being. There are no outstanding differences between males and females, although the beta scores are higher for the latter.

With regard to self-concept, differences are identified between males and females in relation to the four dimensions taken from a PCA: academic, family, physical and social, with males' scores only being higher for the physical dimension. Similar results have been observed in other studies with adolescent Catalan samples (Luna 2010). The dimension that most correlates with present safety is physical self-concept. The same is true of future security, for which the score is lower and very similar to two other dimensions: academic and family self-concept. The regression model based on the four dimensions of self-concept shows that physical self-concept obtains the highest beta score for both present safety and future security. When these results are divided according to gender, we observe that physical self-concept is the most contributing dimension to present safety for both genders, but especially for males. For future security, the dimension that contributes most for males is academic self-concept, and for females it is family self-concept, reflecting the correlations found by gender.

Closely related to the above, some agreement exists regarding the importance of physical appearance with regard to global self-esteem and self-concept during adolescent years (Coleman and Hendry 2003), followed by acceptance by peers, and some way behind, success with academic issues and sports. It would therefore seem that, as far as self-concept is concerned, adolescents and young adults base how they feel about the present on one of the most important building blocks of their self-concept: the physical dimension. Other dimensions take on significance when it comes to expectations about security in the future, academic performance becoming the most important building block for males, and family for females.

In a previous study (Casas et al. 2009b), we observed that there was a moderate ($r=0.512$) correlation between the ESMS and OLS among university students, suggesting the existence of a connection between sense of meaning in own life and personal well-being. In this study we have explored the correlation between the ESMS and present safety and future security, assuming the latter to be an indicator of personal well-being although with less weight than OLS. Although these correlations are much lower ($r=0.356$ for present safety and $r=0.325$ for future security), they are not negligible. The ESMS also functions as a good predictor of present safety and future security, although beta scores and explained variance are lower compared to the regression model developed using the OLS. Again, scores are higher for present safety and for females. These results lead us to conclude that finding a sense of meaning to one's own life is important in guaranteeing high levels of personal well-being probably because it helps individuals to structure their daily actions around the achievement of certain objectives.

As hypothesised in the introduction, freedom of choice and control over one's own life is also connected to satisfaction with security. The connection is, however, not so strong compared to other psychosocial constructs such as the ESMS. When a regression model is performed, the beta score and the percentage of explained variance are considerably higher for present safety than for future security. It would seem that although individuals feeling they have some control over the things they do in their life may contribute to creating positive evaluations in relation to both items, other variables such as OLS play a more determining role in this. Differences are observed between males' and females' evaluations, with the former correlating more with feelings about the present and less with future security.

In relation to the item on freedom of choice and control, we must add that for the purposes of this study, it has been considered an indicator of security of choice and control, a factor which is supposed to contribute to perceptions of security. This is due to the fact that the statement used to introduce this scale places strong emphasis on the control dimension. However, the item also refers to freedom of choice, meaning that this scale might also be measuring aspects related to the factor of inner personal security or security with self-concept described in the introduction. Future studies are needed which include scales exploring the perception of control.

Similar to previous studies conducted on samples of adolescents (see, for instance, Coenders et al. 2005), sympathy and kindness are among the values which obtain higher scores in our study carried out with young people. Notwithstanding this, personality obtains the highest mean. When males' and females' responses are analysed separately, similarly to other studies (Casas et al. 2007a, b) males' display higher mean scores for more materialistic values aspired to (money, power and image), whereas females' scores are higher for the more interpersonal values such as abilities with people, family, solidarity and so on. The reason for such differences is probably to be found in different underlying socialisation processes, which can be very subtle.

All correlations between the 21 studied values aspired to and satisfaction with both present safety and future security are statistically significant, although they range from low to moderate scores. Among the highest correlations with present safety (above 0.2), we find, in this order, value given to enjoying life, optimism, sense of meaning in life and sense of humour. Only two values correlate above 0.2 with future security: enjoying life and optimism. This suggests that in future studies it would be interesting to add a scale to evaluate optimism, as it seems to be a psychosocial variable connected to perceptions of security which we had not originally considered.

Sense of meaning in life once again appears as a factor worth considering when explaining satisfaction with safety in the present and future security through regression models. Sense of humour is also connected to present safety and future security. We might speculate that when things are taken too seriously, the feeling of security might be affected in a negative way as there are many 'objective' circumstances that can lead people to think that insecurity and instability are the most relevant characteristics of modern societies.

Among all the values studied, the best contributor to explaining satisfaction with both present safety and future security is enjoying life, followed by optimism (present safety) and profession (future security). Interestingly, valuing the family acts as a predictor for only future security, whereas valuing sense of humour, sympathy and power only does so for how they feel about the present. Value given to optimism and to power is a predictor for the males' but not the females' model where present safety is concerned. The contrary is also true for value given to kindness, humanity, willpower and profession. It would seem that males' evaluations of present safety are based more on external factors, whereas females' are constructed upon more internal components.

The final regression models for predicting present safety and future security were calculated taking as independent variables those which were previously significant predictors in each of the partial regression models (see Tables 10.5, 10.7, 10.12, 10.14, 10.16 and 10.22). The procedure we followed meant that satisfaction with present safety was considered as a predictor of future security and vice versa. When the model is not differentiated by gender, we observe that these two variables obtain the highest beta scores, confirming the above. We have also calculated this same model without considering those two items and have seen that some variables which were excluded in the model, such as freedom of choice or control over own life, are now included. This suggests that it would be a good idea to use more-sophisticated analysis techniques in the future to determine whether a particular psychosocial construct contributes more significantly to explaining present safety or future security.

The respective regression models explain 41.3% of the variance in the case of present safety and 37.9% in the case of future security, meaning that many other components that could also contribute are missing. In line with the aforementioned results, satisfaction with life achievements is significant in the final model, although only for present safety, and for both present safety and future security with regard to OLS. The four dimensions of self-concept were also included: physical and social self-concept for present safety, and academic, social and family self-concept for future security. Contrary to our expected theoretical model described in the introduction, the ESMS and freedom of choice and control over one's own life drop out of the final model. This leads us to think that although they contribute to explaining satisfaction with present safety and future security when considered in isolation, their combination with all of the variables studied might be more complex than expected, suggesting that the application of non-linear analysis techniques would be desirable in the future. Important differences between genders emerge when the same final model is calculated for males and females separately.

It is important to highlight some limitations of the work carried out in this study. First of all, the study is a cross-sectional one, not longitudinal, so we cannot talk about causal relationships among the variables studied, but only about their correlational nature. In addition, as it constitutes a first approach to studying the relationships between present safety and future security and other related psychosocial constructs, it would be necessary to extend this study to other samples of young people, including those who are not in mainstream secondary educational pathways. The highly abstract content of some of the variables explored in this chapter, especially in reference to the ESMS, makes it difficult to extend this same study to younger samples (under 15), although it would be desirable to do so in future studies.

As anticipated in the translation issues section, we have not been able to reach many conclusions on 'safety' because there is no equivalent word in either the Catalan or Spanish languages. The technique of focus groups could be very helpful in the future to deepen into the understanding and related factors of the construct of 'security' especially if comparing opinions of English-speaking and non-English-speaking adolescents and young people.

One of the conditions for satisfaction with a particular life domain item to be included in the PWI is that it has both an objective and a subjective dimension, and also that it is formulated in such an abstract way as to allow it to be understood through different criteria (Cummins et al. 2003). It is probable that the items relating to present safety and future security represent an even more abstract deconstruction of the more general construct of satisfaction with life as a whole in comparison with others such as, for instance, satisfaction with relationships with other people. This implies that the criteria used to evaluate these two life domains might be very different. With regard to adolescent and youth populations, it is reasonable to think that the criteria used to evaluate present safety and future security differs from that used with adults. Focus groups and in-depth individual interviews may prove very helpful in looking deeper into this question.

Although we are far from being able to reach any definitive conclusions, the results of this study have both theoretical and practical implications. First of all, it makes some contribution to the understanding of what perceptions of security are by first testing its relationships with some psychosocial factors such as self-concept, overall sense of meaning in own life, freedom of choice and control over own life and values aspired to in the future. They have been understood as indicators of inner personal security or security with self-concept, spiritual security, security of choice and control, and security related to aspirational values in the future, respectively.

Secondly, the results obtained offer some contribution to understanding perceptions of security by first testing its relationship with psychosocial factors such as self-concept, overall sense of meaning in own life, freedom of choice and control over own life, and values aspired to in the future. They also shed some light on quality of life studies by contributing to our understanding of the relationships existing between perceptions of security and personal well-being, an area in which few studies have been conducted and which requires further attention from the scientific community. Finally, it widens the perspective of those programmes/policy decisions aimed to enhance the well-being of the population which should also address the issue of security, from the point of view of the perceptions and evaluations of the people involved.

Acknowledgements The authors would like to acknowledge the financial support received from the Spanish Ministry of Education and Science through the National Plan of Scientific Research, Development and Technological Innovation, for this research project with reference SEJ2007–62813/PSIC.

Thanks are also given to Barney Griffiths for the meticulous and hard work done with the translation of this article, and for the clarifications raised to help better explaining our results in English.

References

Australian Unity of Well-being Index. (2006). *The well-being of Australians-income security, Report 15.* Melbourne: Australian Centre on Quality of Life.

Australian Unity of Well-being Index. (2010). *The well-being of Australians-life better/worse, children and neighbourhood, Report 23.* Melbourne: Australian Centre on Quality of Life.

Bar-Tal, D., & Jacobson, D. (1998). A psychological perspective on security. *Applied Psychology: An International Review, 47*(1), 59–71.

Böhnke, P. (2008). Does society matter? Life satisfaction in the enlarged Europe. *Social Indicators Research, 87,* 189–210.

Bowlby, J. (1999). *Attachment and loss* (2nd ed., Vol. I). New York: Basic Books.

Casas, F., Figuer, C., González, M., & Coenders, G. (2003). Satisfaction with life domains and salient values for future: Analyses about children and their parents. In W. Glatzer, S. von Below, & M. Stoffregen (Eds.), *Challenges for quality of life in the contemporary world* (pp. 233–247). Dordrecht: Kluwer.

Casas, F., González, M., Figuer, C., & Coenders, G. (2004). Subjective well-being, values and goal-achievement: The case of planned versus by chance searchers on the Internet. *Social Indicators Research, 66*(1–2), 123–141.

Casas, F., Buxarrais, M. R., Figuer, C., González, M., Tey, A., Noguera, E., & Rodríguez, J. M. (2005). Values and their influence on the life satisfaction of adolescents aged 12 to 16: A study of some correlates. *Psychology in Spain, 9*(1), 21–33.

Casas, F., Figuer, C., González, M., & Malo, S. (2007a). The values adolescents aspire to, their well-being and the values parents aspire to for their children. *Social Indicators Research, 84,* 271–290.

Casas, F., Figuer, C., González, M., Malo, S., Alsinet, C., & Subarroca, S. (2007b). The well-being of 12- to 16-year-old adolescents and their parents: Results from 1999 to 2003 Spanish samples. *Social Indicators Research, 83,* 87–115.

Casas, F., Coenders, G., Cummins, R. A., González, M., Figuer, C., & Malo, S. (2008). Does subjective well-being show a relationship between parents and their children? *Journal of Happiness Studies, 9*(2), 197–205.

Casas, F., González, M., & Bertran, I. (2009a). Personal well-being of parents and their adolescent child. *IX ISQOLS Conference Quality of Life Studies: Measures and Goals for the Progress of Societies,* Florence, 19–23 July 2009.

Casas, F., González, M., Figuer, C., & Malo, S. (2009b). Satisfaction with spirituality, satisfaction with religion and personal well-being among Spanish adolescents and young university students. *Applied Research in Quality of Life, 4,* 23–45.

Casas, F., Sarriera, J. C., Alfaro, J., González, M., Malo, S., Bertran, I., Figuer, C., Abs, D., Bedin, L., Paradiso, A., Weinreich, K., & Valdenegro, B. (2011). Testing the personal well-being index on 12–16 year-old adolescents in 3 different countries with 2 new items. *Social Indicators Research.* doi:10.1007/s11205-011-9781-1.

Coenders, G., Casas, F., Figuer, C., & González, M. (2005). Relationships between parents' and children's salient values for future and children's overall satisfaction. A comparison across countries. *Social Indicators Research, 73,* 141–177.

Coleman, J. C., & Hendry, L. B. (2003). *Psicología de la adolescencia [Psychology of adolescence].* Madrid: Morata.

Csikzentmihalyi, M. (1997). *Finding flow: The psychology of engagement with everyday life.* New York: Basic Books.

Cummins, R. A. (1996). The domains of life satisfaction: An attempt to order chaos. *Social Indicators Research, 38,* 303–328.

Cummins, R. A., & Gullone, E. (2000). Why we should not use 5-point Likert scales: The case for subjective quality of life measurement. *Proceedings, Second International Conference on Quality of Life in Cities* (pp. 74–93). Singapore, National University of Singapore.

Cummins, R. A., Eckersley, R., Van Pallant, J., Vugt, J., & Misajon, R. (2003). Developing a national index of subjective well-being: The Australian unity well-being index. *Social Indicators Research, 64*, 159–190.

Cummins, R. A., Woerner, J., Tomyn, A., Gibson, A., & Knapp, T. (2005). *The well-being of Australians personal relationships. Report 14, Part B.* Melbourne: Australian Centre on Quality of Life.

Dew, T., & Huebner, E. S. (1994). Adolescents' perceived quality of life: An exploratory investigation. *Journal of School Psychology, 32*, 185–199.

Diener, E. (1994). El bienestar subjetivo. [Subjective well-being]. *Intervención Psicosocial, 3*(8), 67–113.

Diener, E., & Fujita, F. (1995). Resources, personal strivings, and subjective well-being: A nomothetic and idiographic approach. *Journal of Personality and Social Psychology, 68*, 926–935.

Diener, E., & Lucas, R. E. (2000). Subjective emotional well-being. In M. Lewis & J. M. Haviland (Eds.), *Handbook of emotions* (2nd ed., pp. 325–337). New York: Guilford.

Diener, E., Emmons, R. A., Larsen, R. J., & Griffin, S. (1985). The satisfaction with life scale. *Journal of Personality Assessment, 49*, 71–75.

Diener, E., Suh, E., & Oishi, S. (1997). Recent studies on subjective well-being. *Indian Journal of Clinical Psychology, 24*, 25–41.

Fordyce, M. W. (1988). A review of research on the happiness measures: A sixty second index of happiness and mental health. *Social Indicators Research, 20*, 355–381.

García, F., & Musitu, G. (1999). *Autoconcepto Forma-5 (A.F.5). [Self-concept 5-Form].* Madrid: TEA Editions.

Huebner, E. S. (1991). Correlates of life satisfaction in children. *School Psychology Quarterly, 6*, 103–111.

Huebner, E. S. (2004). Research on assessment of life satisfaction of children and adolescents. *Social Indicators Research, 66*, 3–33.

Huebner, E. S., & Alderman, G. L. (1993). Convergent and discriminant validation of a children's life satisfaction scale: Its relationship to self-and teacher-reported psychological problems and school functioning. *Social Indicators Research, 30*, 71–82.

Javaloy, F. (coord.) (2007). *Bienestar y felicidad de la juventud española. [Well-being and happiness of the Spanish youth].* Madrid: Observatorio de la Juventud en España.

Kasser, T., & Ryan, R. M. (1996). Further examining the American dream: Differential correlates of intrinsic and extrinsic goals. *Personality and Social Psychology Bulletin, 2*, 280–287.

La Guardia, J., Ryan, R., Couchman, C. E., & Deci, E. (2000). Within-person variation in security of attachment: A self-determination theory perspective on attachment, need fulfillment, and well-being. *Journal of Personality and Social Psychology, 79*(3), 367–384.

Lacković-Grgin, K., Grgin, T., Penezić, Z., & Sorić, I. (2001). Some predictors of primary control of development in three transitional periods of life. *Journal of Adult Development, 8*(3), 149–160.

Lau, A., Cummins, R. A., & McPherson, W. (2005). An investigation into the cross-cultural equivalence of the personal well-being index. *Social Indicators Research, 72*, 403–430.

Leone, C., & Burns, J. (2000). The measurement of locus of control: Assessing more than the meets the eye? *The Journal of Psychology, 134*(1), 63–76.

Luna, X. (2010). *Personal well-being and school satisfaction in adolescence.* Master's thesis, University of Girona, Girona.

Maslow, A. H. (1970). *Motivation und personality* (2nd ed.). New York: Harper & Row.

Mukherjee, R. (1989). *The quality of life: Valuation in social research.* New Delhi/Newbury Park: Sage.

Rosenberg, M. (1979). *Conceiving the self.* New York: Basic Books.

Rotter, J. B. (1966). Generalized expectancies for internal versus external control of reinforcement. *Psychology Monographs, 80*, 1–28.

Ryff, C. D. (1989a). Beyond Ponce de Leon and life satisfaction: New directions in quest of successful aging. *International Journal of Behavioral Development, 12*, 35–55.

Ryff, C. D. (1989b). Happiness is everything, or is it? Explorations on the meaning of psychological well-being. *Journal of Personality and Social Psychology, 57*, 1069–1081.

Schwartz, S. H. (1992). Universals in the content and structure of values: Theoretical advances and empirical tests in 20 countries. In M. P. Zanna (Ed.), *Advances in experimental social psychology* (Vol. 25, pp. 1–65). New York: Academic.

Seligson, J. L., Huebner, E. S., & Valois, R. F. (2003). Preliminary validation of the brief multidimensional students' life satisfaction scale (BMSLSS). *Social Indicators Research, 61*, 121–145.

Struch, N., Schwartz, S. L., & Van der Kloot, W. A. (2002). Meanings of basic values for women and men: A cross-cultural analysis. *Personality and Social Psychology Bulletin, 28*(1), 16–28.

Tomyn, A., & Cummins, R. A. (2011). The subjective well-being of high school students: Validating the personal well-being index-school children. *Social Indicators Research, 101*, 405–418.

Veenhoven, R. (2005). Apparent quality-of-life in nations: How long and happy people live. *Journal of Happiness Studies, 71*, 61–86.

Wills-Herrera, E., Orozco, L. E., Forero-Pineda, C., Pardo, O., & Andovona, V. (2011). The relationship between perceptions of insecurity, social capital and subjective well-being: Empirical evidences from areas of rural conflict in Colombia. *The Journal of Socio-Economics, 40*, 88–96.

Wridt, P. (2010). A qualitative GIS approach to mapping urban neighborhoods with children to promote physical activity and child-friendly community planning. *Environment and Planning B: Planning and Design, 37*(1), 129–147.

Yiengprugsawan, V., Seubsman, S., Khamman, S., Lim, S. S. Y., & Sleigh, A. C. (2010). Personal well-being index in a national cohort of 87,134 Thai adults. *Social Indicators Research, 98*, 201–215.

Chapter 11
Security and Well-Being in the Triple Frontier Area of Latin America: Community Awareness of Child Trafficking, the Smuggling of Persons and Sex Tourism

Dave Webb and Lia Rodriguez de La Vega

1 Introduction

Our goals for this descriptive chapter can be summarised as follows:

First, we discuss the key concepts of human trafficking, smuggling of persons, sexual exploitation and sex tourism in the context of security and quality of life (QOL) studies. From the perspective of the victim who experiences a loss of personal liberty and exposure to significant physical and mental abuse, it is not hard to imagine how the personal security and quality of life of these victims is negatively affected.

Second, given the absence of coverage of this specific topic in the QOL literature, this chapter bridges the gap. The reader will quickly recognise that the area is vast, and so we can only offer broad coverage of the field with this chapter. Following a brief review of relevant literature, we introduce the geographic region of interest for this work, the Triple Frontier in Latin America, highlighting how its position facilitates serious crime and specifically, those crimes associated with the trade in humans. Furthermore, because we recognise that many readers may not be familiar with these crimes, we present the reader with two case testimonies highlighting the nature of the victim's lived experience. We feel that presenting these case testimonies, albeit they are not a part of our research, is useful in that they enable the reader to understand a little more of the world of the victim.

D. Webb (✉)
University of Western Australia, 35 Stirling Highway, Crawley, WA 6009, Australia
e-mail: dave.webb@uwa.edu.au

L.R. de La Vega
La Matanza University/Lomas de Zamora University, Buenos Aires, Argentina
e-mail: liadelavega@yahoo.com

D. Webb and E. Wills-Herrera (eds.), *Subjective Well-Being and Security*,
Social Indicators Research Series 46, DOI 10.1007/978-94-007-2278-1_11,
© Springer Science+Business Media B.V. 2012

Third, having set the scene, we then present findings from a research project of which the second author was a part. One of the purposes of the research project was to explore how much knowledge individuals living in the region have in regard to human trafficking, the smuggling of persons and sex tourism. Major crimes such as these occur not in a vacuum, but rather in a regional context within which communities play a vital role whether advertently or inadvertently in support of the groups carrying out these crimes, or more positively, in opposition to them. In this light, the education of communities is seen as a necessary element in their eradication.

Fourth, following analysis of the data obtained from a section of the above-mentioned project, we synthesise the information presented and suggest ways in which knowledge within communities can be enhanced to ensure that community members feel more competent and willing to give voice and act in ways that make the region less attractive to criminals and thus, more secure for inhabitants. Though it was not tested in the reported study, consistent with the literature, we argue that greater security in the region achieved through grass roots intervention would logically lead to enhanced QOL and well-being for all.

Finally, we present suggestions for future research and conclude our chapter with a call to our colleagues to contribute to the expansion of knowledge in the field. Such a call also amplifies the plea of Antonio Maria Costa, Executive Director of the United Nations Office of Drugs and Crime (UNODC 2009), for social scientists in academia and governments to work more closely with UNODC (*and others*[1]) in the development of evidence-based anti-slavery policy.

2 Key Concepts of Interest in This Chapter

2.1 Quality of Life

A significant body of literature exploring many facets of quality of life (QOL) research exists. The literature in the field encompasses research on well-being (e.g. Diener 2000; Cummins et al. 2003), life satisfaction (e.g. Cummins 1996) and happiness (e.g. Veenhoven 2000), and indeed, it is evident from a review of these that the above terms are often employed interchangeably in reference to well-being. Ryan and Deci (2001) point out that much of the work essentially derives from two perspectives: 'the hedonic approach to well being, which focuses on happiness and defines well being in terms of pleasure attainment and pain avoidance; and the eudaimonic approach, which focuses on meaning and self realization and defines well being in terms of the degree to which a person is fully functioning (P241)'.

On initial consideration, it might appear that of the two approaches, the eudaimonic perspective is most pertinent to this discussion on human trafficking. Clearly,

---

[1] Text in brackets added by authors.

we are not exploring what it means to lead a fulfilled life, but rather how, as a consequence of being trafficked for the purpose of sexual exploitation, the potential for the victims of these crimes to lead a fulfilled life is adversely affected. Indeed, many sources refer to human trafficking as a form of modern-day slavery (e.g. Bales 2007; Kara 2009), and the relationship between slavery and reduced quality of life is not up for debate. Indeed, whilst no empirical studies specifically exploring slavery and well-being exist, we are aware from the literature of the importance and complexity of the opposite, i.e. freedom, in respect to well-being (e.g. Veenhoven 2000; Conticini and Hulme 2007). Furthermore, it is clear, given the suffering from physical and psychological abuse experienced by victims of the crimes against persons discussed in this chapter (Bruch 2004), that the hedonic view is also relevant, that is to say, where little pleasure can be experienced by those who suffer severe physical and psychological abuse at the hands of their perpetrators. In this respect, in articulating the interrelatedness between both approaches, Ryan et al. (2008) argue that 'positive affect and pleasure are both correlates and consequences of living well, that is to say, of eudaimonia (P141)'. Similarly therefore, we consider as a working frame of reference the relevance of both hedonic and eudaimonic conceptualisations in this chapter on human trafficking and sexual exploitation.

When discussing quality of life, in general it is proposed that one is thinking at the aggregate level; in other words, one is offering a judgement of how one feels about one's life assessed across multiple life domain areas (Cummins et al. 2003): standard of living, health, achievements in life, personal relationships, community connectedness, how safe one feels and future security. Of these, the last two domains emphasising safety and security are central to this study though we can't of course discount the relevance of the others.

Consider for example the situation of a 14-year-old female who has been trafficked from her home country and is now held captive in a foreign land to be prostituted to tourists. Being held captive often includes living in depraved conditions, sometimes under lock and key; having little access to health care, education or other opportunities that are generally open to other young girls; seclusion from the possibility of making friends, a form of psychological abuse; physical abuse by both traffickers and clients and an overall fear that escape would lead to subsequent violence to her family members elsewhere. Unfortunately, this scenario is only too common and not simply the subject matter of blockbuster movies. It is indeed hard to comprehend the insecurity and negative quality of life that someone exposed to such conditions must experience. Our discussion on well-being in this chapter is contextual rather that an integral aspect of the descriptive research we report on later. In a sense, we are asking the reader to consider our ideas in situ, that is, by imagining how the experience of being trafficked impacts negatively on the well-being of victims. In the final paragraphs of this chapter, we offer some suggestions for future research, and amongst these we highlight the need for studies to explore empirically the impact of being trafficked on well-being. We turn now to a brief review of the relevant security literature.

2.2 Human Security

To explore the dizzying complexity of security, Rothchild (1995) takes a macro view to present security both vertically and horizontally in a geometric space. Vertically, security extends downwards from the security of nations to include the security of groups and individuals, and upwards from the security of nations to include the security of the international system and biosphere. The horizontal plane focuses on security type – individuals, nations, systems etc. – and the locus of responsibility for security extending in 'all directions from national states upwards to international institutions and downwards to regional and local governments as well as sideways to NGO's, public opinion and the press, and to the abstract forces of nature or of the market (P55)'.

The above perspective is useful in that it locates responsibility for security not just with one party but with many. We present the same view later in this chapter when we highlight the necessity for a 'whole of community' systemic involvement in combating the crimes of trafficking, smuggling of persons and the sexual exploitation of children.

Rothchild is not alone in her explication of the concept of security, indeed, focussing on the individual. Alkire (2003) provides a useful working definition that considers 'life fulfilment' which the reader will recall is central to eudaimonic well-being. Alkire offers that:

> The objective of human security is to safeguard the vital core of all human lives from critical pervasive threats, in a way that is consistent with long-term human fulfilment. (P2)

Furthermore, in respect to the individual, no unanimous agreement concerning the sources of insecurity from which an individual has to be protected exists. Some commentators (e.g. Hampson et al. 2002; cf. Alkire 2003) discuss a vision of human security encompassed under the perspective 'freedom from fear', which has, at its base, the elimination of the use of force and violence (and the threat of its use) from daily life. Others (e.g. King and Murray 2001; cf. Alkire 2003) suggest human security must be characterised by a broader concept, summarised in the phrase 'freedom from want'. In this second perspective, the basic needs of the individual in terms of their economic, food, social and health security needs are considered. Indeed, Sen (1999) underscores the important link between both 'freedom from fear' and 'freedom from want' in his seminal work on 'Development as Freedom' (cf. Acharya 2001).

Historical attention to issues of human security dates back to the nineteenth century with the establishment of international humanitarian law and the International Red Cross (Morillas-Bassedas 2007). Nevertheless, Alkire (2003) notes that the phrase 'human security' is most often associated with the 1994 Human Development Report (UNDP 1994) which highlights that the key premises of human security include a joint focus on freedom from fear and freedom from want, as well as an emphasis on the four essential characteristics of human security, notably: (1) recognition of the *universal applicability* of human security, (2) recognition that the components of human security are *interdependent*, (3) a suggested *preference for prevention* rather than the later need for intervention and (4) a *people-centredness* including exercise of choice, access to markets and social opportunities and whether individuals live in conflict or peace (UNDP 1994; cf. Alkire 2003).

It is worth noting that the two freedoms, freedom from fear and freedom from want that lie at the heart of the United Nations, are essentially about freedom from abuse in the case of the former, and in the case of the latter, freedom from poverty. Consequently, the notion of security, as we see it, bears close relation with both direct and/or indirect forms of abuse which we discuss below from a human rights position. To put this discussion into context, the persons of interest in this chapter include the victims of smuggling or trafficking who have been exposed to violent physical and psychological abuse at the hands of their perpetrators. In particular, though not exclusively, the victims are children, predominantly females with an average age of between 12 and 17 years. Consequently, it is clear that such child victims have suffered one or more fundamental rights abuses according to Article 1, UN Convention on the Rights of the Child (UNICEF 2010). The above-referenced UN legislation highlights across 6 theme areas 54 articles drawn up to specifically protect and manage the rights of the child, that is, the rights of the child to be free and protected from amongst others: child labour (Article 32), sexual exploitation (Article 34), sale and abduction (Article 35), other forms of exploitation (Article 36) and torture and deprivation (Article 37). It is our position that any violation of these rights represents a direct abuse of an aspect of the quality of life of the child or young person in question.

Having now introduced the concepts of human trafficking, smuggling of persons and sexual exploitation, we now move to discuss these in greater detail. We feel it worth pointing out to the reader that sexual exploitation does not necessarily stand in contrast to the smuggling and the trafficking of persons, but rather, sexual exploitation is often the consequence of these. Thus, a victim can be said to be 'trafficked for the purpose of sexual exploitation'. Indeed, the UNODC global report on human trafficking (UNODC 2009) highlights that 79% of victims are trafficked for the purpose of sexual exploitation (P6).

2.3 Human Trafficking

Key on the agenda of the 2000 Millennium Summit was the recognition by world leaders that an essential value for the twenty-first century was freedom – freedom from fear and freedom from want. However, the then Secretary-General Mr. Kofi Annan notes that such freedom is denied to millions around the world. He elaborates:

> I believe the trafficking of persons, particularly women and children, for forced and exploitative labour, including for sexual exploitation, is one of the most egregious violations of human rights that the United Nations now confronts. It is widespread and growing. It is rooted in social and economic conditions in the countries from which the victims come, facilitated by practices that discriminate against women and driven by cruel indifference to human suffering on the part of those who exploit the services that the

victims are forced to provide. The fate of these most vulnerable people in our world is an affront to human dignity and a challenge to every State, every people and every community. (UNODC 2004, Piv)

Consequently, Mr Kofi Annan urged Member States 'to ratify not only the United Nations Convention against Transnational Organized Crime, but also the Protocol to Prevent, Suppress and Punish Trafficking in Persons, Especially Women and Children, which can make a real difference in the struggle to eliminate this reprehensible trade in human beings (UNODC 2004, Piv)'. Article 3a of the protocol states that:

> Trafficking in persons is understood as the capture, the transport, the reception of persons resorting to the use of force or other forms of constraint, kidnapping, fraud, deceit, abuse of power or any situation of vulnerability or to the concession or receipt of payments or benefits to obtain the consent of a person who has authority on another for intentions of exploitation. This exploitation will include as minimum, the exploitation of the foreign prostitution or other forms of sexual exploitation, labor or forced services, slavery or similar practices of slavery, bondage or the extraction or organs (UNODC 2004, P42).

Though Kara (2009) suggests that the above definition is not without confusion, we can distinguish three basic elements that allow us to understand the process that victims of human trafficking go through: (a) capture and displacement,[2] (b) the deprivation of their freedom and (c) their exploitation. In this way, the Protocol of Palermo (complementary to the Convention of the United Nations against Transnational Organized Crime) distinguishes amongst the modalities of exploitation which include sexual exploitation, forced labour or services, slavery or practices similar to slavery, servitude or the removal of organs (UN Palermo Protocol 2000 Article 3a).

2.4   Smuggling of Persons

The crimes of trafficking in persons and the smuggling of persons have received considerable media attention in recent years. Though both involve the movement of people, the difference between them is not well understood. In contrast to the definition of human trafficking, the smuggling of persons is defined by Article 3a of the UN Protocol against the Smuggling of Migrants by Land, Sea and Air (UN Palermo Protocol 2000) as:

> the procurement, in order to obtain, directly or indirectly, a financial or other material benefit, of the illegal entry of a person into a State Party of which the person is not a national or a permanent resident.

Iselin and Adams (2003) articulate the main differences between the smuggling of persons and human trafficking in terms of a number of key areas including:

• The question of consent: Generally, in almost all instances of people smuggling, the individual being smuggled has consented to illegally crossing a border (P4). In terms

---

[2] If the victim moves inside the same country, it is referred to as internal trafficking in persons. If the victim moves outside it, it is referred to as international trafficking in persons.

of human trafficking, generally there is no consent, and where consent exists, such consent is usually obtained by fraud or coercion. With respect to children, consent is irrelevant since a person under the age of 18 years cannot in law give such consent.

- The recruitment process: Generally, persons looking to be smuggled will approach the recruiter, whereas with human trafficking, it is often the trafficker that makes the first approach.
- Arrival at the destination: First, the smuggling of persons always involves a trans-border crossing whereas human trafficking can also take place domestically within a country. Second, where a border crossing is involved, smuggled persons are generally free to make their own way after crossing the border whereas trafficked persons are often accompanied by a 'minder' and enslaved.
- The role of violence: Generally, because traffickers need to force their victims to a state of compliance, violence is often present. In the case of smuggling, because the relationship is one where the services of the smuggler are sought out by the person desiring to be smuggled, no force is necessary, and hence violence is often absent.[3]
- Potential profits: With smuggling, there is usually a one-off payment made between the person smuggled and the smuggler. For the most part, no other revenue avenues are present. In the case of human trafficking, the trafficker has a number of revenue opportunities including those associated with cost recuperation and from the sale of the services offered by the victim.

It should be noted that the above is an oversimplification of what in reality is a complex area of law. Indeed, many nuances exist in law, making absolute identification before the commission of one of these acts very difficult. The main ambiguities centre on consent, force and exploitation. However, for the purpose of this chapter, the above overview serves to provide the non-expert reader with some understanding of the main differences between the trafficking in persons and the smuggling of persons.

2.5 Commercial Sexual Exploitation of Children and Sex Tourism

We commence this section by reminding the reader that the commercial sexual exploitation of children (CSEC) is one of the primary outcomes of human trafficking. Thus, we discuss human trafficking and sexual exploitation hand in hand. Recall, the UNODC (2009) global report on the trafficking in persons identifies that about 79% of all victims are trafficked for the purpose of sexual exploitation (P6). We next explore the commercial sexual exploitation of children more precisely in the context of sex tourism.

The commercial sexual exploitation of children is in direct contravention to Article 34 of the UN Convention on the Rights of the Child (UNICEF 2010) which

---

[3] Trafficking is considered a crime against persons, and smuggling is considered a crime against the State.

highlights that State Parties undertake to protect children from all forms of sexual exploitation and sexual abuse. For these purposes, State Parties are responsible for preventing:

- The inducement or coercion of a child to engage in any unlawful sexual activity
- The exploitative use of children in prostitution or other unlawful sexual practices
- The exploitative use of children in pornographic performances and materials

The commercial sexual exploitation of children comes in many forms including situations of prostitution/paid sexual intercourse, child pornography, trafficking with sexual intent, early or forced marriages and the commercial sexual exploitation of children and adolescents (CSECA) in travel and tourism. In respect to the latter, child sex tourism has been defined by ECPAT (2010) as:

> the commercial sexual exploitation of children by men or women (women represent less than 5% of offenders) who travel from one place to another, usually from a richer country to one that is less developed, and there engage in sexual acts with children, defined as anyone aged under 18.

Child sex tourism extends to include the offer of children's services to tourists, in general foreigners, including also the organisations that offer these services and the network of children who satisfy these types of demands, implying generally some form of payment (in money or in kind).

An exhaustive search of the literature reveals no indication of the overall size of the global sex tourism industry. However, that the industry is of significant size is unanimous (e.g. Orndorf 2010; Cotter 2009).

In respect to the commercial sexual exploitation of children in a travel and tourism context, Sotello (cf. Save the Children Sweden 2005) identifies that both domestic and overseas visitors can be involved. Essentially, the exploiter comes in one of two persona: (1) the *situational* exploiter, who does not travel with the intention of having sexual relations with children but seizes the opportunity and availability to do it in the place of destination and (2) the *preferential* exploiter, who uses all the means he has at hand to obtain information and access to the service of sex with children in destinations all over the world (CSEC 1996).

The situational exploiter turns out to be easily influenced by the advertising and information that circulate in the place of destination, which implies that his conduct will be influenced by such factors as (1) the promotion of a destination as 'suitable' or 'favourable' towards this activity, (2) the local acceptance of the offence of sex with children and (3) the perception of impunity in the place of destination. To all these factors, we need to add those who offer tourism or non-tourism services that favour or facilitate sexual contact with children. The preferential exploiter, on the other hand, modifies his destination choice according to the severity of both legislation and prosecution systems in countries of interest (Save the Children Sweden 2005).

Having explored in the above sections the literature on well-being, security, human trafficking, the smuggling of persons and child exploitation and introduced the context of sex tourism, we turn our attention now to the geographic location of interest to this chapter, namely the Triple Frontier which is located at the intersection of Argentina, Brazil and Paraguay.

3 The Triple Frontier (Argentina, Brazil, Paraguay)

The Triple Frontier area refers to the transit zone enclave joining three cities from three countries: Ciudad del Este (Paraguay[4]), Puerto Iguazú (Argentina) and Foz de Iguaçú (Brazil). The area is also home to Iguazú falls, ranked 5th in the 7 nature wonders of the world listing and a UNESCO world heritage destination since 1984, making the area a haven for tourism. However, beyond the magnificence and beauty of this natural paradise lies a sinister side.

With no holds barred, Robinson (1999, cf., Sverdlick 2005, P87) elaborates:

> The anus of the earth is cut into the jungle on the Paraguay side of the Parana River, a home-away-from-home for the South American drug cartels, Chinese Triads, Japanese Yakuza, Italian gangsters, Russian gangsters, Nigerian gangsters and Hezbollah terrorists, and is called Ciudad del Este.... A city of 200,000 hustlers, whores, hoodlums, revolutionaries, thugs, drug traffickers, drug addicts, murderers, racketeers, pirates, mobsters, extortionists, smugglers, hit men, pimps and wannabes.

Increasingly, the Triple Frontier has become a centre for international organised crime and illegal trade, and furthermore, it is considered one of the most dangerous areas in Latin America (MUNUC 2010). Examples of international organised crime and illegal trade carried out in the region include the illegal trade of goods, illegal immigration, money laundering, corruption, smuggling, weapons and drug trafficking and terrorism (Sverdlick 2005) as well as the trafficking of humans for domestic servitude, forced labour and sexual exploitation (The Protection Project), and including prostitution for the purpose of fuelling the sex tourism industry. These crimes are reportedly mostly carried out by international crime organisations from Columbia, Brazil, China, Lebanon, Italy, Russia, Nigeria, Cote d'Ivoire, Japan and Ghana with strong support coming from business executives, military leaders and politicians in the region (Hudson 2003).

What makes the region so attractive to criminals is a combination of several factors working together in conjunction: the region's geographic location being at an intersection of three countries, poor border control, significant poverty, the absence of clear and legitimate alternative economic opportunities and the natural features of the environment attracting amongst others a constant flow of domestic and international visitors. In terms of numbers, Sverdlick (2005) reports that

---

[4] Puerto Iguazú (population 32,038, INDEC 2001), Foz de Iguaçú (population 311,336, IBGE 2001) and Ciudad del Este (population 223,350, Department of Alto Parana, Paraguay) (Dirección Nacional de Estadísticas, Encuestas y Censo de Paraguay 2002).

'The Friendship International Bridge connecting Ciudad del Este (Paraguay) with Foz de Iguazú (Brazil) carries in excess of 40,000 persons daily, and up to 60,000 people daily during weekends (P89)'. Also of attraction is that Ciudad del Este is reportedly the third largest duty-free zone in the world with a daily trade amounting to some US$12 million (Sverdlick 2005).

4 Human Trafficking, the Smuggling of Persons and Sexual Exploitation in the Triple Frontier

According to UNICEF reports, globally over 100 million children have been abandoned, with 40 million being accounted for by Latin America alone (Forselledo 2001, Inter-American Children's Institute). Castanha (2001) reports that nearly 65% of the children who live on the streets of Latin-American capitals are in some respect involved in sexual exploitation. Of these, 50% are said to have been involved in some form of prostitution.

The Inter-American Children's Institute indicates that besides the marginality of women and children, poverty also plays a central role in the advancement of sexual exploitation. Indeed, this view is widely supported by other researchers (e.g. Kane 1998; Lau 2008; Silva 2009). A CEPAL, UNICEF and SECIB (2001) collaborative report (c.f. Instituto Interamericano del niño 2003) highlights that the reduction of poverty is lower in homes with children and teenagers. Also, what regional development has seen has not been sufficient to reduce the increase in the number of those that live in this condition. Consequently, many families living in these conditions have been forced in to the precarious situation of having to generate an income in any way they can, including having children contribute to the family's survival. Where this results in travel away from home, it potentially exposes the children to different forms of abuse and exploitation to which they have not been prepared or educated.

The Triple Frontier has been the subject of a number of academic studies that have explored human trafficking in the region (e.g. Sprandel 2007; Silva 2009). Sprandel examined government and institutional programmes in existence to combat trafficking and highlighted the need for an even greater focus on implementation. Alternatively, Silva examined poverty and low health in rural areas of Argentina, and whilst not a focal aspect of her work, she highlights the relationship between a reduction in these with an increase in the incidence and likelihood of child sexual exploitation and trafficking. In addition, others have emphasised the link between the major crime activities of drugs and arms trafficking and also terrorism with human trafficking (e.g. Hudson 2003; Sverdlick 2005). Furthermore, numerous NGO-led studies have been carried out in the region.[5]

---

[5] Specifically, we refer to a study carried out by Save the Children in conjunction with IOM. Also, Luna Nueva, an NGO from Paraguay, has been actively involved in supporting victims of sexual exploitation and has collaborated with the IOM in another study.

Migration officers based in Puerto Iguazú estimate that 20% of the victims of trafficking in the region are under the age of 18 years, affirming that often the recruitment in the area is made by a relative or known person who charges between 1,000 and 1,500 pesos for the capture and the transfer of the victim. The International Work Organization (IWO) estimates that in the Triple Frontier, at least 3,500 boys and girls under the age of 18 are exposed to this situation (Salviolo 2010).

Finally, a study carried out by researchers from the Johns Hopkins University (The Protection Project) indicates that whilst Latin-American governments have taken several measures to offer assistance and protection to victims of trafficking, such efforts have been hindered by the lack of adequate resourcing, the corruption of government officials and weakness in combative legislation and/or in their application.

In the following section, we provide a brief overview of the regulatory and policy mechanisms in place.

5 Regulations and Public Policy

We focus our attention in this section on legislation, key to combating the smuggling of persons and human trafficking in the Triple Frontier area.[6]

In this regard, of relevance is the Protocol of Ouro Preto and the Protocol of Asunción concerning the promotion and protection of human rights in the Mercosur[7] and associated countries (Carvalho et al. 2004). It is only in more recent years that the synchronisation of penal legislation between Mercosur countries has become a priority of leaders. Of note is the Protocol of Judicial Mutual Assistance in Penal Matters for the Mercosur, used by Argentina, Brazil and Paraguay, who, together with Bolivia and Chile, signed the General Plan of Cooperation and Reciprocal Coordination for Security (1999) in the Mercosur Region, and the Republic of Bolivia and the Republic of Chile. The objective of the above agreement is the coordination of efforts of all relevant bodies in the fight against organised crime including the smuggling of persons and human trafficking.

Specifically in terms of child smuggling, the exchange of information concerning missing children is promoted between the Departments of Immigration, the Security forces and/or Police in the region. The exchange of information mainly concerns the actions taken at international borders as well as at other potential exit points such as airports, rail, bus and shipping ports. Such actions include the formation and management of a database which forms a part of the System of Security Exchange of Information of the Mercosur (SSEI).

---

[6] For a comprehensive list of regulatory mechanisms, we refer interested readers to Carvalho et al. (2004).

[7] The Common Market of the South (Mercosur) is a custom union, created by the signing of the Asunción Treatment, and it is formed by Argentina, Brazil, Paraguay and Uruguay. The associated countries are Chile, Colombia, Ecuador and Perú. Bolivia and Venezuela are in the process of incorporation to the market.

In June 2000, the Common Market's (Mercosur) Council approved a complement initiative to this plan, specifically for the trafficking of children. The referred to initiative determines that member countries should ensure that the content contained within the Convention of the Rights of Children and of the Inter-American Convention on the International Restitution of Minors is in full force (Carvalho et al. 2004). Implicit too is the need for Member States to commit to taking the necessary actions to ensure its fulfilment and enforcement. This complement to the plan determines the intensification of police and immigration department activity in the revision of the required legal documentation for children, in particular when they travel unaccompanied by their parents or other legal persons who have legitimate charge over them. Such action thereby works towards guaranteeing that the children do not become victims of human trafficking and that Member States will maintain close coordination between all relevant security departments when an irregular situation is detected (Carvalho et al. 2004).

In terms of regional politics, the Southern Child Initiative aims at promoting a joint Mercosur State effort geared towards fulfilling the International Convention of the Rights of Children and to the adjustment of national legislation to any relevant policy. In this context, a legislative database concerning the trafficking of persons, the smuggling of persons and the sexual exploitation and sale of children has been developed. Such action enables comparison between State responses and the subsequent promotion of necessary reform (Argentine Committee for the Follow up and Application of the International Convention on the Rights of Children 2008).

The National Secretariat of Childhood, Adolescence and Family (NSCAF), Ministry of Social Development in Argentina, has developed a series of initiatives as a part of an overall framework to combat child sexual exploitation in the Triple Frontier (NSCAF 2008). In the context of meetings organised by the NSCAF in the city of Puerto Iguazú, Province of Misiones (Argentina), specifically with respect to child sexual exploitation, an Agreement of Cooperation was countersigned between the Republic of Argentina, the Federal Republic of Brazil and the Republic of Paraguay (NSCAF 2008). Parallel to this, a Protocol of Common Intervention was signed in respect to the victims of child sexual and labour exploitation, and a common communications campaign to highlight various prevention initiatives has been designed in three languages (Spanish, Portuguese and Guaraní) with material distributed in these respective countries (NSCAF 2008).

Finally, in June 2008, the city of Buenos Aires (Argentina) hosted the First International Congress for the region on the trafficking of persons and child pornography. The event, organised by the Argentine Department of Justice, Security and Human Rights, resulted in the development of a number of key outcomes to advance thinking within the region (ACNUR 2008).[8]

---

[8] The congress highlighted the importance of the event itself as part of a regional policy on the subject, the need for a multidisciplinary approach to combatting human trafficking and child pornography, the importance of developing specific laws about relevant key issues in each country within the region, the importance of gender consideration and the importance of enabling refugee status for victims who return to their country of origin (ACNUR 2008).

6   The Experience of Victims

In this section, we present two short case testimonies[9] obtained from trafficking victims who were fortunate to be rescued. The testimonies portray the typical experiences of child victims all over the world. For clarification, we add that they are not in any way a part of, or related to, the research we report on later in this chapter. We include them here simply so that the reader can better imagine the lived experience of victims. We ask the reader to consider the obvious impact of the described situations on the security and well-being of these victims, and, similarly, to recognise that the full severity of the victim's situation is often understated for reasons of fear and self-preservation.

Case A

When I was 13 my family sold me to a 40-year-old man from Argentina who raped me continually. I eventually fell pregnant and had a baby girl. The man took my baby and abandoned me in the city. That same day, 5 men approached me and asked why I was crying. They told me they would take care of me and keep me safe. I had nowhere else to go, so I went with them. Nothing happened that first night. The next day, the men paid for my train ticket, and took me to a town 7 hours away. When we arrived, they took me to an apartment, locked me up, and then raped and beat me over and over again. They brought many different men to me and forced me to have sex with them. They made me cook and clean the apartment, and would beat me if it wasn't good enough. Finally, one of the neighbours called the police. I was being raped by a 'client' when the police raided the apartment, rescued me and took me to the shelter. I was 14 years old.

Case B

I met Jorge about six months ago. We became friends, and used to go out for coffee together. One morning at 8 am he called me and asked to meet for coffee. At first I refused because it was too early. But he kept asking, so finally I gave in and went to meet him. When I arrived, he gave me an open can of drink for energy. The next thing I remember is waking up in a strange city, and realising I had been drugged and raped. Jorge kept me drugged whilst he drove me from Paraguay to Brazil. Whenever I would come round and ask where he was taking me, he would beat and rape me.

We drove to a village where Jorge sold me to a couple in their fifties. The couple took my papers, my phone and all my money. For 3 days, I could not eat or sleep. The couple kept me locked up, and forced me to have sex with men without protection. Whenever I refused they would beat me. After a week, I managed to steal my phone and call my boyfriend. I explained what had happened, and he called the police who organized a raid. The police arrested the couple, freed me, and found three other girls in the house who had been kept there for the past three years.

---

[9] These case studies have kindly been provided to the authors for inclusion in this chapter by the A21 Campaign. For the protection of victims of human trafficking in the care of the A21 Campaign, all person and place names and details pertaining to specific cases are always changed.

The insecurity and the vulnerability of the above victims can clearly be 'heard' in each of the above presented testimonies. It is not our intention to shock the reader; indeed, it is difficult to convey in text the reality of the circumstances experienced by many victims. It takes many years, if at all, for victims to come to terms with the abuse that they have experienced. Consequently, many are understandably reluctant to speak openly with others about their experiences even long after they escape and/ or have been rescued.

7   Community Involvement

It is harder to bring the criminals involved in carrying out these crimes to justice when conditions in the region act unwittingly in support of them. In this light, complex as it is, we reinforce that it is only when all parties come together collaboratively to combat these crimes that we are likely to see any real progress being made. In an environment that is highly attractive to tourists, this includes not only parents, schools, government officials and NGOs but also the wider community including particularly those businesses that directly interact with domestic and international tourists.

Examples of effective community collaboration can be seen elsewhere in the world. For example, in South-East Asia, a tourist area notorious for the existence of human trafficking and child sexual exploitation (Blackburn et al. 2010), a partnership model is being followed by The Grey Man, a nonprofit organisation located in Australia dedicated to the eradication of human trafficking and the exploitation of children (The Grey Man 2010). Operating in Thailand and Cambodia, The Grey Man has proactively been engaged in prevention and rehabilitation efforts in conjunction with local representatives since 2004. These include amongst others community development projects, the goal of which is to improve living circumstances in an effort to reduce the likelihood of children being sold as a form of income. Furthermore, in conjunction with local law enforcement agencies, The Grey Man assists in the rescue of children from brothels and then subsequently assists placing them in shelters that offer various forms of post-rescue support including repatriation (where appropriate), health care, education and job training.[10]

Before of course the participation of the wider community can be obtained and an effective strategy put in place, a necessary first step is to assess the local situation and particularly the existing level of knowledge of all community members and groups in respect to these crimes.

---

[10] Further information on The Grey Man organisation can be obtained by writing to them at the address provided for The Grey Man in the Reference section of this paper. A similar example exists in Brazil between the Atlantic Hotel International (AHI) network – the second hotel network in Brazil – and the WCF (World Childhood Foundation) Institute, Brazil. Together they designed a Code of Conduct. In addition, AHI provided training to its employees and proactively advertised in support of the protection of children against sexual exploitation. The AHI also supports social projects that contribute money for the cause (ECPAT and Save the Children 2007).

8 Research Study

As we have indicated, the magnitude of the problem together with situational complexities clearly highlights that to fully address the situation not only requires the involvement of multiple parties, but moreover, the development of a more cooperative shared action response. As a foundation for such a response, we contend that it is important to ascertain the level of awareness that exists within the region concerning the trafficking, smuggling and sexual exploitation of children. We argue that it is necessary to develop a good understanding of these issues because it is not the responsibility of government departments and law enforcement agencies alone to tackle these crimes. We next describe a study and present findings from a large-scale project carried out in the region between 2007 and 2008.

In 2007, as an aspect of their work in the region, The Latin American Migratory Studies Centre (CEMLA), funded by the International Organization for Migrations (IOM) and Save the Children (OIM-CEMLA-Save the Children 2008), carried out a large but simple descriptive field study in the three named cities of the Triple Frontier.[11] The principal aim of the project was to explore what was known about these crimes by citizens, tourism (hotel) operators and other social agents living in the region. In addition to ascertaining the state of understanding in regards to associated criminal activity, the bigger picture, which will be reported on in another publication, also included: who was involved, the locus of responsibility in terms of combating these crimes and whether respondents had personally taken any action in respect to these crimes, i.e. whether they had reported anyone engaged in the crimes. The study reported on here follows the implementation of a survey to a convenience sample of 1,465 people. In the following sections, we report on the within-region 'knowledge' component since consistent with our thoughts presented earlier, it is clear that for the fight against these crimes to be successful, the involvement of all citizens in the region is necessary.

9 Study Implementation

The fieldwork upon which this chapter is based was carried out in the Triple Frontier area between October 25 and 27, 2007. The surveys were written in Spanish for participants in Argentina and Paraguay and Portuguese for participants in Brazil. Data collection was carried out by trained locals in each of the respective cities to ensure that they not only had the linguistic abilities required, but also that they were familiar with each respective region and its peculiar dynamics. All persons involved in data collection were fully trained on both the subject matter and the survey instrument by representatives from CEMLA.

---

[11] Prevención de la Trata, Tráfico y Explotación Sexual Comercial de niños, niñas y adolescentes en viajes y turismo en la Triple Frontera: Paraguay, Argentina y Brasil, Encarnación (Paraguay) y Posadas (Argentina).

The findings presented in the following section are representative of specific sections of the survey. As a reminder, in this chapter we focus specifically on knowledge regarding human trafficking, the smuggling of persons and sexual exploitation within the local community.

10   Survey Items and Results

In order to obtain an understanding of the profile of respondents, relevant descriptive statistics can be seen in Table 11.1. A review of the table reveals a fairly heterogenous sample across the main demographic areas of age, gender, level of education achieved, location of residence and marital status.

To explore the level of knowledge in the region about the crimes in question, respondents were asked to respond (Yes/No) to whether they knew what trafficking in persons, the smuggling of persons and child sex tourism was. For elaboration, they were then asked to provide a description of each. To enable the cross-tabulation of data, all categories for the non-dichotomous question were recoded such that all non-response replies were coded as '0' and all legitimate response descriptions were recoded as '1'.

A cross-tabulation analysis performed at the overall level revealed that only 22% of respondents stated that they knew what was meant by 'trafficking in persons' (Pearson Chi-square 892.343, df 2, $P = .000$), whereas for the smuggling of persons and sex tourism, the affirmative response percentages were 61% (Pearson Chi-square 942.853, df 2, $P = .000$) and 41% (Pearson Chi-square 987.975, df 2, $P = .000$), respectively.

The above picture changes dramatically by location of residence. For Puerto Iguazú (Argentina), a cross-tabulation analysis for trafficking in persons reveals 59% of respondents (289 where sample $n = 493$) knew what this was (Pearson Chi-square 167.303, df 6, $P = .000$); for the smuggling of persons and sex tourism, the affirmative response percentages were 59% (Pearson Chi-square 293.320, df 2, $P = .000$) and 30% (Pearson Chi-square 337.067, df 2, $P = .000$), respectively.

For Foz de Iguaçú (Brazil), the picture is both clouded and revealing. First, the picture is clouded in that in the Portuguese language (spoken in Brazil), only one term is used for both the offences of 'the smuggling of persons' and 'human trafficking' (tráfico de pessoas). Thus, any direct comparison against the Spanish-speaking samples from Puerto Iguazú (Argentina) and Ciudad del Este (Paraguay) is difficult. Nonetheless, asked about 'tráfico de pessoas', which, recall, means both the smuggling of persons and human trafficking, a cross-tabulation analysis reveals 80% of respondents (i.e. 379 where sample $n = 475$) indicated that they knew what this was (Pearson Chi-square 167.303, df 6, $P = .000$). For sex tourism, the affirmative response percentage was 65% (Pearson Chi-square 262.571, df 2, $P = .000$). Second, the picture is revealing in that, when probed for more detail,[12] the Brazilian respondents (Foz de Iguaçú) were clear in

---

[12] Once the respondent descriptions had been identified, they were qualitatively grouped in accordance with identified themes. These themes are representative of the 7 category responses shown in Table 11.2.

Table 11.1 Descriptive statistics for the total sample

Demographics		Count	Layer N (%)	Cumulative (%)
Age	Not provided	0	0.0	0.0
	1 > 18 years	202	13.9	13.9
	19 > 24 years	276	19.0	32.9
	25 > 39 years	460	31.7	64.6
	40 > 49 years	236	16.3	80.9
	50 > 59 years	148	10.2	91.0
	60 > 69 years	107	7.4	98.4
	70+ years	23	1.6	100.0
Gender	Not stated	0	0.0	0.0
	Male	718	49.0	49.0
	Female	747	51.0	100.0
Level of education achieved	Not stated	23	1.6	1.6
	No education	61	4.2	5.8
	Primary school not completed	245	16.7	22.5
	Completed primary school	257	17.5	40.0
	High school not completed	313	21.4	61.4
	High school completed	346	23.6	85.0
	Further education not completed	132	9.0	94.0
	Further education completed	88	6.0	100.0
Location of residence	Not stated	0	0.0	0.0
	Puerto Iguazú (Argentina)	493	33.7	33.7
	Foz de Iguaçu (Brazil)	475	32.4	66.1
	Ciudad del Este (Paraguay)	487	33.2	99.3
	Other than these towns	10	0.7	100.0
Marital status	Not stated	7	0.5	0.5
	Single	657	44.8	45.3
	Married	578	39.5	84.8
	Divorced	64	4.4	89.1
	Co-habiting	83	5.7	94.8
	Widowed	70	4.8	99.6
	Other	6	0.4	100.0

their understanding that both the smuggling of persons and the trafficking in persons (based on the use of the single term) involved the illegal transportation of individuals from one place to another. Indeed, a cross-tabulation analysis (Table 11.2[13]) reveals the greater certainty in this regard relative to the two neighbouring country samples. Of course, we acknowledge that it is possible that this is an artefact of a combined understanding. That said, we are led to believe that the incidence of human trafficking is greater than that of the smuggling of

---

[13] Note that the questions were asked in the relevant local language, and they are presented in English in Table 11.2 for the convenience of the reader only. Therefore, the wording would have differed between 'trafico de personas' for the Spanish-speaking respondents and 'tráfico de pessoas' for the Portuguese-speaking respondents. Subsequent interpretation would have differed as described.

Table 11.2 Cross-country comparison of understanding of trafficking (Argentina and Paraguay) and single term 'trafico' for Brazil

		Do you know what is meant by trafficking of persons?							
Count		Don't know	Sale of children for sex	Trickery/ lying	Illegal activity (needs reporting)	Illegal transport of persons	Use of children as sex merchandise for tourists	Other	Total
Place of residence	Puerto Iguazu	219	20	7	19	185	7	36	493
	Foz de Iguac	118	12	3	8	301	5	28	475
	Ciudad del Este	279	25	18	6	119	5	35	487
	Other	3	0	0	1	6	0	0	10
Total		619	57	28	34	611	17	99	1465

Chi-square tests

	Value	df	Asymp. sig. (2-sided)
Pearson Chi-square	182.740[a]	18	0.000
Likelihood ratio	184.707	18	0.000
Linear-by-linear association	15.762	1	0.000
N of valid cases	1,465		

[a]7 cells (25.0%) have expected count less than 5. The minimum expected count is .12

persons in Brazil. Also, a number of campaigns to raise awareness to the offence of trafficking in persons have run throughout the country (MCTP 2010), and hence we feel it likely that the point of reference is in fact trafficking in persons and not the smuggling of persons. We present this as an issue in need of further exploration later in this chapter.

For Ciudad del Este (Paraguay), a similar cross-tabulation analysis for trafficking in persons reveals 44% of respondents (216 where sample $n = 487$) knew what this was (Pearson Chi-square 167.303, df 6, $P = .000$); for the smuggling of persons and sex tourism, the affirmative response percentages were 44% (Pearson Chi-square 336.636, df 2, $P = .000$) and 29% (Pearson Chi-square 353.384, df 2, $P = .000$), respectively.

Closer examination of the cross-tabulation output reveals that a significant number of the respondents, who indicated that they knew what trafficking in persons, the smuggling of persons and child sex tourism was, were unable to elaborate further by providing a description of each when requested to do so. At the overall level for trafficking in persons, this equated to 31% of those who said they knew what trafficking in persons was, for the smuggling of persons 17% and child sex tourism 21%.

Again at the individual location of residence level, the picture is equally revealing. For Puerto Iguazú (Argentina), with respect to trafficking in persons, the smuggling of persons and child sex tourism, the percentages are 31%, 19% and 24%, respectively. For Foz de Iguaçú (Brazil), with respect to child sex tourism, the percentage was 20%. Recall that we are unable to comment on the position with respect to the smuggling of persons and trafficking in persons for the reasons we outlined earlier. Though disappointing, this is an important revelation since it highlights the need to not only differentiate in particular between the trafficking in persons and the smuggling of persons, but also to be able to convey this through educational campaigns such as those currently being developed and implemented as an extension of the CEMLA study. Finally, for Ciudad del Este (Paraguay), with respect to trafficking in persons, the smuggling of persons and child sex tourism, the percentages are 34%, 20% and 21%, respectively, presenting a similar picture to that of both of the other cities (with the proviso of limited comparison with Foz de Iguaçú as highlighted).

To explore the data in greater depth, a 2-step clustering technique was carried out to establish whether homogenous groupings existed within the sample. Three such clusters resulted. Following this, a profile of these clusters was obtained for each of the stated (Yes/No) vs. demonstrated (response descriptions offered) knowledge variables for each of trafficking in persons, the smuggling of persons and child sex tourism (Tables 11.3 and 11.4).

Table 11.3 reveals how the sample comprising each of the three clusters responded to the questions shown on the left side of the table. Note that the first three questions starting from the top reflect the dichotomous Yes/No question, and these are followed by questions asking respondents to elaborate further by providing a description for each of trafficking, the smuggling of persons and child sex tourism. Clearly proportionately, the knowledge level of cluster 3 is the highest and 1 the lowest.

Table 11.3 Chi-square cluster results by stated and demonstrated knowledge

Variables	Cluster 1 n=678	Percentage	Cluster 2 n=210	Percentage	Cluster 3 n=577	Percentage	Significance Chi-square	Total n =	Percentage	Percentage demonstrated Vs stated knowledge
Stated Knowledge of trafficking – Yes/No	54	8.00	47	22.40	217	37.60	P=0.000	318	21.71	
Stated Knowledge of smuggling - Yes/No	186	27.40	147	70.00	558	96.70	P=0.000	891	60.82	
Knowledge of child sex tourism – Yes/No	56	8.30	105	50.00	442	76.60	P=0.000	603	41.16	
Demonstrated knowledge of trafficking	38	5.60	27	12.90	151	26.20	P=0.000	216	14.74	67.93
Demonstrated knowledge of smuggling	140	20.60	63	30.00	544	94.30	P=0.000	747	50.99	83.84
Demonstrated knowledge of child sex tourism	36	5.30	16	7.60	431	74.70	P=0.000	483	32.97	80.10

Table 11.4 A comparison of clusters according to specified demographics

Variables	Cluster 1 n=678	Percentage	Cluster 2 n=210	Percentage	Cluster 3 n = 577	Percentage	Significance Chi-square	Total n =	Percentage
Age									
1>18 years	119	17.60	21	10.00	62	10.70	$P=0.000$	202	13.79
19>24 years	128	18.90	34	16.20	114	19.80	$P=0.000$	276	18.84
25>39 years	199	29.40	61	29.00	200	34.70	$P=0.000$	460	31.40
40>49 years	90	13.30	53	25.20	93	16.10	$P=0.000$	236	16.11
50>59 years	76	11.20	20	9.50	52	9.00	$P=0.000$	148	10.10
60>69 years	50	7.40	16	7.60	41	7.10	$P=0.000$	107	7.30
70+ years	14	2.10	3	1.40	6	1.00	$P=0.000$	23	1.57
Missing	2	0.30	2	1.00	9	1.60	–	13	0.89
Gender									
Female	330	48.70	106	50.50	311	53.90	$P=0.18$	747	50.99
Male	348	51.30	104	49.50	266	46.10	$P=0.18$	718	49.01
Location of residence									
Puerto Iguazú (Argentina)	264	38.90	72	34.30	157	27.20	$P=0.000$	493	33.65
Foz de Iguaçú (Brazil)	67	9.90	115	54.80	293	50.80	$P=0.000$	475	32.42
Ciudad del Este (Paraguay)	341	50.30	22	10.50	124	21.50	$P=0.000$	487	33.24
Education level achieved									
Don't know/Won't answer	3	1.30	6	2.90	8	1.40	$P=0.000$	17	1.16
No education	39	5.80	9	4.30	13	2.30	$P=0.000$	61	4.16
Incomplete primary education	111	16.40	46	21.90	88	15.30	$P=0.000$	245	16.72
Complete primary education	150	22.10	31	14.80	76	13.20	$P=0.000$	257	17.54
Incomplete High school	159	23.50	41	19.50	113	19.60	$P=0.000$	313	21.37
Completed High school	134	19.80	46	21.90	166	28.80	$P=0.000$	346	23.62
Incomplete Higher education	46	6.80	18	8.60	68	11.80	$P=0.000$	132	9.01
Completed Higher education	30	4.40	13	6.20	45	7.80	$P=0.000$	88	6.01

(continued)

Table 11.4 (continued)

Variables	Cluster 1 n=678	Percentage	Cluster 2 n=210	Percentage	Cluster 3 n=577	Percentage	Significance Chi-square	Total n =	Percentage
Marital status									
Don't know/Won't answer	2	0.30	0	0.00	5	0.90	P=0.000	7	0.48
Single	346	51.00	91	43.30	220	38.10	P=0.000	657	44.85
Married	210	31.00	98	46.70	270	46.80	P=0.000	578	39.45
Divorced	23	3.40	8	3.80	33	5.70	P=0.000	64	4.37
Co-habiting	51	7.50	4	1.90	28	4.90	P=0.000	83	5.67
Widow	41	6.00	8	3.80	21	3.60	P=0.000	70	4.78
Other	5	0.70	1	0.50	0	0.00	P=0.000	6	0.41

The above findings, when considered together, indicate that at an aggregate level across the three clusters,[14] the level of knowledge is disappointingly low (Table 11.3). More specifically, only 22% (rounded) indicated that they knew what trafficking in persons was as opposed to 61% (rounded) for the smuggling of persons and 41% (rounded) for child sex tourism. Furthermore, in terms of trafficking in persons, only 68% of those persons who said they knew what it was could provide a description. For example from Table $11.3 = (216/318)*100$ and 84% and 80%, respectively, for the smuggling of persons and child sex tourism.

Closer scrutiny of the table reveals too that in each case, and more severely so for cluster 2, stated knowledge exceeded the ability of respondents to demonstrate their knowledge by providing a description of what was meant by each of the crimes in question. For example, with respect to cluster 2, 50% of respondents in this cluster indicated that they knew what child sex tourism was, yet only 7.6% were able to provide a description. Proportionately, therefore, only 15.2% of those who said they knew what sex tourism was could provide a description. These results are reflective not only of poor knowledge but also an exaggerated level of knowledge with respect to this cluster. Cluster 3 was most accurate in this regard with 70%, 99% and 97% for trafficking in persons, the smuggling of persons and child sex tourism, respectively.

To explore the clusters in even greater detail, further analysis was carried out to identify whether the three clusters could be more closely profiled when examined with the demographic variables of age, gender, location of residence, education level achieved and marital status. Of these, age, location of residence, education level achieved and marital status all revealed significant differences (Table 11.4).

Table 11.4 provides a more detailed breakdown of level of knowledge by the demographics of age, gender, location of residence, education level achieved and marital status. First, no significant gender differences are evident. However, significant differences are revealed for age, location of residence, education level achieved and marital status. In terms of developing a coordinated and targeted educational campaign response, arguably, the most workable variables to employ are the location of residence of the respondent and age. In terms of location of residence, if we focus our attention on cluster 2 in respect to child sex tourism, recall that in this group only 15.2% of those who said they knew what child sex tourism was could provide a description (Table 11.3). Next, if we consider that the majority in cluster 2 are representative of those respondents living in Foz de Iguaçú, we can say that a targeted campaign in this region focussing on raising knowledge in regard to child sex tourism would be beneficial. In support, this is not unreasonable since this location is representative of the Brazil side of Iguazú falls, the major world heritage tourism location and the second most visited of Brazil's national parks receiving 1.07 million visitors annually (Janer 2010). Unfortunately, no current information regarding visitor numbers to the Argentine side of the falls could be located at the time of writing; however, 330,000 persons visited in 1986 (UNEP

---

[14] We wish to highlight to readers that the three clusters do not correspond to the three geographic regions.

WCMC 1990), and it would not be unreasonable to suggest that this number has today increased to a number similar to Brazil since many visitors report visiting both sides of the falls.

Beyond the above, we can't ignore that cluster 2 only represents 14.33% (210) of the overall sample of 1,465 persons, and so we need to look elsewhere to ensure that a targeted campaign directed to Foz de Iguaçú is appropriately directed and that it has the greatest reach potential. In this regard, cluster 3 representing a further 39.4% of the sample (577) would also benefit from any such campaign locally directed. Furthermore, in regard to Foz de Iguaçú, it may be recalled that for reasons of language limitation, Brazilian respondents were not able to differentiate between the smuggling of persons and trafficking in persons in any detail. Clearly, therefore, there is room for additional education in this regard targeted to the same audience. Consequently, focussing on the trafficking of persons and the exploitation of persons for the purpose of sex tourism would be a useful strategy at raising awareness in this region.

Turning our attention to cluster 1 (Table 11.4), we can see that the largest group of respondents ($n = 341$) in this cluster have, as their place of residence, Ciudad del Este (Paraguay). Table 11.3 informs that the two areas of minimal knowledge for respondents comprising this cluster are the trafficking of persons and child sex tourism. Indeed, of the 678 persons comprising cluster 1, only 8% (54) indicated that they knew what the trafficking of persons was, and only 5.6% (38) of the overall population of this cluster were able to provide a description. Similarly, in terms of child sex tourism, only 8.3% (56) indicated that they knew what child sex tourism was, and only 5.3% (36) of the overall population of this cluster were able to provide a description. The exceedingly low levels of knowledge for this cluster suggest that a similarly directed education campaign targeted to Ciudad del Este (Paraguay) would be useful. In this regard, a translation of the same campaign directed to Foz de Iguaçú articulated to highlight the specifics of human trafficking would suffice and would furthermore ensure that costs are kept to a minimum. Relevant authorities would benefit from coordinating their efforts in this regard. Of further potential usefulness when designing such a campaign would be to recognise that approximately 50% of the population representing clusters 1–3 fall within the age grouping of 19–39. Consequently, a campaign designed to draw the attention and interest of young adults is most likely to have the most significant behavioural impact on this group.

Before closing this overview of findings, though the focus thus far has been on residents living in Paraguay (Ciudad del Este) and Brazil (Foz de Iguaçú), Argentine (Puerto Iguazú) respondents are well represented in all three clusters ($n = 264, n = 72,$ $n = 157$). Consequently, a tripartite sharing of campaign resources between authorities in all three countries would likely result in the greatest impact in terms of overall region knowledge.

Finally, with respect to 'education level achieved' and 'marital status', whilst significant differences have been identified (Table 11.4), there is no suggestion that either of these would be useful in designing a campaign targeted at improving local knowledge regarding the discussed crimes. Separate cross-tabulation analysis confirms this suggestion.

11 Final Considerations

Prior to describing the empirical component of this chapter, we presented the reader with two case studies to enable the reader to build a picture of what life for the young victims of trafficking is like. We did this primarily because from our experience, few people are aware of the serious negative security and well-being impacts of these crimes.

In the definitions presented for both security and well-being, we highlighted the importance of freedom from needs and wants in terms of security and being able to lead a self-realised, fully functioned life of meaning and pleasure and absence of pain. In our discussion, we have drawn the reader's attention to how the suffering experienced by the victims of these crimes detracts in every respect from their potential to lead what might vaguely be described as a life fulfilled. Enslavement, deprivation of liberty and of genuine friendships and being subject to ongoing extreme physical and psychological abuse as well as many other forms of exploitation are clearly all counterproductive in this regard. What is most important in the fight to end what Mr Kofi Annan (Ex-Secretary-General United Nations) described as 'one of the most egregious violations of human rights that the United Nations now confronts' and as 'a challenge to every State, every people and every community (UNODC 2004, Piv)' are the collective efforts of all parties.

Having argued that the responsibility for tracking these crimes needs to be shared between multiple parties, what will now be clear to the reader is that whilst the focus here is about the plight of the most vulnerable members of society, i.e., children, ultimately, this has a bearing on the quality of life of communities in general. Certainly, it would seem almost morally inappropriate to discuss on the one hand community quality of life if on the other we fail to protect the security and well-being needs of society's most vulnerable members. As a starting point, assessing knowledge, raising community awareness and putting forward a call for action are paramount.

An extensive study, funded by the IOM and Save the Children, and implemented by CEMLA in the Triple Frontier region of Latin America, reveals that though some knowledge regarding the trafficking and smuggling of persons as well as the commercial sexual exploitation of children for the sex tourism trade exists, considerable room for improvement is evident.

In this regard, we have offered suggestions as to where targeted awareness and educational campaign efforts can be directed. However, we point out that these are simply the tip of the iceberg. Beyond these, additional efforts are needed at every level of civil society commencing at the grass roots level. In terms of awareness, both parents and children need to be educated about the potential dangers involved in their children pursuing risky behaviours such as chasing promising job offers away from the security of the home. Similarly, this responsibility needs also to be taken up in schools, and indeed we suggest that there is a place for open discussion on personal safety, security and well-being within the national curriculum. Furthermore, businesses play a significant role in all societies, and clearly, there is a substantial need for those businesses involved in offering goods and services not only to local nationals but also to tourists to contribute towards the eradication of these crimes. As an example, many organisations globally have accepted the challenge to join the fight against the sexual exploitation of children for the purpose of sex tourism by signing a code of conduct referred to simply as 'The Code'. The code sets out six criteria to which all signatories must adhere:

1. To establish an ethical policy regarding commercial sexual exploitation of children
2. To train the personnel in the country of origin and travel destinations
3. To introduce a clause in contracts with suppliers, stating a common repudiation of commercial sexual exploitation of children
4. To provide information to travellers by means of catalogues, brochures, in-flight films, ticket slips, home pages, etc.
5. To provide information to local 'key persons' at the destinations
6. To submit an activity report annually

At the time of writing, signatory partners in both Argentina and Brazil to The Code exist, but to the best of our knowledge, no signatories exist in Paraguay (The Code 2010).

Similarly, more needs to be done to promote uptake by all organisations involved in the travel and tourism value chain both in the country of origin as well as in Argentina, Brazil and Paraguay, and of course beyond. Membership offers educational opportunities for signatories to directly participate in reducing the incidence of the crimes discussed in this chapter. Furthermore, membership can also be seen as an opportunity for signatories to promote their efforts in this regard as a part of their overall corporate social responsibility programmes. Indeed, we would go so far as to suggest that industries should insist on the need for organisations to become a member to obtain a licence to do business.

With respect to action at the State and government level, the Mercosur and associated countries have clearly made advances both in terms of regulation and in the development of public policy pertaining to their implementation. These achievements are to be recognised and applauded. In addition, it is also necessary to continue with the development of new measures and the deepening of others. For this, it is necessary to insist that a more systemic approach to the matter be considered in models of development that imply recognition of the child not only as a person with rights but as a person particularly vulnerable to situations of physical and psychological abuse. Such models of development would not only give explicit recognition to the social position of the child in the society of which she/he is a member, but it would also recognise their need for access to education and healthcare and, indeed, the broader familial circumstances in which the child is situated. Clearly these are complex matters, and they take us beyond the specific realms of this chapter. Nonetheless, we note them here as worthy of future research attention.

In terms of the prevention of crime and the detection and prosecution of offenders once a crime has been committed, many models of best practice exist amongst police, security and immigration services. We suggest the need for greater collaboration at all levels and the need for a forum for sharing.

Consequently, with the above we have advanced the need for a joint consolidated effort across a network of interested parties including the home, school, business, civil society and at the official government level in all three countries. Advancing the efforts that are already in place, we propose the establishment of an Observatory of Human Trafficking in the region. Such an observatory would act as an environment for the sharing of information and debate, policy making and the education and training through workshops and seminars of persons involved both directly and indirectly in the fight against these crimes. These persons would include security, crime enforcement and immigration officials; other State-level decision makers; NGO staff; teachers; hotel staff and tourism site staff, e.g. national parks as well as others involved directly in the travel and tourism business and others as identified. Clearly, costs would be involved in achieving the desired goals. In this regard, it must be seen as an integral infrastructure necessity for the region as a whole. It would not be unrealistic to imagine, in addition to government support, seeking commercial backing for such a venture.

In this chapter, we have barely touched the surface on this issue; clearly, there is much more that remains to be said. Our research efforts will continue, and we hope that others will join us by designing research programmes in their own environments that contribute not only to eradicating all forms of modern-day slavery but also towards providing a more secure existence and a better quality of life for all, whether victims of human trafficking, smuggling of persons, sexual exploitation, sex tourism or otherwise.

In terms of potential future research, we offer the following suggestions:

We have identified how, for the Brazilian sample, a single term is used to denote both the trafficking and the smuggling of persons (tráfico de pessoas). We propose that more substantive research to determine in greater detail what is understood by this term would be useful in advancing the fight against trafficking in this country and the wider region.

At the macro regional level, research of direct relevance in terms of security and quality of life could include exploring the connection between reducing the commercial sexual exploitation of children, human trafficking and other serious criminal activities such as the trafficking of weapons and drugs and money laundering as well as the structure of criminal networks and their overall impact on security and quality of life in the region.

Still at the regional level, also of value would be to explore the extent to which the quality of life of the most vulnerable members of a community; for example children who are at risk of sexual and economic exploitation can be considered a powerful indicator of the general well-being of a community. Further research could investigate whether improving the quality of life and security needs of vulnerable children might lead to an improvement in the general levels of community well-being.

Tailby (2001) highlights that when people move through multiple transit points and countries, the required level of organisation and the need for local support increases. This is of course an issue of key significance in the Triple Frontier. Such support could include corrupt officials involved for reasons of personal gain to local citizens who simply turn a blind eye out of fear or ignorance. In this regard, steps to address corruption at all levels need to be taken. These could include enforced transparency through the adoption of advanced technological systems and processes, as well as at the base level, ensuring that similarly transparent hiring and remuneration policies are in place. We are not so naïve to suggest that these will address any evident corruption, but we recognise them as important and in need of attention. Consequently, a programme of research exploring models of best practice and their potential transferability would be advantageous.

At a simple level in this chapter, we have advocated the need for greater regional awareness and the importance of education programmes designed to change attitudes and behaviours in respect to the focal crimes discussed here. Studies that explore models of best practice and their effectiveness from the micro individual to Mondo industry level would be of significant benefit in destabilising the support environment within which these criminal networks thrive. The aforementioned studies could also usefully extend to include an assessment of their impact on enhanced perceived security as well as individual and community well-being.

The risk of trafficking is greatest in regions with significant unemployment. Holding the goal to reduce the incidence and risk of children falling victim to trafficking, of value would be studies exploring the efficacy of establishing microfinance funded local community enterprises.

Similarly, studies exploring the community quality of life impact of such programmes would provide a useful basis from which their transferability could be identified.

Finally, at the micro individual level, to the best knowledge of the authors, no prior empirical study exploring the impact of trafficking on the quality of life of victims, the victim's family and friends and, dare we say, traffickers has been conducted. These likewise would provide a timely contribution to the quality of life literature. Consistent with Tyldum (2010), we advocate carrying out such studies on former victims, which albeit subject to recall bias, will nonetheless be very useful in advancing knowledge regarding the well-being impacts of these crimes. Clearly, to attempt to carry out such research on current victims, not only would the researcher find access difficult, but as Tyldum highlights: '....to collect information about ongoing abuse, exploitation and coercion.....and then not act to improve their situation is likely to ruin any belief the victim had in humanity, or even hope of being rescued (P4)'.

In addition to the research suggestions we present above, many other useful possibilities exist (see Tyldum 2010 for example). We hope with the above that our colleagues likewise feel compelled to embark on research that will contribute towards the eradication of this hideous crime against humanity.

Acknowledgements We wish to acknowledge The Latin American Migratory Studies Centre (CEMLA) for providing permission to publish this work. We also wish to acknowledge The A21 Campaign and The Grey Man for providing case material reported on in this chapter.

References

Acharya, A. (2001). Human security: East versus West. *International Journal, 56*(3), 442–460.

Alkire, S. (2003). Concepts of human security. In L. C. Chen, S. Fukuda-Parr, & E. Seidensticker (Eds.), *Human insecurity in a global world* (pp. 15–39). Cambridge: Harvard University Press.

Bales, K. (2007). *Ending slavery: How we free today's slaves.* Berkley: University of California Press.

Blackburn, A. G., Taylor, R. W., & Davis, J. E. (2010). Understanding the complexities of human trafficking and child sexual exploitation: The case of Southeast Asia. *Women & Criminal Justice, 20*(1), 105–126.

Bruch, E. M. (2004). Models wanted: The search for an effective response to human trafficking. *Stanford Journal of International Law, 40*(1), 1–46.

Carvalho, H., Romero, A., & Sprandel, M. (2004). *La explotación sexual comercial de niños, niñas y adolescentes en las legislaciones de Argentina, Brasil y Paraguay: alternativas de armonización para el MERCOSUR.* Asunción: OIT/Programa IPEC Sudamérica.

Castanha, N. (2001). *Hacia la definición de una norma modelo sobre abuso y explotación sexual de niños, niñas y adolescentes en las Américas.* Documento interno del Instituto Interamericano del Niño. Montevideo: Instituto Interamericano del Niño.

Conticini, A., & Hulme, D. (2007). Escaping violence, seeking freedom: Why children in Bangladesh migrate to the street. *Development and Change, 38*(2), 201–227.

Cotter, K. M. (2009). Combatting child sex tourism in Southeast Asia. *Denver Journal of International Law and Policy, 37*(3), 493–512. http://law.du.edu/documents/djilp/37No3/combating-child-sex-tourism-southeast-asia-kelly-m-cotter.pdf. Accessed September 17, 2011.

Cummins, R. A. (1996). The domains of life satisfaction: An attempt to order chaos. *Social Indicators Research, 38*, 303–332.

Cummins, R. A., Eckersley, R., Pallant, J., Van Vugt, J., & Misajon, R. (2003). Developing a national index of subjective well being: The Australian unity well being index. *Social Indicators Research, 64*, 159–190.

Diener, E. (2000). Subjective well-being: The science of happiness and a proposal for a national index. *The American Psychologist, 55*, 34–43.

Dirección General de Estadísticas, Encuestas y Censos de Paraguay. Censo 2002. http://www.dgeec.gov.py/index.htm. Accessed April 2, 2010.

ECPAT (2010). End child prostitution, child pornography and the trafficking of children for sexual purposes. CSEC terminology. http://www.ecpat.net/EI/Csec_cst.asp. Accessed October 27, 2010.

ECPAT & Save the Children (2007). Good business practices. Successful cases for the prevention of sexual exploitation in children and adolescents in Latin America. http://ceidas.org/documentos/Centro_Doc/prevencion.empresas.ecpat.stc.2007.pdf. Accessed August 15, 2010.

Forselledo, A. G. (2001). Niñez en situación de calle. Un modelos de prevención de las fármaco dependencias basado en los derechos humanos. *INFANCIA. Boletín del Instituto Interamericano del Niño, 69*, 236.

Hampson, F. O., Daudelin, J., Hay, J. B., Martin, T., & Reid, H. (2002). *Madness in the multitude: Human security and world disorder.* Ottawa: Oxford University Press.

Hudson, R. (2003). *Terrorist and organized crime groups in the Tri-Border area (TBA) of South America: A report prepared by the federal research division, Library of Congress*, Washington, DC – 20540–4840 under an interagency agreement with the United States government. http://www.loc.gov/rr/frd/pdf-files/TerrOrgCrime_TBA.pdf. Accessed July 4, 2010.

Instituto Brasileño de Geografía y Estadística (IBGE). Censo 2001. http://www.ibge.gov.br/loja-virtual/fichatecnica.php?codigoproduto=8929. Accessed April 2, 2010

Instituto Interamericano del niño. (2003). *La explotación sexual de niños, niñas y adolescentes en América Latina.* Montevideo: Instituto Interamericano del Niño.

Instituto Nacional de Estadística y Censo (INDEC) (Argentina). Censo 2001. http://www.indec.mecon.ar/. Accessed April 2, 2010.

320 D. Webb and L.R. de La Vega

Iselin, B., & Adams, M. (2003). *Distinguishing between human trafficking and people smuggling: UN Office of Drugs and Crime*, Regional Centre for East Asia and the Pacific, Bangkok. http://www.embraceni.org/wp-content/uploads/2006/06/Distinguishing%5B1%5D1.pdf. Accessed July 7, 2010.

Janer, A. (2010). *The national parks of Brazil*. http://www.ecobrasil.org.br/publique/media/Brazil%20National%20Parks%20mar%202010.pdf. Accessed July 8, 2010.

Kane, J. (1998). *Sold for sex*. Aldershot: Arena.

Kara, S. (2009). *Sex trafficking: Inside the business of modern slavery*. New York: Columbia University Press.

King, G., & Murray, C. (2001). Rethinking human security. *Political Science Quarterly, 116*(4), 585–610.

Lau, C. (2008). Child prostitution in Thailand. *Journal of Child Health Care, 12*, 144–155.

MCTP (2010). Movimento contra o trafico de pessoas. http://www.traficodepessoas.org.br/index.html. Accessed November 8, 2010.

Model United Nations of the University of Chicago (MUNUC). *Bringing law, stability, and infrastructure to the Triple Border Area*. http://munuc.uchicago.edu/munucxvii/pdfs/OAS_A.pdf. Accessed July 13, 2010.

Morillas-Bassedas, P. (2007). Génesis y evolución de la expresión de la seguridad humana. Un repaso histórico. *Revista CIDOB d'Afers Internacionals, 76*, 47–58.

National Secretariat of Childhood, Adolescence and Family (NSCAF) – Ministry of Social Development in Argentina. (2008). *Third periodic report on the convention on the rights of the child in virtue of its 44 article*. http://www.derechoseducacion.org.ar/derechos/images/pdf/informe_estado_al_comite_onu08.pdf. Accessed August 11, 2010.

OIM-CEMLA-Save the Children (2008). *Prevención de la trata, tráfico y explotación sexual comercial de niños, niñas y adolescentes en viajes y turismo en la Triple Frontera: Paraguay*, Argentina y Brasil, Encarnación (Paraguay) y Posadas (Argentina). Unpublished report.

Orndorf, M. (2010). The secret world of child sex tourism: Evidentiary and procedural hurdles of the 'protect act'. *Penn State International Law Review, 28*(4), 789–814.

Robinson, J. (1999). *The merger: How organized crime is taking over the world*. New York: Simon & Schuster.

Rothchild, E. (1995). What is security? The quest for world order. *Daedalus, 124*(3), 53–98.

Ryan, R. M., & Deci, E. L. (2001). On happiness and human potentials: A review of research on hedonic and eudaimonic well-being. *Annual Review of Psychology, 52*, 141–166.

Ryan, R. M., Huta, V., & Deci, E. (2008). Living well: A self-determination theory perspective on eudaimonia. *Journal of Happiness Studies, 9*, 139–170.

Salviolo, C. (2010). *Trata y explotación de niños. CASACIDN*. http://www.casacidn.org.ar/leer.php/120. Accessed May 29, 2010.

Save the Children Sweden. (2005). *Sistematización de las iniciativas regionales para la prevención del turismo sexual infantil en América Latina: Hacia una estrategia regional*. Lima: Save the Children. Suecia. http://white.oit.org.pe/ipec/documentos/sist_prevencion_turismo_sexual.pdf. Accessed May 28, 2010.

Sen, A. (1999). *Development as freedom*. New York: Knopf.

Silva, M. A. (2009). Poverty and health in Argentina. *Social Medicine, 4*(2), 98–108.

Sprandel, M. (2007). Trafficking in persons: Advances in institutionalization and in critical thinking. In E. Sydow, & M. L. Mendonça (Eds.), *Human rights in Brazil 2007: A report by network for social justice and human rights* (pp. 129–137). São Paulo: Social network for justice and human rights- Heinrich Böll Foundation. http://www.social.org.br/relatorioingles2007.pdf#page=129. Accessed July 6, 2010.

Sverdlick, A. (2005). Terrorists and organised crime entrepreneurs in the 'triple frontier' among Argentina, Brazil, and Paraguay. *Trends in organised crime, 9*(2), 84–93.

Tailby, R. (2001). *Organised crime and people smuggling/trafficking to Australia*. Trends and issues in crime and criminal justice no. 208. http://aic.gov.au/documents/7/F/E/%7B7FE1BB81-D038-4C1E-A34D-8453FAAC6D2F%7Dti208.pdf. Accessed October 26, 2010.

The A21 Campaign (2011): http://www.thea21campaign.org/. Accessed September 17, 2011.
The Code (2010). www.thecode.org. Accessed July 8, 2010.
The Grey Man (2010). www.thegreyman.org. Accessed October 27, 2010.
The protection project. Escuela de estudios internacionales avanzados. Universidad John Hopkins. Trata de personas, en especial mujeres y niños en los países de América. Un informe regional del alcance del problema y la respuesta gubernamental y no gubernamental. http://www.iin.oea.org/iin/cad/sim/pdf/mod2/Tráfico%20UnivrJohnHopkins.pdf. Accessed May 29, 2010.
Tyldum, G. (2010). Limitations in research on human trafficking. *International Migration, 48*(5), 1–13. doi:10.1111/j.1468-2435.2009.00597.x
UNDP. (1994). *United Nations Development Program. Human development report.* New York: Oxford University Press.
UNEP & WCMC. (1990). *Iguazú national park and national reserve.* http://sea.unep-wcmc.org/sites/pa/0386q.htm. Accessed July 13, 2010.
Veenhoven, R. (2000). The four qualities of life: Ordering concepts and measures of the good life. *Journal of Happiness Studies, 1,* 1–39.

Documents

ACNUR (2008). *Conclusions and recommendations of the first Mercosur and associated states international congress on human trafficking and child pornography.* http://www.acnur.or/biblioteca/pdf/6442.pdf. Accessed April 3, 2010.
An agenda for peace. Preventive diplomacy, peacemaking and peace-keeping. *Report of the Secretary-General pursuant to the statement adopted by the Summit Meeting of the Security Council* on January 31, 1992. http://www.un.org/docs/SG/agpeace.html. Accessed May 22, 2010.
Argentine committee for the follow up and application of the international convention on the rights of children (2008). http://www.casacidn.org.ar/indice.php/32. Accessed April 19, 2010.
CEPAL, UNICEF, & SECIB (2001). *Building equity form childhood and adolescence in Iberoamérica.* Santiago de Chile: CEPAL, UNICEF, SECIB.
CSEC World Congress (1996). *Sex exploiter.* Submitted by ECPAT. http://csecworldcongress.org/PDF/en/Stockholm/Background_reading/Theme_papers/Theme%20paper%20Sex%20Exploiter%201996_EN.pdf. Accessed July 1, 2010.
First act to follow-up the subnational plan for the eradication of child labour in the countries of the Mercosur and Chile. (2002). http://white.oit.org.pe/ipec/documentos/decla_primeracta_segui_ti_bbaa2002.pdf. Accessed June 28, 2010.
Inter-American convention on the international restitution of minors. http://www.oas.org/juridico/spanish/tratados/b-53.html. Accessed June 11, 2010.
Protocol of Asunción. http://www.mercosur.int/msweb/Normas/normas_web/Decisiones/ES/CMC_2005–06–19_NOR-DEC_17_ES_Prot-DD-HH-MCS.PDF. Accessed June 16, 2010.
Protocol of judicial mutual assistance in penal matters for the Mercosur (1996). http://www.oas.org/juridico/mla/sp/traites/sp_traites-mla-mercosur-1996.html. Accessed June 28, 2010.
Protocol of Ouro Preto, the protocol of Asunción on the commitment with the promotion and protection of human rights of the Mercosur and associated states (1991). http://www.mercosur.org.uy/innovaportal/file/721/1/CMC_1994_PROTOCOLO%20OURO%20PRETO_ES.pdf. Accessed June 6, 2010.
Protocol of Ushuaia on democratic commitment in the Mercosur, the Republic of Bolivia and the Republic of Chile (1998). http://www.sre.gob.mx/dgomra/mercosur/documentos/Ushuaia_98.doc. Accessed June 21, 2010.
UNODC (2004). United Nations convention against the transnational organized crime and the protocols thereto, New York. http://www.unodc.org/documents/treaties/UNTOC/Publications/TOC%20Convention/TOCebook-e.pdf. Accessed July 1, 2010.

UNODC (2009). United Nations office on drugs and crime: Global report on trafficking in persons, Feb 2009. P7. http://www.unodc.org/documents/human-trafficking/Global_Report_on_TIP.pdf. Accessed October 25, 2010.

UNICEF – United Nations Convention on the Rights of the Child (2010). http://www.unicef.com. au/Unicef/SchoolRoom/ForChildrenandYoungPeople/LearnMoreandGetInvolved/ ChildrensRights/TheUNConventionontheRightsoftheChild/tabid/126/Default.aspx. Accessed June 30, 2010.

UN Palermo Protocol (2000) – United Nations convention against transnational organized crime. http://www.uncjin.org/Documents/Conventions/dcatoc/final_documents/383e.pdf. Accessed July 8, 2010.

Index